Klaus J. Zülch

Atlas of the Histology of Brain Tumors

Histologischer Atlas der Hirntumoren

Atlas d'histologie des tumeurs cérébrales

Atlas histológico de los tumores cerebrales

Гистологический атлас опухолей мозга человека

脳腫瘍組織図譜

Springer-Verlag New York Heidelberg Berlin 1971

Klaus Joachim Zülch, Professor of Neurology and Director of the Division of General Neurology at Max-Planck-Institute for Brain Research, D-5000 Köln-Merheim

With 100 Figures

ISBN 0-387-05274-7 Springer-Verlag New York Heidelberg Berlin
ISBN 3-540-05274-7 Springer-Verlag Berlin Heidelberg New York

Universitätsdruckerei H. Stürtz AG Würzburg

Preface

In most cases the neurosurgical approach to the treatment of brain tumors is still the method of choice. Microscopic examination and classification are of central importance in this regard. In addition, the experimental production of brain tumors has entered a new and very productive phase in which the comparison of these neoplasms with those in man is of basic significance.

This book is submitted because of the desire for a central atlas of brain tumors and for the reasons stated above. We were able to utilize the majority of photographs from the "Handbuch der Neurochirurgie", thereby keeping the cost low. In order to make this work readily useable, the legends — which followed Springer's issue of the UICC atlas but were expanded to include the japanese language — were translated into six languages. The work remains an atlas since only a brief chapter was devoted to a scientific introduction. For additional information we refer to "Brain Tumors" (in German and English) or to volume III of the "Handbuch der Neurochirurgie" for more detailed data. I hope that the daily routine of microscopic classification used in our institute has resulted in a practical and useful work.

I am most grateful to Drs. J. M. BRUCHER/Louvain, J. CERVOS-NAVARRO/Berlin, K. HIZAWA/Tokushima-shi, at present Köln, G. R. JOHNSON/Columbus (Ohio), at present Köln, B. MAIR/London, D. J. PANTSCHENKO/Kiew, K. SATO/Tokyo, at present Köln, J. P. SERRA/Goyania, at present Köln, T. SHIRAI/Chiba, at present Köln, J.-D. TOLEDO/Bilbao, E. TOLOSA/Barcelona for their translations, to Dr. H.-D. MENNEL for his constant help with the preparation, to Mrs. M. GÖLDNER and Mr. H. GÖLDNER for their technical assistance during my scientific work for the past twenty years, and to Dr. H. GÖTZE and Springer-Verlag for their generous layout and excellent quality of this book.

Köln 1971 K. J. ZÜLCH

Vorwort

Noch immer ist die neurochirurgische Behandlung der Hirntumoren für die meisten Fälle die Methode der Wahl. Damit hat die mikroskopische Untersuchung und Klassifikation ihre zentrale Stellung behalten. Auch ist die experimentelle Erzeugung von Hirntumoren in eine neue, äußerst erfolgreiche Phase getreten, wo der Vergleich mit den menschlichen Blastomen von grundlegender Wichtigkeit ist.

Damit besteht weiterhin der Bedarf nach einem zentralen Atlaswerk über die Hirntumoren beim Menschen, das im folgenden vorgelegt wird. Wir konnten aus dem Handbuch der Neurochirurgie die Mehrzahl der hier zusammengestellten Bilder übernehmen, wodurch der Preis sich wesentlich senken ließ. Um das Werk schnell benutzbar zu machen, wurden die Legenden — der Springer-Ausgabe des UICC-Atlas folgend, aber um die japanische Sprache vermehrt — in sechs Sprachen gegeben. Als wissenschaftliche Einleitung wurde nur ein kurzes Kapitel gegeben, das Werk sollte ein Atlas bleiben. Zur weiteren Information stehen ,,Die Hirngeschwülste" (in deutscher und englischer Sprache) zur Verfügung, als ausführliche Materialsammlung auch der Band III des ,,Handbuches für Neurochirurgie". Ich hoffe, daß aus der Alltagsarbeit des Klassifizierens am Mikroskop, wie sie heute noch in unserem Institut geübt wird, ein praktisch brauchbares Werk entstanden ist.

Den Herren J. M. Brucher/Louvain, J. Cervos-Navarro/Berlin, K. Hizawa/Tokushima-shi, z.Zt. Köln, G. R. Johnson/Columbus (Ohio), z.Zt. Köln, B. Mair/London, D. J. Pantschenko/Kiew, K. Sato/Tokyo, z.Zt. Köln, J. P. Serra/Goyania, z.Zt. Köln, T. Shirai/Chiba, z.Zt. Köln, J.-D. Toledo/Bilbao, E. Tolosa/Barcelona bin ich zu großem Dank für die Übersetzung der Legenden verpflichtet, Herrn H.-D. Mennel für seine unermüdliche Hilfe bei der Vorbereitung, schließlich Frau M. und Herrn H. Göldner für ihre über die letzten zwanzig Jahre währende technische Unterstützung meiner wissenschaftlichen Arbeiten. Herrn Dr. H. Götze und dem Springer-Verlag schulde ich Dank für die großzügige Anlage und die vorzügliche Ausstattung dieses Buches.

Köln 1971 K. J. Zülch

Avant-Propos

Le traitement neuro-chirurgical reste la méthode de choix pour la plupart des cas de tumeurs cérébrales. C'est pourquoi l'examen microscopique et la classification microscopique ont gardé une importance primordiale. En outre, l'induction de tumeurs expérimentales, qui est entrée dans une phase nouvelle et pleine de succès, permet d'établir des comparaisons d'un intérêt fondamental avec les blastomes humains.

Il est donc souhaitable de réaliser un atlas des tumeurs cérébrales humaines, comme celui proposé dans ce volume. La plupart des illustrations ont pu être reprises du «Handbuch der Neurochirurgie», ce qui a permis d'en réduire sensiblement le prix. Afin de rendre cet ouvrage rapidement utilisable, les légendes sont imprimeés en six langues, suivant l'édition de l'atlas de l'UICC avec traduction supplémentaire en japonais. Le chapitre qui sert d'introduction scientifique est bref, car l'ouvrage doit rester un atlas. Dans le livre intitulé «Les tumeurs cérébrales» (édité en allemand et en anglais), on trouvera des informations complémentaires, de même qu'il existe dans le volume III du «Handbuch für Neurochirurgie» un inventaire complet et détaillé de notre matériel.

Cet atlas est l'émanation de nos efforts quotidiens de classification microscopique que nous poursuivons encore aujourd'hui dans notre institut. J'espère qu'il se révélera utile et pratique à l'usage.

Je suis très profondément reconnaissant envers MM. J. M. Brucher/Louvain, J. Cervos-Navarro/Berlin, K. Hizawa/Tokushima-shi, provisoirement à Cologne, G. R. Johnson/Columbus (Ohio), provisoirement à Cologne, B. Mair/London, D. J. Pantschenko/Kiew, K. Sato/Tokyo, provisoirement à Cologne, J. P. Serra/Goyania, provisoirement à Cologne, T. Shirai/Chiba, provisoirement à Cologne, J.-D. Toledo/Bilbao, E. Tolosa/Barcelona, qui ont assuré la traduction des légendes. Je remercie également M. H.-D. Mennel pour son aide constante lors de la préparation, Mme et M. H. Göldner pour leur collaboration technique dans mes travaux scientifiques durant ces vingt dernières années, ainsi que le Dr. H. Götze et les éditions Springer pour leur contribution généreuse et la présentation très soignée de cet ouvrage.

Cologne 1971 K. J. Zülch

Prefacio

El tratamiento neuroquirurgico es todavia el metodo de elección para la mayor parte de los tumores del cerebro, por eso la investigación y clasificación microscopicas encuentranse en primer plano. Tambien la producción experimental de tumores cerebrales ha entrado en una nueva fase y así su comparación con los observados en el ser humano es de capital importancia.

De este modo surgió el deseo de confeccionar este Atlas de tumores cerebrales que aquí presentamos.

Tomamos del «Handbuch der Neurochirurgie» muchas de las fotografias, de este modo fué posible conseguir un precio bajo de impresión y para poder ser la publicación facilmente difusible y útil, todo texto, así como los piés de las fotografias son dados en seis idiomas de modo parecido al Atlas UICC editado por la Springer, aumentado con la lengua japonesa.

Dedicamos solo un pequeño capítulo a la investigación pués el libro debe permanecer con las características de un Atlas.

Para mayores informaciones hay el «Hirngeschwülste» (en alemán e inglés) y con más detalle en el tomo III del «Handbuch für Neurochirurgie».

Esperamos que esta obra sea de utilidad práctica para el trabajo diario de los que se dedican a la clasificación de los tumores, como aún hoy se hace en nuestro Instituto.

Damos nuestras mas expresivas gracias a los Sres.: J. M. Brucher/Louvain, J. Cervos-Navarro/Berlin, K. Hizawa/Tokushima-shi/Köln, G. R. Johnson/Columbus (Ohio)/Köln, B. Mair/London, D. J. Pantschenko/Kiew, K. Sato/Tokyo/Köln, J. P. Serra/Goyania/Köln, T. Shirai/Chiba/Köln, J.-D. Toledo/Bilbao, E. Tolosa/Barcelona por la tradución correspondiente.

Al Sr. H. D. Mennel por su constante ayuda en la preparación de la obra.

A la Sra. y Sr. H. Göldner por su continua colaboración en nuestros trabajos cientificos por más de veinte anos.

Al Sr. H. Götze y a la Editora Springer-Verlag tambien las gracias por su generosa contribución y primorosa impresión de este libro.

Köln 1971

K. J. Zülch

Предисловие

В большинстве случаев нейрохирургическое лечение опухолей мозга все еще остается методом выбора и поэтому микроскопическому исследованию и классификации этих опухолей придается первостепенное значение. В новую и исключительно плодотворную фазу вступила также проблема экспериментальных опухолей мозга и особенно важным представляется сравнительное их изучение с опухолями мозга человека.

В связи с этим и подготовлен настоящий атлас опухолей мозга человека. Большинство представленных здесь иллюстраций взято из «Handbuch der Neurochirurgie», что позволило значительно удешевить издание. Для большей доступности и эффективного использования мы по примеру атласа, составленного Международным Противораковым Союзом и вышедшем в издательстве Шпрингер, приводим подписи к иллюстрациям на шести языках, добавив также и японский язык. Настоящая книга остается в основном атласом и лишь в небольшой главе дается научное введение. Более подробные сведения можно почерпнуть в книге «Опухоли мозга» (на немецком и английском языках), а исчерпывающие данные в третьем томе «Handbuch der Neurochirurgie». Хочу надеяться, что эта книга, в которой изложен опыт микроскопической классификации опухолей мозга, накопленный в нашем институте, найдет полезное практическое применение.

За переводы подписей к иллюстрациям выражаю глубокую благодарность докторам J. M. Brucher (Лувен), J. Cervos-Navarro (Берлин), K. Hizawa (Токусима, Кёльн), G. R. Johnson (Колумбус, Кёльн), B. Mair (Лондон), Д. И. Панченко (Киев), K. Sato (Токио, Кёльн), P. Serra (Гояния, Кёльн), T. Shirai (Чиба, Кёльн), J.-D. Toledo (Бильбао), E. Tolosa (Барселона).

Я также благодарю за помощь в подготовке книги д-ра H.-D. Mennel, за двадцатилетнюю техническую помощь в моей научной работе г-жу M. Göldner и г-на H. Göldner, за помощь в построении и великолепное оформление книги д-ра H. Götze и издательство Springer.

Кёльн, 1971 К. И. Цюльх

序

今なお、神経外科的療法は脳腫瘍の多くの症例に最適の方法である。その際、脳腫瘍の顕微鏡的検索とそれに基く分類が主要な役割を果している。さらに、近時脳腫瘍の実験的研究の進展はめざましく、実験的脳腫瘍とひとのそれを比較することは欠くことの出来ないものとなった。

このような理由から、ひとの脳腫瘍に関する図譜を作製することが必要となり、本書が執筆されるにいたった。われわれは神経外科学叢書 (Handbuch der Neurochirurgie) にすでに掲載された写真を多数引用することが出来たので、この図譜の価格を下げることが可能となった。さらに、この図譜を手軽に利用出来るようにするため、Springer 出版社より先に出した UICC 図譜につづいて、図譜の説明を日本語によるものを追加して6ケ国語ですることとした。本書をあくまで図譜にとどめるために、学問な記載は簡潔なものとした。さらに詳細な報告を望まれる場合は、神経外科学叢書の第3巻から資料を集めて出来た「脳腫瘍」(ドイツ語および英語版) を御参照いただきたい。われわれの研究所で日頃行っている脳腫瘍の顕微鏡的分類から、実際に臨床にたづさわる方々に役立つものが出来ると考えている。

翻訳をされた J. M. BRUCHER/Louvain, J, CERVOS-NAVARRO/Berlin, K. HIZAWA/Köln・徳島、G. R. JOHNSON/Köln・Columbus (Ohio), B. MAIR/London, D. J. PANTSCHENKO/Kiew, K. SATO/Köln・東京、J. P. SERRA/Köln・Goyania, T. SHIRAI/Köln・千葉、J-D. TOLEDO/Bilbao, E. TOLOSA/Barcelona, の諸博士に、さらに資料整理を手伝われた H-D. MENNEL 博士、そしてこの20年間私の研究に技術的援助を続けられた GÖLDNER 氏夫妻に深く感謝します。

又、H. GÖTZE 博士と Springer 出版社には、先見の明ある企図と、この図譜の実現のためにはらわれた努力に敬意を表します。

1971年

Köln にて
K. J. ZÜLCH

Contents

Inhaltsverzeichnis

Table des matières

Indice

Содержание

目　次

Introduction

A surgically excised tumor is examined microscopically to obtain information which can lead to a prognosis of the life expectancy of the patient. A histological classification is prerequisite to this. Therefore, there have been attempts to classify the tumors of the various organs on the basis of their microscopic morphology for over a century. The postoperative survival time is then correlated with the type of tumor. By this procedure the "malignancy" of a particular tumor is determined. Thus, certain microscopic characteristics for slowly and rapidly growing tumors have been established.

As a result of nearly 50 years of work in the classification of intracranial tumors, we are now able to differentiate distinctly the individual groups. We know not only the frequently appearing architectures and cell types but also the many variations in stromal architecture and cellular elements. We have also recognized for the past 30 years that the regressive changes which may often be extensive are specific for a particular tumor type. Consequently, one is able to diagnose precisely tumor tissue undergoing regressive changes.

Historical

The classification of brain tumors goes back to Virchow (1846), the discoverer of glia. His classification was purely descriptive and was improved by Borst (1902) in his tumor atlas. The basic principle of classification from the time of Johannes Müller (1838) consisted in the comparison of individual tumor types with the developmental stages of the cells. This principle was applied to brain tumors for the first time by Pick and Bielschowsky (1911) and by Ribbert (1918) and reached its peak in the precise investigations of Bailey and Cushing (1926/30). Bailey and Cushing were able to analyse the tumor cells by applying modern silver impregnating techniques and to compare them with normal cells and their stages of development during cell maturation; the knowledge concerning normal cells was previously established by German and Spanish histologists. This classification which was at first very complicated was later modified. Thus, today there exists a corrected classification which incorporates the various changes proposed by Penfield and Bergstrand and our own experience. This scheme classifies all the neurosurgically occurring tumors into 25 types. The average postoperative survival time based on the records of the large American and European clinics was incorporated into this classification (Cushing, Olivecrona, Tönnis, Mayo-Clinic).

In addition to this scheme, there are others throughout the world which are based on the same principle. For example, there is the scheme of Del Rio Hortega which is preferred in the Latin American countries. It was briefly described by Polak.

Only a slight modification of this basic scheme is found in the atlas by Russell and Rubinstein where only brief mention is made of the postoperative prognosis. Likewise, the same principles are employed in the atlas by Roussy-Oberling although it does not contain any reference to the prognosis.

The most important classification, besides that of Bailey and Cushing, has been that of Kernohan which contains information concerning malignancy. Kernohan combined the histological classification according to the cell type with a biological classification which graded malignancy and differentiated it into four stages. Kernohan's classification has been widely adopted in the English speaking countries.

Our classification (1951, 1956, 1965), which recognized 25 varieties of intracranial tumors, was the result of daily collaborative work with the neurosurgeons. It was the basis for the German and English publications of "Brain Tumors" and for the detailed description of all the recognized forms of brain tumors and their variations which appeared in the "Handbuch der Neurochirurgie" (vol. III. Springer, Heidelberg 1956). This scheme was also the basis for "Farbatlas der Hirntumoren" published with the support of the firms AGFA and LEITZ and for the contribution in the "Lehrbuch der pathologischen Anatomie" by KAUFMANN.

The aim of our introduction to the classification is to describe the intracranial tumors so simply that they could be diagnosed with anilin stained paraffin sections, since this corresponds to the routine techniques of general pathologists and neuropathologists. It is possible to diagnose intracranial tumors in the majority of cases by this method.

One must not, however, minimize the difficulties which exist and must concede that for perhaps 10 to 20% of the cases the classification of intracranial tumors is still a *fine art*. This can be learnt only from long years of experience. One has to know, especially, the cell form and architecture of a tumor, and, likewise, how the varieties occur or develop through regressive changes. These variations have been described in detail and illustrated in the "Handbuch der Neurochirurgie" but for everyday work it is too detailed and explanatory. Also, its use is limited since many users are restricted in their knowledge of the German language. Our small book of "Brain Tumors" does not contain the number of illustrations necessary for one to be able to learn the details of diagnosis.

The purpose of this atlas is to supplement the *complete text* of the *small textbook* by means of a *large number of typical photographs of tumors and their variations*. The pictures are explained only briefly. For a detailed description one should consult the "Brain Tumors" or the "Handbuch für Neurochirurgie". Since many of the illustrations used in this atlas are from vol. III of the "Handbuch für Neurochirurgie", it has been possible to keep the cost low and yet provide a photographic atlas.

Confusion in the Terminology

In the last 10 years we have experienced that the individual schools concerned with the terminology of intracranial tumors are unable to come to a common agreement; the definitive proof of this being the Cologne International Tumor Symposium in 1961. There still exists a "verbal confusion", a lack of understanding, in the terminology. This impedes the statistical studies of clinicians who want to investigate the value of a certain method of treatment (operation, radiation treatment, cytotoxic treatment).

Consequently, we have referred to the classification of the "Unio Internationalis Contra Cancrum" (UICC) in order to establish a basis for the present work. The UICC showed that through compromise one is able, for the most part, to standardize the various nomenclatures if one compares the frequently used names and definitions and then explains the synonyms. These, then, have to be illustrated and defined by means of pictures from the large tumor-atlas of world literature.

Moreover, according to the wish of the UICC, one school should not be favored over another; one proceeds "pragmatically", utilizing only frequently used and well recognized names even though they may no longer be scientifically correct. In addition the better synonyms should be mentioned.

This is illustrated for example by the "hypernephroma". Every general pathologist and clinician is acquainted with what is meant by this tumor concept even though the term is not scientifically correct and should be improved. Besides the name hypernephroma, the atlas of the UICC also contains modern terms.

The classification scheme of the UICC (Springer-Verlag, Berlin-Göttingen-Heidelberg, 1965) described almost all of the tumors occurring in the human body but only dealt with their morphology. Also, the tumors seen in neurosurgery were grouped together and each was illustrated by a photograph. This atlas is not sufficient for learning how to diagnose intracranial tumors. Its significance lies much more in its attempt to standardize the nomenclature. Therefore, it is only logical that this first general work of the UICC must be completed by means of individual publications dealing with the tumors of the different organ systems.

The following contribution attemps to fulfil this goal for *intracranial tumors*. In the classification, we have followed the suggestions of the UICC even where we were of a different scientific point of view and had, up until now, utilized another order or grouping. Individual groups were completed as far as it was possible since some of these groups are still being debated by the UICC. Then in accordance with the proceedings of the UICC, the acknowledged synonyms were included and thus the work of this society was, essentially, furthered. This can be seen, for example, in our description of the "monstrocellular sarcoma".

The Prognosis

A morphological classification is of little value to the clinician if it does not include a prognosis concerning the postoperative survival period. This had been achieved for the BAILEY-CUSHING scheme after 30 years of work and was given for each group (1965). Here the surgeon seeks eventual precision and clearly arranged data. This was the reason for the success of KERNOHAN'S proposal of a classification which was based on 4 grades of malignancy. It also paralleled the view of old pathology which expressed the malignancy of a tumor by such terms as "benign", "semibenign", "semimalignant", or, finally, "ma-

Scheme I. *Modified grading for tumors of the brain and related structures*

Tumors	Grade I benign	Grade II semibenign	Grade III semimalignant	Grade IV malignant
Gangliocytoma				
isomorphous	+	+		
polymorphous			+	
Ependymoma				
isomorphous	+	+		
polymorphous			+	
Plexuspapilloma				
isomorphous	+			
polymorphous			+	
Astrocytoma				
isomorphous		+		
polymorphous			+	
Oligodendroglioma				
isomorphous		+		
polymorphous			+	
Glioblastoma				+
Spongioblastoma				
isomorphous	+			
polymorphous			+	
Medulloblastoma				+
Pinealoma				
isomorphous	+			
anisomorphous		+		
polymorphous			+	
Neurinoma				
amitotic	+			
polymitotic			+	
Meningeoma				
amitotic/oligomitotic	+			
polymitotic			+	
Angioblastoma (LINDAU)	+			
Sarcoma				+
Pituitary adenoma				
isomorphous	+			
polymorphous		+		
Craniopharyngioma	+			

lignant"; that is, a four grade classification. KERNOHAN'S classification, however, was not entirely complete. It had to be modified for everyday use and adapted to recent discoveries within our profession. Upon analysis of the data and clinical aspects for the individual tumor groups it became evident that no tumor group possessed all four grades of malignancy. Instead they generally contained two or, at most, three grades of malignancy.

From a practical standpoint it was of *special significance* that the grades of malignancy be standardized thus permitting comparisons. An oligodendroglioma of grade III had to correspond in its biological activity or behavior to that exhibited by a plexus papilloma, also of grade III malignancy.

We attempted such an improved "classification of grading" in 1961 and presented it for discussion to the International Tumor Symposium in Cologne. Then, after further experimental work a useful scheme evolved and was confirmed, electronmicroscopically, in a comprehensive work with W. WECHSLER.

We considered it important to indicate, especially, the "transitional stages" of malignancy such as those long recognized with the astrocytoma. Here we know that perhaps 10% of all cases have either malignant parts or, have developed to malignancy (ZÜLCH and TELTSCHAROW, 1948). We found, too, that in addition to the isomorphous groups the "polymorphous oligodendroglioma" (1955) shows distinctly higher tendencies toward

Scheme II. Classification of brain tumours and their different degrees of malignancy

Degree of malignancy	Prognosis after "total" removal	Tumours	
		extracerebral	intracerebral
Grade I benign	Cure or survival of 5 and more years at least	Neurinomas Meningeomas Pituitary Adenomas Craniopharyngeomas	Gangliocytomas (temporo-basal) Ependymomas of the ventricles Plexuspapillomas Spongioblastomas Angioblastomas (LINDAU)
Grade II semibenign	Postoperative survival time: 3—5 years	Pituitary Adenomas, polymorphous	Gangliocytomas of other location Ependymomas (cerebral) Astrocytomas, isomorphous Oligodrendrogliomas, isomorphous Pinealomas, anisomorphous
Grade III semimalignant	Postoperative survival time: 2—3 years	Meningeomas, polymitotic Neurinomas, polymitotic	Gangliocytomas, polymorphous Ependymomas, polymorphous Plexuspapillomas, polymorphous Astrocytomas, polymorphous Oligodendrogliomas, polymorphous Pinealomas, polymorphous
Grade IV malignant	Postoperative survival time: 6—15 month	Sarcomas	Glioblastomas Medulloblastomas Primary Sarcomas

malignancy. We then turned our attention to observations concerning the malignant forms within the spongioblastomas (1968/1969), the plexus papillomas, the neurinomas, the pinealomas and the gangliocytomas. These transitional forms of malignancy were included in the classification scheme. Thus, all of the various tumor types could be compared with one another. Now the groups provide the *same prognosis for a brain tumor* in as far as it is possible on the basis of details obtained from a microscopic examination of the morphology.

Morphology and Clinical Malignancy

It should briefly be pointed out that predictions concerning the behavior of a tumor are further modified by its "clinical malignancy", as shown in the following scheme:

Scheme III. *"Clinical" malignancy of intracranial tumors = Biological (histological) malignancy plus*

1. Volumen auctum
2. Mass movements with hernias
   temporal / cerebellar } pressure cone
3. Action on c.s.f. pathway: hydrocephalus
4. Action on arteries (infarcts!)
5. Action on vital centers: hypothalamus, mesencephalon, medulla oblongata etc.

The "clinical malignancy" of a tumor can be defined only by the clinician himself after he has reviewed all of his experience in the individual case. Morphology is able to provide only concepts concerning the "genuine growth" of a tumor and through the tumor's morphological classification which is based on the experiences of earlier generations it is also able to indicate the biological behavior of specific groups.

I hope that this atlas of classification of intracranial tumors fulfils *everyday needs*. I also express the hope that it aids us all in the standardization of the nomenclature of intracranial tumors and permits a better understanding between morphologists and clinicians throughout the world. Only then will it be possible to consider questions pertaining to therapy, *statistically unobjectionable*, and to produce comparable results. To begin with, the terms applied must be clear and easily translated into the concepts of another classification. Secondly, the knowledge about all of the known variants of a tumor must be surmised from the classification. Thirdly, the variants must be able to be analyzed with the corresponding staining method or impregnation. This is demonstrated in the present atlas.

The classification of intracranial tumors is not always simple since they often do not have a "pure" cell population. Here, the old basis of "classical pathology" applies: a potiori fit denominatio, the classification is related to the *most frequently* occurring cell type.

Of course, it is difficult for the morphologist to classify correctly when he receives only *a small piece of tissue* for examination; the results of morphological classification improve with the *larger pieces of tissue* which the surgeon sends. This is our request to the surgeons.

The hope of the atlas is to provide a morphological and biological classification of the intracranial tumors and assist the surgeon in his work.

Bibliography p. 258.

Einleitung

Eine operierte Geschwulst wird mikroskopisch untersucht, um Vorstellungen über die Prognose der Lebenserwartung des Patienten zu gewinnen. Voraussetzung dafür ist eine histologische Klassifikation. Deshalb versucht die Morphologie seit über einem Jahrhundert, die Geschwülste der verschiedenen Organe nach den mikroskopischen Gewebsbildern zu klassifizieren. Die postoperative Überlebenszeit wird dann mit der Geschwulstart in eine Korrelation gesetzt. Daraus wird das „Wachstum" dieser Geschwulst bestimmt. Darüber hinaus gibt es auch gewisse mikroskopische Merkmale für langsames oder beschleunigtes Wachstum einer Geschwulst.

Fast 50 Jahre der Arbeit an der Klassifikation der intrakraniellen Tumoren brachten als Ergebnis, daß wir die einzelnen Gruppen sehr genau differenzieren können. Wir kennen die am häufigsten auftretenden Architekturen und die Zelltypen, wir kennen aber auch die vielen Varianten in der Grundarchitektur und in den Zellelementen. Eine Erkenntnis der letzten 30 Jahre ist, daß auch die regressiven Vorgänge oft weitgehend für eine Geschwulst spezifisch sind. Man kann daher auch aus dem regressiv veränderten Geschwulstgewebe noch recht exakte Diagnosen stellen.

Historisches

Die Klassifikation der Hirntumoren geht auf VIRCHOW (1846), den Entdecker der Glia zurück. Die von ihm geschaffene Einteilung war rein deskriptiv und wurde von BORST (1902) in seinem Geschwulstatlas verfeinert. Das grundlegende Prinzip der Klassifikation bestand seit JOHANNES MÜLLER (1838) in dem Vergleich der einzelnen Geschwulstformen mit den Entwicklungsstufen der Zellen. Dieses Prinzip wurde von PICK und BIELSCHOWSKY (1911) und von RIBBERT (1918) erstmals für Hirngeschwülste angewandt, fand aber seinen Höhepunkt erst in den genauen Untersuchungen von BAILEY und CUSHING (1926/30). Diese konnten die Zellen der Tumoren mit den modernen Silbermethoden analysieren und mit den Normalzellen und ihren Entwicklungsstufen während der Zellreifung vergleichen, die aus den Arbeiten der deutschen und spanischen Normalanatomie bekannt waren. Die zunächst sehr komplizierte Einteilung wurde später verdichtet. Heute ist ein nach verschiedenen Änderungsvorschlägen von PENFIELD und BERGSTRAND und aufgrund eigener Erfahrungen korrigiertes Einteilungsschema verfügbar, das mit etwa 25 Typen alle innerhalb der Neurochirurgie vorkommenden Geschwulstformen zu klassifizieren versteht. Für die Geschwulstgruppen dieser Klassifikation ist die durchschnittliche postoperative Lebenserwartung aus den Ergebnissen der großen amerikanischen und europäischen Kliniken gut bekannt (CUSHING, OLIVECRONA, TÖNNIS, Mayo-Clinic).

Neben diesem Schema sind noch weitere — auf dem gleichen Prinzip aufgebaute — Klassifikations-Schemata in der Welt gebräuchlich, z.B. das von DEL RIO HORTEGA, das in den lateinamerikanischen Staaten bevorzugt wird. Es wurde kürzlich noch einmal von POLAK beschrieben.

Nur geringe Abweichungen finden sich auch in dem Atlas von RUSSELL und RUBINSTEIN, wo allerdings die postoperative Prognose kaum beschrieben wird. Auf den gleichen Grundsätzen baute sich auch der Atlas von ROUSSY-OBERLING auf, der allerdings ebenfalls keine Hinweise zur Prognose enthält.

Am wichtigsten ist aber neben der Einteilung von BAILEY und CUSHING die Klassifikation von KERNOHAN geworden. Sie enthält bereits eine Information über die Malignität. KERNOHAN kombinierte die *histologische* Einteilung nach dem Zelltyp mit einer *biologischen* Gradeinteilung der Malignität und unterschied dabei 4 Stufen. Die Einteilung KERNOHANs hat in den englisch sprechenden Ländern große Verbreitung gefunden.

Die eigene Klassifikation (1951, 1956, 1965) mit 25 Unterarten intrakranieller Tumoren war aus der täglichen Zusammenarbeit mit den

Neurochirurgen, d.h. aus der Praxis des Alltags entstanden. Sie war die Grundlage für die deutsche und die englische Ausgabe der „Hirngeschwülste", ebenso wie für die ausführliche Beschreibung aller bekannten Bilder der Hirngeschwülste und ihrer Varianten im „Handbuch der Neurochirurgie", Band III, Springer/Heidelberg 1956. Schließlich war auch der mit der Unterstützung der Firmen AGFA und LEITZ herausgegebene „Farbatlas der Hirntumoren" und der Beitrag im „Lehrbuch der pathologischen Anatomie" von KAUFMANN (1958) auf diesem Schema aufgebaut.

Dabei war es das Ziel unserer Anleitung zur Klassifikation, die intrakraniellen Tumoren so vereinfacht zu beschreiben, daß sie bereits am Anilin-gefärbten Paraffinschnitt diagnostiziert werden konnten, da dies der Routinetechnik der allgemeinpathologischen und neuropathologischen Institute entspricht. Tatsächlich gelingt so die Diagnose der intrakraniellen Tumoren in einer großen Zahl von Fällen.

Man darf aber die noch bestehenden Schwierigkeiten nicht bagatellisieren und muß zugeben, daß für etwa 10—20% der Fälle die Klassifikation der intrakraniellen Tumoren auch heute noch eine *große Kunst* ist. Diese lernt man nur durch jahrelange Erfahrung. Besonders muß man die zahlreichen Varianten eines Tumors in Zellform und Architektur genau kennen, ebenso wie die Abarten, die durch regressive Vorgänge entstanden sind. Diese Varianten wurden seinerzeit ausführlich im Handbuch der Neurochirurgie beschrieben und abgebildet. Dieser Beitrag war als ein wissenschaftliches Nachschlagewerk gedacht. Für die praktische Arbeit des Alltags war die Beschreibung damit etwas zu breit. Vielen Benutzern erschwert auch die mangelnde Kenntnis der deutschen Sprache die Benutzung unseres Handbuchbeitrages. Unser kleines Buch über die „Hirngeschwülste" wiederum hatte zu wenig Abbildungen, um daraus die Diagnostik im einzelnen erlernen zu können.

Ziel der Herausgabe dieses Atlas war daher, den *ausreichenden Text* des *kleinen Lehrbuches* durch eine *große Zahl von typischen Bildern der Tumoren und ihrer Varianten zu ergänzen*. Die Bilder sollten aber nur durch einen kurzen Text erläutert werden. Für die ausführliche Beschreibung soll auch weiter das Handbuch bzw. „Die Hirngeschwülste" zur Verfügung stehen. Die Mehrzahl der Abbildungen dieses Atlas stammt aus dem Band III des Handbuches der Neurochirurgie; dadurch konnte ein sehr breites Bildwerk ohne zusätzliche Aufwendungen für die Reproduktion veröffentlicht werden.

Die Verwirrung in der Terminologie

In den letzten 10 Jahren haben wir aber die Erfahrung gewonnen, daß sich die einzelnen Schulen über die Terminologie der intrakraniellen Tumoren nicht einigen konnten; das bewies endgültig das Kölner Internationale Tumor-Symposion 1961. Es besteht immer noch eine „Sprachverwirrung", ein Mangel an Verständigung in der Terminologie. Dies erschwert jede statistische Arbeit der Kliniker, wenn sie den Wert einer bestimmten Behandlungsart (Operation, Strahlenbehandlung, cytostatische Behandlung) untersuchen wollen.

Wir haben daher auf die Klassifikation der „Unio Internationalis Contra Cancrum" zurückgegriffen und der vorliegenden Bearbeitung zugrunde gelegt. Die UICC ging bei ihrem Vermittlungsversuch von der Feststellung aus, daß man verschiedene Nomenklaturen am ehesten vereinheitlichen kann, wenn man die häufig gebrauchten Namen und Definitionen nebeneinanderstellt und durch Synonyme erklärt. Diese müssen dann durch Bilder aus den großen Tumor-Atlanten der Weltliteratur definiert und illustriert werden.

Dabei sollte nach dem Willen der UICC nicht *eine* Schule bevorzugt werden; man ging „pragmatisch" vor, verwandte nur die häufig gebrauchten, aber jedem bekannten Namen, auch wenn sie wissenschaftlich nicht mehr haltbar waren. Es wurden dann aber bessere Synonyme erwähnt.

Dies sei am Beispiel des „Hypernephroms" erläutert. Jedem Allgemeinpathologen und Kliniker ist bekannt, was mit diesem Geschwulstbegriff gemeint ist, obwohl er wissenschaftlich nicht zutreffend ist und verbessert werden sollte. Wir finden daher in dem Atlas der UICC neben diesem Begriff des Hypernephroms modernere Termini.

Das Klassifikationsschema der UICC (Springer-Verlag, Berlin-Göttingen-Heidelberg, 1965) umfaßte fast alle im menschlichen Körper vorkommenden Tumoren, gab aber nur einen ersten Anhalt über die Morphologie. Auch die in der Neurochirurgie vorkommenden Geschwülste wurden zusammengestellt und je durch ein Bild erläutert. Dieser Atlas reichte nicht aus, um die Diagnostik der intrakraniellen Tumoren zu lernen. Seine Bedeutung liegt vielmehr nur in dem Versuch, die Nomenklatur zu vereinheitlichen. Daraus ergibt sich logisch, daß dieses erste Übersichtswerk der UICC durch Einzelveröffentlichungen über die Tumoren der verschiedenen Organsysteme ergänzt werden muß.

Der folgende Beitrag versucht diese Aufgabe für die *intrakraniellen Tumoren* zu verwirklichen. Wir haben uns bei der Klassifikation an die Vorschläge der UICC gehalten, auch dort, wo wir wissenschaftlich selbst anderer Ansicht waren und bisher eine andere Reihenfolge oder Gruppierung verwandt haben. Doch wurden einzelne Gruppen ergänzt, soweit die UICC diese in ihr Schema noch nicht übernommen hat, weil sie umstritten sind. Es wurden dann entsprechend dem Vorgehen der UICC die bekannten Synonyme mitgeteilt und

Schema I. *Malignitätsstufen („Grading") der neuroektodermalen Hirntumoren*

Tumoren	Grad I benigne	Grad II semibenigne	Grad III semimaligne	Grad IV maligne
Gangliocytome				
isomorph	+	+		
polymorph			+	
Ependymome				
isomorph	+	+		
polymorph (selten)			+	
Plexuspapillome				
isomorph	+			
polymorph (sehr selten)			+	
Astrocytome				
isomorph		+		
polymorph			+	
Oligodendrogliome				
isomorph		+		
polymorph			+	
Glioblastome				+
Spongioblastome				
isomorph	+			
polymorph (selten)			+	
Medulloblastome				+
Pinealome				
isomorph	+			
anisomorph		+		
polymorph			+	
Neurinome				
amitotisch	+		+	
polymitotisch				
Meningeome				
amitotisch/oligomitotisch	+		+	
polymitotisch				
Angioblastome (Lindau)	+			
Sarkome				+
Hypophysenadenome				
isomorph	+			
polymorph		+		
Craniopharyngeome	+			

damit die Arbeit dieser Gesellschaft grundlegend weitergeführt. Das sieht man z.B. an unserer Beschreibung des „monstrocellulären Sarkoms".

Die Prognose

Eine morphologische Klassifikation bleibt aber für den Kliniker nur von geringem Wert, wenn sie nicht eine Prognose über die postoperative Überlebensdauer enthält. Diese war für das Bailey-Cushingsche Schema in 30 Jahren erarbeitet worden und für jede Gruppe angegeben (1965). Hier sucht der Chirurg nach möglichst präzisen und übersichtlichen Angaben. Und dies war sicher der Grund für den großen Erfolg des Kernohanschen Vorschlages einer Einteilung nach 4 Graden der Malignität. Es stand auch in Parallele zu dem Vorgehen der alten Pathologen, die die Malignität eines Tumors durch Begriffe wie „benigne", „semibenigne", „semimaligne" oder schließlich „maligne" ausdrückten, d.h. eine vier-Grad-Einteilung. Dieses Klassifikationsschema ist aber von KERNOHAN niemals bis ins einzelne durchgeführt worden. Es mußte für den Alltagsgebrauch modifiziert und der neuen Entwicklung unseres Faches angepaßt werden. Die globalen Angaben über die einzelnen Tumorgruppen wurden ergänzt und die Erfahrung berücksichtigt, daß nicht bei *jeder* Tumorgruppe 4 Stufen der Malignität bestehen, sondern gewöhnlich nur 2 oder höchstens 3 (Schema I).

Für den praktischen Gebrauch war von *besonderer Bedeutung*, die Gradstufen der Malignität zu vereinheitlichen und dadurch vergleichbar zu machen. Ein Oligodendrogliom des Malignitätsgrades III mußte in der biologischen Wertigkeit dem Verhalten eines Plexuspapilloms des gleichen Malignitätsgrades III entsprechen (Schema II).

Einen solchen Versuch der „Gradeinteilung" haben wir verbessert 1961 auf dem Internationalen Tumor-Symposion in Köln zur Diskussion gestellt. Aus der weiteren praktischen Arbeit ist dann ein brauchbares Schema entstanden, das kürzlich in einer Übersichtsarbeit mit W. WECHSLER auch elektronenmikroskopisch begründet wurde.

Wir halten es für wichtig, besonders auf die „Übergangsstufen" der Malignität hinzuweisen, wie sie beim Astrocytom seit langem bekannt waren. Hier wußte man, daß etwa 10% aller Fälle entweder maligne Partien haben, oder aber im Begriffe sind, maligne zu entarten

Schema II. *Klassifikation der Hirntumoren und ihre Stellung in einer vierstufigen Malignitätsskala*

Malignitätsstufe	Prognose	Tumoren	
		extracerebral	intracerebral
Grad I benigne	Heilung oder Überlebenszeit von 5 und mehr Jahren	Neurinome Meningeome Hypophysenadenome Kraniopharyngeome	Gangliocytome (temporobasal) Ependymome (ventriculär) Plexuspapillome Spongioblastome Angioblastome
Grad II semibenigne	Überlebenszeit: 3 bis 5 Jahre	Hypophysenadenome, polymorph	Gangliocytome (übrige) Ependymome (Großhirn, paraventriculär) Astrocytome, isomorph Oligodendrogliome, isomorph Pinealome, anisomorph
Grad III semimaligne	Überlebenszeit: 2 bis 3 Jahre	Meningeome (polymitotisch) Neurinome (polymitotisch)	Gangliocytome, polymorph Ependymome, polymorph Plexuspapillome, polymorph Astrocytome, polymorph Oligodendrogliome, polymorph
Grad IV maligne	Überlebenszeit: 6 bis 15 Monate	Sarkome	Pinealome, polymorph Glioblastome Medulloblastome (Retinoblastome) Primäre Sarkome

(ZÜLCH und TELTSCHAROW, 1948). Wir fanden auch, daß neben der „isomorphen" Gruppe auch „polymorphe Oligodendrogliome" (1955) mit einer deutlich höheren Malignität vorkommen. Wir verwerteten dann Beobachtungen über maligne Formen bei den Spongioblastomen (1968/1969), den Plexuspapillomen, den Neurinomen, den Pinealomen und Gangliocytomen. Diese Übergangsstufen der Malignität wurden in das Schema der Klassifikation eingefügt und dabei alle Tumorstufen miteinander vergleichbar gemacht. *Jetzt* geben die Gruppen die *gleiche Prognose für eine Hirngeschwulst*, soweit sich derartige Angaben überhaupt von einem Morphologen aufgrund der mikroskopischen Untersuchung machen lassen.

Morphologische und klinische Malignität

Es muß allerdings kurz darauf hingewiesen werden, daß solche Voraussagen über das Verhalten des Wachstums weitgehend durch die „klinische Malignität" eines Tumors modifiziert werden, wie das folgende Schema beweist:

Schema III. „*Klinische*" *Malignität eines intrakraniellen Tumors = Biologische (histologische) Malignität plus*

1. Volumen auctum
2. Massenverschiebung
   mit Hernien {temporaler / cerebellärer} Druckconus
3. Einwirkung auf Liquorbahn: Hydrocephalus occlusus
4. Einwirkung auf Gefäße: Infarkt
5. Einwirkung auf vitale Zentren: Hypothalamus, Mesencephalon, Medulla oblongata etc.

Die „klinische Malignität" kann aber nur vom Kliniker selbst unter Berücksichtigung aller seiner Erfahrungen mit dem Einzelfall definiert werden. Der Morphologe kann nur Vorstellungen über das „genuine Wachstum" eines Tumors vermitteln und durch seine morphologische Klassifikation auf die Erfahrungen früherer Generationen auch über das biologische Verhalten bestimmter Gruppen hinweisen.

Ich hoffe, daß dieser Atlas der Klassifikation der intrakraniellen Tumoren sich für den *Alltag* als brauchbar erweist. Ich drücke auch die Hoffnung aus, daß er uns allen bei der Vereinheitlichung der Nomenklatur der intrakraniellen Tumoren hilft und damit eine bessere Verständigung zwischen Morphologen und Klinikern in der Welt ermöglicht. Nur dann wird es gelingen, Fragen der Therapie *statistisch einwandfrei* zu bearbeiten und Ergebnisse vergleichbar zu machen. Denn erstens müssen die verwandten Termini verständlich sein und leicht in die Begriffe einer anderen Klassifikation übersetzt werden können. Zweitens muß bei der Klassifikation die Kenntnis aller bekannten Varianten einer Geschwulst vorausgesetzt werden. Drittens müssen diese Varianten mit den entsprechenden Methoden der Färbung oder Imprägnation analysierbar sein. Das wird im vorliegenden Atlas gezeigt.

Die Klassifikation der intrakraniellen Tumoren ist nicht immer einfach, weil sie oft nicht eine „reine" Zellpopulation haben. Hier gilt der alte Grundsatz der „klassischen Pathologie": a potiori fit denominatio, die Klassifikation hängt ab von dem am *häufigsten* vorkommenden Zellelement.

Für den Morphologen ist es allerdings schwer, korrekt zu klassifizieren, wenn er nur *kleinste Gewebestücke* zur Untersuchung bekommt: Die Resultate der morphologischen Klassifikation verbessern sich in dem gleichen Maße, in dem der Neurochirurg *größere Gewebsteile* zur Untersuchung einsendet, dies ist unsere Bitte an den Operateur.

Den Atlas begleitet die Hoffnung, daß er die morphologische und biologische Klassifikation der intrakraniellen Tumoren ermöglicht und damit den Neurochirurgen in seiner Arbeit unterstützt.

Literatur S. 258.

Introduction

L'examen microscopique d'une tumeur opérée est destiné à donner une estimation de la survie du patient. C'est dans ce but qu'on établit une classification histologique. Aussi, depuis un siècle, les morphologistes s'efforcent de grouper les tumeurs des différents organes selon leur aspect microscopique. On établit ensuite une corrélation entre la survie post-opératoire et chacun des types tumoraux et l'on détermine alors leur «vitesse de croissance». On peut en outre établir certains critères microscopiques correspondant à la croissance lente ou rapide d'une tumeur.

Depuis près de 50 ans, les travaux sur la classification des tumeurs intra-crâniennes ont permis d'en distinguer de façon très précise les différents groupes. Nous connaissons non seulement les architectures et les types cellulaires les plus fréquents, mais aussi leurs nombreuses variantes. Durant ces 30 dernières années, nous avons appris également que les phénomènes régressifs ont souvent un caractère très spécifique pour chaque type tumoral, de telle sorte qu'il est encore possible de porter un diagnostic exact malgré les altérations régressives d'un tissu tumoral.

Historique

C'est à VIRCHOW (1846) que l'on doit la découverte de la glie et la classification des tumeurs cérébrales. Les subdivisions qu'il créa étaient purement descriptives, mais BORST (1902) les précisa davantage dans son atlas des tumeurs. Depuis JOHANNES MÜLLER (1838), le principe fondamental de classification reposait sur la comparaison des différentes formes tumorales aux stades de développement des cellules. Ce principe fut appliqué pour la première fois aux tumeurs cérébrales par PICK et BIELSCHOWSKY (1911) et par RIBBERT (1918), mais il obtint son couronnement grâce aux observations attentives de BAILEY et CUSHING (1926/1930). Ces auteurs analysèrent les cellules tumorales par les méthodes argentiques modernes et purent ainsi les comparer aux cellules normales et à leurs stades de maturation, bien connus depuis les travaux d'anatomie normale des écoles allemande et espagnole. Leur classification, qui était initialement très compliquée, fut condensée par la suite. Aujourd'hui, grâce aux différentes améliorations proposées par PENFIELD et par BERGSTRAND et sur la base de notre propre expérience, nous disposons d'un nouveau schéma de classification, qui répartit en 25 types toutes les formes tumorales observées en neurochirurgie. Pour chacun de ces types tumoraux, on connaît la durée moyenne de survie post-opératoire grâce aux données fournies par les grands centres américains et européens (CUSHING, OLIVECRONA, TÖNNIS, Mayo-Clinic).

A côté de ce schéma, il existe encore d'autres classifications basées sur le même principe. Par exemple, celle de DEL RIO HORTEGA, dont POLAK vient encore de donner une brève description, est utilisée de préférence dans les pays d'Amérique latine.

Il n'y a également que peu de différences dans l'atlas de RUSSELL et RUBINSTEIN, où néanmoins le pronostic post-opératoire est à peine envisagé. Sur le même principe repose également l'atlas de ROUSSY-OBERLING, qui ne fournit pas non plus d'indications sur le pronostic.

A côté de la classification de BAILEY et CUSHING, la plus importante est celle de KERNOHAN, qui contient déjà une information sur la malignité. KERNOHAN combina la subdivision *histologique* selon le type cellulaire avec une graduation *biologique* de la malignité et distingua ainsi 4 degrés. Cette classification de KERNOHAN a reçu une forte diffusion dans les pays de langue anglaise.

Notre classification personnelle (1951, 1956, 1965), qui comporte 25 types de tumeurs intra-crâniennes, est le fruit d'une collaboration permanente avec les neurochirurgiens et de la pratique quotidienne. Elle a servi de base à l'élaboration de notre livre «Tumeurs cérébrales» édité en allemand et en anglais, ainsi qu'à la description détaillée de tous les aspects connus des tumeurs cérébrales et de leurs variantes dans le «Handbuch der Neurochirurgie» (vol. III. Springer, Heidelberg 1956). Enfin, sur le même schéma, nous avons publié un «Atlas en couleurs des tumeurs cérébrales» grâce à l'aide des firmes Agfa et Leitz, et nous avons apporté notre contribution dans le «Handbuch der pathologischen Anatomie» de KAUFMANN (1958).

En présentant notre classification, nous avons tenu à simplifier la description des tumeurs intra-crâniennes, de telle sorte qu'on puisse déjà les diagnostiquer sur des coupes à la paraffine colorées à l'aniline, méthode de routine utilisée dans les instituts d'anatomie pathologique et de neuropathologie. Par cette simple technique, il est possible, en effet, de reconnaître un grand nombre de tumeurs intra-crâniennes.

Il importe toutefois de ne pas minimiser les difficultés et de préciser que, dans 10 à 20% des cas, la classification des tumeurs intra-crâniennes exige des *connaissances spéciales*. C'est ce qu'on apprend après plusieurs années d'expérience. En particulier, il faut connaître exactement les nombreuses variantes cellulaires et architecturales de chaque tumeur ainsi que leurs variétés dues aux phénomènes régressifs. Nous en avons décrit et illustré les détails dans le «Handbuch der Neurochirurgie», qui fut conçu comme un manuel scientifique de référence. Cependant, pour la pratique quotidienne, les descriptions qu'il contient sont un peu trop étendues. En outre, pour beaucoup d'utilisateurs, une connaissance insuffisante de la langue allemande rendait difficile l'usage de notre «Handbuch». D'autre part, dans notre petit traité sur «les tumeurs cérébrales», le nombre restreint d'illustrations ne permettait plus d'étudier en détail le diagnostic.

En rassemblant dans cet atlas un grand nombre d'illustrations typiques des tumeurs et de leurs différentes variétés, nous avons voulu fournir un complément à notre *petit traité*, dont le texte était suffisant. Le commentaire de chaque figure est assez bref, car on peut en trouver une description complète dans notre «Handbuch» ou dans notre traité sur «les tumeurs cérébrales». Etant donné que la plupart des images de cet atlas proviennent du volume III du «Handbuch für Neurochirurgie», il a été possible de l'illustrer abondamment en limitant les frais au minimum.

Confusion de la terminologie

Durant les dix dernières années, nous avons constaté que l'accord n'était pas unanime entre les différentes écoles à propos de la terminologie des tumeurs intra-crâniennes. Le Symposium international de Cologne sur les tumeurs, en 1961, l'a clairement démontré. Il persiste encore toujours une confusion de mots et une incompréhension d'ordre terminologique, qui rendent difficile l'établissement de statistiques par les cliniciens désireux d'apprécier la valeur de tel ou tel traitement (chirurgie, radiothérapie, cytostatiques).

Nous nous sommes donc tourné vers la classification établie par l'Union Internationale contre le Cancer et nous avons abandonné la systématisation que nous avions établie. Dans une tentative de conciliation, l'UICC estima qu'on pouvait en premier lieu unifier les différentes nomenclatures en juxtaposant les appellations et définitions les plus courantes et en les considérant comme synonymes. Il faudrait alors les définir et les illustrer au moyen d'images extraites des grands atlas de tumeurs de la littérature mondiale.

Ainsi, selon le vœu de l'UICC, aucune école ne serait avantagée; on procéderait de façon «pragmatique», uniquement en apparentant les noms les plus courants et bien connus de tous, même s'ils ne sont plus valables scientifiquement, et l'on se bornerait à indiquer le meilleur synonyme.

Comme exemple, citons l'«hypernéphrome». Chaque anatomopathologiste et chaque clinicien savent bien de quelle tumeur il s'agit quand on utilise cette dénomination, qui pourtant n'est pas juste et devrait être modifiée. Aussi, dans l'atlas de l'UICC, on peut trouver des appellations plus modernes à côté de ce terme «hypernéphrome».

Le schéma de classification de l'UICC (Springer-Verlag, Berlin-Göttingen-Heidelberg, 1965) comprenait presque toutes les tumeurs pouvant survenir dans le corps humain, mais il ne procurait qu'une indication élémentaire sur la morphologie. De même, les tumeurs rencontrées en neurochirurgie étaient inventoriées et chacune d'elles était illustrée par une figure. Par cet atlas, il n'est pas possible d'apprendre le diagnostic des tumeurs intra-crâniennes. Son rôle est plutôt de tenter l'unification de la nomenclature. C'est pourquoi, il paraît nécessaire de compléter ce premier travail d'ensemble de l'UICC par des publications séparées sur les tumeurs des différents organes.

Par le présent ouvrage, nous avons tenté d'accomplir cette mission en ce qui concerne les *tumeurs intra-crâniennes*. Nous avons maintenu la classification proposée par l'UICC, même si, d'un point de vue scientifique, nous étions partisan d'une autre conception et habitué jusqu'à présent à une autre façon de classer et de grouper. Néanmoins, nous avons ajouté certains groupes, pour autant que l'UICC ne les ait pas encore adoptés dans son schéma parce qu'ils sont discutables. Conformément à la proposition de l'UICC, nous avons mentionné les synonymes connus et nous avons ainsi contribué à approfondir le travail fourni par cette association. A ce propos, signalons par exemple notre description du «sarcome monstrocellulaire».

Schéma I. *Graduation modifiée pour les tumeurs du cerveau et des structures annexes*

Tumeurs	Grade I bénin	Grade II semi-bénin	Grade III semi-malin	Grade IV malin
Gangliocytome				
isomorphe	+	+		
polymorphe			+	
Ependymome				
isomorphe	+	+		
polymorphe			+	
Papillome des plexus				
isomorphe	+			
polymorphe			+	
Astrocytome				
isomorphe		+		
polymorphe			+	
Oligodendrogliome				
isomorphe		+		
polymorphe			+	
Glioblastome				+
Spongioblastome				
isomorphe	+			
polymorphe			+	
Médulloblastome				+
Pinéalome				
isomorphe	+			
anisomorphe		+		
polymorphe			+	
Neurinome				
amitotique	+			
polymitotique			+	
Méningiome				
amitotique/oligomitotique	+			
polymitotique			+	
Angioblastome (LINDAU)	+			
Sarcome				+
Adénome hypophysaire				
isomorphe	+			
polymorphe		+		
Crânio-pharyngiome	+			

Le pronostic

Pour le clinicien, une classification morphologique présente peu d'intérêt lorsqu'elle n'apporte aucun pronostic sur la durée de la survie post-opératoire. Dans la classification de BAILEY et CUSHING, les études de 30 années ont permis de déterminer ce pronostic pour chacun des groupes tumoraux (1965). Le chirurgien peut y trouver des renseignements aussi précis et généraux que possible. C'est aussi ce qui fit certainement le grand succès de la proposition de KERNOHAN d'adopter une subdivision en quatre degrés de malignité. KERNOHAN s'alignait ainsi sur la pratique ancienne des anatomo-pathologistes de désigner le degré de malignité d'une tumeur par les termes «bénin», «semi-bénin», «semi-malin» ou «malin». Cependant, ce schéma de classification n'a pas été appliqué par KERNOHAN jusque dans les détails. Pour pouvoir l'utiliser couramment, il fallait le modifier et l'adapter aux progrès récents de nos connaissances. Des données plus complètes furent rassemblées pour *chacun* des groupes tumoraux qui, comme l'expérience l'a montré, ne présentent habituellement que deux ou au maximum trois degrés de malignité au lieu de quatre.

Pour des raisons pratiques, il était *particulièrement important* d'unifier les degrés de malignité afin de pouvoir les comparer entre eux. Un oligodendrogliome de grade III devait présenter le même comportement biologique qu'un papillome des plexus de grade III également.

Au cours de la discussion, lors du Symposium international de Cologne sur les tumeurs en 1961, nous avons proposé une formule améliorée de «graduation». Après en avoir fait l'expérience dans la pratique, nous avons élaboré, à l'occasion d'un travail d'ensemble en collaboration avec W. WECHSLER, un schéma utilisable qui est basé également sur les données de la microscopie électronique.

Il est important d'attirer l'attention sur l'existence de «degrés de transition» de malignité. Cette notion était connue depuis longtemps pour les astrocytomes, qui, dans 10% des cas environs, présentent des portions

Schéma II. *Classification des tumeurs cerébrales et leurs différents degrés de malignité*

Degré de malignité	Pronostic après exérèse "totale"	Tumeurs	
		extra-cérébrales	intra-cérébrales
Grade I bénin	Guérison ou au moins survie de 5 ans et plus	Neurinome Meningiome Adénome hypophysaire Crânio-pharyngiome	Gangliocytome (temporo-basal) Ependymome des ventricules Papillome des plexus Spongioblastome Angioblastome (LINDAU)
Grade II semi-bénin	Survie post-opératoire: 3 à 5 ans	Adénome hypophysaire polymorphe	Gangliocytome (autres localisations), Ependymome (cérébral) Astrocytome isomorphe Oligodendrogliome isomorphe Pinéalome anisomorphe
Grade III semi-malin	Survie post-opératoire: 2 à 3 ans	Méningiome polymitotique Neurinome polymitotique	Gangliocytome polymorphe Ependymome polymorphe Papillome polymorphe des plexus Astrocytome polymorphe Oligodendrogliome polymorphe Pinéalome polymorphe
Grade IV malin	Survie post-opératoire: 6 à 15 mois	Sarcome	Glioblastome Médulloblastome (Rétinoblastome) Sarcome primitif.

malignes ou sur le point de l'être (Zülch et Teltscharow, 1948). Depuis lors, nous avons observé aussi qu'il existe, à côté du groupe «isomorphe», des «oligodendrogliomes polymorphes» (1955) dont la malignité est nettement plus élevée. Nous avons décrit aussi des formes malignes de spongioblastome (1968/1969), de papillome des plexus, de neurinome, de pinéalome et de gangliocytome. Ces degrés intermédiaires de malignité furent inclus dans le schéma de classification, de telle sorte que tous les grades tumoraux soient comparables. De cette façon, *le pronostic est identique pour les différentes tumeurs* cérébrales rassemblées dans chaque groupe, du moins dans la mesure où il est permis à un morphologiste de fournir un tel renseignement sur la base d'un examen microscopique.

Malignité morphologique et clinique

Il faut rappeler brièvement que la «malignité clinique» d'une tumeur peut différer considérablement de l'estimation de sa vitesse de croissance, comme le montre le schéma suivant:

Schéma III. *Malignité «clinique» des tumeurs intra-crâniennes = malignité biologique (histologique) plus:*

1. croissance du volume
2. déplacements en masse, avec hernies: cône de pression { temporal / cérébelleux }
3. action sur la voie du L.C.R.: hydrocéphalie
4. action sur des artères (infarctus!)
5. action sur des centres vitaux: hypothalamus, mésencéphale, etc.

C'est uniquement le clinicien lui-même qui, dans chaque cas particulier, peut définir «la malignité clinique» à la lumière de toute son expérience. Le morphologiste peut seulement donner une estimation de la «croissance propre» d'une tumeur et, par sa classification morphologique et grâce à l'expérience fournie par les générations précédentes, il peut aussi fournir une indication sur le comportement biologique d'un groupe déterminé.

J'espère que cet atlas sur la classification des tumeurs intra-crâniennes se montrera utile dans la *pratique courante.* Je souhaite également qu'il puisse nous aider tous dans l'unification de la nomenclature des tumeurs intra-crâniennes et rendre plus facile la compréhension entre les morphologistes et les cliniciens dans le monde. C'est alors seulement que les problèmes thérapeutiques pourrons faire l'objet d'études statistiques irréprochables et que l'on pourra comparer entre eux les différents résultats.

Il est donc nécessaire en premier lieu que les termes conformes soient clairement définis et qu'ils puissent être traduits facilement dans le langage d'une autre classification. En deuxième lieu, une classification doit comprendre toutes les variantes connues de chaque tumeur. En troisième lieu, il doit être possible d'analyser ces variantes par les techniques appropriées de coloration et d'imprégnation, comme nous le montrons dans cet atlas.

La classification des tumeurs intra-crâniennes n'est pas toujours facile, car elles ne sont pas souvent constituées d'une population cellulaire «pure». Ici intervient le vieux principe de la «pathologie classique»: a potiori fit denominatio; la classification repose sur le type cellulaire *le plus abondant.*

Sans aucun doute, le travail de classification du morphologiste est rendu difficile lorsqu'il ne dispose que de *très petits fragments de tissu.* Les résultats de l'analyse morphologique seront d'autant meilleurs que les fragments de tissu envoyés par le neurochirurgien seront *plus volumineux.* Tel est le souhait que nous adressons au chirurgien.

Cet atlas porte en lui l'espoir de rendre possible la classification morphologique et biologique des tumeurs intra-crâniennes et d'aider ainsi le neurochirurgien dans son œuvre.

Bibliographie voir p. 258.

Introducción

Cuando un tumor es operado se examina microscópicamente a fin de tener un pronóstico del tiempo de vida del paciente.

Condición para eso es una clasificación histológica.

Por este motivo la morfología busca hace más de un siglo clasificar los tumores de varios organos de acuerdo con el aspecto microscópico del tejido, y el tiempo de sobrevivencia de los post-operados y entonces colocar en correlación la especie del tumor, determinándose así el crecimiento del tumor.

Además hay ciertos criterios microscópicos para determinar el crecimiento rápido o lento del tumor.

Casi 50 años de trabajo en la clasificación de tumores intracraneanos nos dió como resultado el poder diferenciar con mucha precisión los distintos grupos.

Conocemos la arquitectura y los tipos celulares mas frecuentes y conocemos también las diferentes variantes de la arquitectura básica y de las propias células.

El conocimiento de los últimos 30 años hizo que procesos regresivos también sean incluidos como específicos de un tumor cuando llevan a un diagnóstico bien exacto con sólo observar el tejido tumoral regresivamente modificado.

Datos históricos

La clasificación de tumores cerebrales remonta a VIRCHOW (1846), descubridor de la glia. La división hecha por él era puramente descriptiva y fué perfeccionada por BORST (1902) en su Atlas de Tumores. El principio básico de la clasificación existe desde JOHANNES MÜLLER (1838) en su comparación de las diferentes formas de tumor con los grados de diferenciación de las células, este principio fué efectuado por primera vez por PICK y BIELSCHOWSKY (1911) y por RIBBERT (1918) para tumores cerebrales, pero su auge sólo fué obtenido en los examenes exactos de BAILEY y CUSHING (1926/1930).

Estos AA. pudieron analizar las células por los métodos modernos argénticos y compararlas con las células normales y sus grados de desenvolvimiento durante la maduración celular que habían sido estudiados a través del conocimiento de la anatomía normal, por la escuelas alemana y española.

La clasificación al principio muy complicada fué más tarde simplificada.

Hoy existe un esquema de clasificación, basado en varias sugestiones hechas por PENFIELD y BERGSTRAND y en la experiencia propia, esquema éste que clasifica todas las formas de tumores en cerca de 25 tipos, que se presentan en neurocirugía.

Para los grupos de tumores de esta clasificación, se conocen bien el tiempo de vida post-operatorio medio, según resultados de las grandes clínicas americanas y europeas.

Al lado de este esquema son usados tambien mundialmente otras clasificaciones construídas en el mismo principio, por ejemplo la de RIO HORTEGA, que es preferida en los países latinoamericanos, reeditada y ligeramente modificada recientemente por POLAK.

Pocas excepciones son encontradas tambien en el Atlas de RUSSELL y RUBINSTEIN, donde por otro lado el pronóstico post-operatorio casi no está descrito.

En los mismos principios se basa también el Atlas de ROUSSY-OBERLING en el que tampoco encontramos casi indicaciones sobre el pronóstico.

Importante también al lado de la clasificación de BAILEY y CUSHING es la clasificación de KERNOHAN que contiene ya una información acerca de la malignidad. KERNOHAN combina la clasificación *histológica* de acuerdo con el tipo celular, con una división de grado *biológico* de malignidad en cuatro grados.

La clasificación de KERNOHAN encontró en los paises de lengua inglesa gran difusión.

La clasificación nuestra (1951, 1956, 1965) con 25 subtipos de tumores intracraneanos fué el resultado del trabajo mútuo diario con los neurocirujanos, esto es, originada de la práctica diagnóstica.

Ella fué la base para la publicación alemana e inglesa de los «Tumores cerebrales» así como para la descripción detallada de todos los cuadros conocidos de los tumores cerebrales y sus variantes en el Tomo III del Manual de Neurocirugía (Springer/Heidelberg, 1956) finalmente dió lugar tambien a la publicación del «Atlas en Colores de los tumores cerebrales» publicado con la ayuda de AGFA y LEITZ, contribución al libro didáctico de Anatomía Patológica de KAUFMANN (1958).

Así pués, nuestra meta fué describir tan simplificadamente los tumores intracraneanos que estos pudiesen ser diagnosticados con cortes de parafina teñidos por anilinas como corresponde a la rutina de todo Servicio de Patología General y Neuropatología.

De este modo se consigue dar el diagnóstico de casi todos los tumores intracraneanos.

Con todo, no se puede menospreciar la dificuldad que todavia existe en un 10 a 20% de casos haciendo que el diagnóstico sea, a vezes, un *verdadero arte*, aprendido solo a través de muchos años de experiencia.

Es necesario conocer exactamente las innumerables variantes de un tumor tanto en células como en su arquitectura y también las aberraciones que se derivan de procesos regresivos.

Estas variantes fueron descritos detalladamente en el Manual de Neurocirugía, siendo esta contribución concebida como una obra cientifica de consulta.

Para el trabajo cotidiano tal vez fué demasiado extenso y para muchos que la utilizan es también una dificultad la falta de conocimientos de la lengua alemana.

Nuestro pequeño libro sobre los tumores cerebrales contenía pocas ilustraciones para que se pudiese aprender a diagnosticar.

Asi nació el objetivo de este «Atlas»: completar a través de *gran número de fotografías típicas de tumores y sus variantes el texto suficiente del pequeño libro didáctico.* Las fotografías pero, tienen que ser descritas suscintamente. Para la descripción detallada deberá ser consultado el libro de «Tumores cerebrales» el Manual de Neurocirugía.

La mayoría de las ilustraciones de este Atlas son sacadas del Tomo III del «Manual de Neurocirugía» de este modo fueron reducidos los gastos consiguiendo una obra bien ilustrada.

La confusión en la terminología

En los últimos 10 años tuvimos la experiencia de que las varias escuelas no concordaban entre sí sobre la terminología de los tumores intracraneanos siendo probado definitivamente por el Simposium internacional de tumores celebrado en Colonia (1961).

Existe aún una «confusión verbal», una falta de comprensión en la terminología. Esto dificulta todo trabajo estadístico de los clínicos, cuando quieren examinar una determinada forma de tratamiento (operación, radiación, citostáticos).

Recurrimos a la clasificación de la «Unio Internationalis Contra Cancrum» sobre la que basamos el presente trabajo.

La UICC parte de que se pueden unificar las diferentes nomenclaturas más rápidamente si se colocan las definiciones y los nombres más usados, uno al lado del otro, declarándolos sinónimos. Esto tendría que ser hecho a través de grandes atlas, definidos e ilustrados por la literatura mundial.

Según voluntad de la UICC ninguna escuela debe tener preferencia, actuando «pragmáticamente» y empleando únicamente los nombres más conocidos de todos, aunque cientificamente ya no sean exactos. En este caso, sin embargo, se citaron sinónimos más adecuados.

Tomemos, a modo de ejemblo, el hipernefroma. Todo patologo general y clnico, sabe lo que quiere decir este termino, a pesar de no ser cientificamente correcto. En el Atlas de UICC encontramos por ello, al lado de esta denominación otras más modernas.

La clasificación de la UICC (Springer-Verlag, Berlin-Göttingen-Heidelberg, 1965) describe casi todos los tumores posibles de encontrar en el cuerpo humano, dando sólo una orientación previa sobre la morfologia. Los tumores corrientes en neurocirugía vienen descritos también a través de una sola fotografía de cada uno de ellos.

Este Atlas no es suficiente para aprender a diagnosticar tumores intracraneanos pués su finalidad es más bien el de unificar la nomenclatura. De ahí que esta obra de la UICC deba ser completada con publicaciones por separado sobre diferentes órganos o sistemas.

Esta nuestra publicación contribuye a ello, en el capítulo de los *tumores intracraneales.*

Seguimos para la clasificación las sugestiones dadas por la UICC incluso en los puntos en que científicamente somos de otra opinión y preferíamos otra clasificación. Pero fueron completados aquellos groupos que la UICC no habia tenido en cuenta en su esquema, por ser dudosos.

Los sinónimos conocidos fueron escritos siguiendo el procedimiento de la UICC y así el trabajo de esta sociedad fué continuado fundamentalmente. Esto se ve, por ejemplo, en nuestra descripción de los sarcomas monstrocelulares.

Pronóstico

Una clasificación morfológica es de poco valor para el clínico si no asocia un pronóstico sobre la sobrevivencia post-operatoria. Esta fué elaborada en 30 años de trabajo con el esquema de BAILEY-CUSHING y mencionada para cada grupo (1965).

El cirujano busca los datos más claros y precisos posibles y esto fué seguramente el éxito de la clasificación de KERNOHAN al

Esquema I. *Modificación de los grados de tumores del cerebro y correlación de estructuras*

Tumores	Grado I benigno	Grado II semibenigno	Grado III semimaligno	Grado IV maligno
Gangliocitoma				
isomorfo	+	+		
polimorfo			+	
Ependimoma	+	+		
isomorfo				
polimorfo			+	
Papiloma de los plexos				
isomorfo	+			
polimorfo			+	
Astrocitoma				
isomorfo		+		
polimorfo			+	
Oligodendroglioma				
isomorfo		+		
polimorfo			+	
Glioblastoma				+
Espongioblastoma				
isomorfo	+			
polimorfo			+	
Méduloblastoma				+
Pinealoma				
isomorfo	+			
anisomorfo		+		
polimorfo			+	
Neurinoma				
amitótico	+			
polimitótico			+	
Meningeoma				
amitótico/oligomitótico	+			
polimitótico			+	
Angioblastoma (LINDAU)	+			
Sarcoma				+
Adenoma pituitario				
isomorfo	+			
polimorfo		+		
Craniofaringeoma	+			

hacer 4 grados de malignidad lo que corresponde al procedimiento de los antiguos patólogos al expresar un tumor a través de los terminos: benigno, semibenigno, semimaligno y maligno esto es, uno de los cuatro grados de la división.

Esta clasificación con todo no fué llevada hasta los menores detalles por KERNOHAN.

Necesitó ser modificada para el uso cotidiano y ser adaptada al nuevo desenvolvimiento de nuestra especialidad.

Los datos globales sobre grupos de tumores fueran completados y la experiencia enseñó que *no siempre* hay cuatro grados de malignidad más si comunmente dos y lo máximo tres.

Para el uso práctico fué de *especial importancia* unificar la graduación de malignidad y hacerla así comparable.

Un oligodendroglioma de grado de malignidad III tenía que corresponder en su valor biológico al comportamiento de un papiloma de los plexos del mismo grado de malignidad.

Una tal tentativa de «división en grados» la presentamos nosotros mejorada en 1961 para discusión en el simposio coloniense internacional de tumores.

Del trabajo práctico subsiguiente surgió un sistema aprovechable y que recientemente en un trabajo más general con W. WECHSLER fué también fundamentado con el microscopio electrónico.

Creemos de importancia aludir especialmente a los grados intermedios de malignidad tales como eran conocidos desde tiempo en el astrocitoma.

Sabíase que cerca de 10% de todos los casos o tenían partes malignas o estaban a un paso de la malignidad (ZÜLCH y TELTSCHAROW, 1948).

Encontramos también que al lado del grupo de los isomorfos aparecian «oligodendrogliomas polimorfos» (1955) con una malignidad aumentada.

Aprovechamos estas observaciones sobre formas malignas en los espongioblastomas (1968—1969), en los papilomas de los plexos, en los neurinomas, en los pinealomas y en los gangliocitomas.

Estos grados de transición de malignidad fueron encajados en la clasificación y así todos

Esquema II. *Clasificación de los tumores cerebrales y su lugar en una escala de cuatro grados de malignidad*

Grado de malignidad	Pronóstico después de la extirpación «total»	Tumores extracerebrales	Tumores intracerebrales
Grado I benigno	Cura o por lo menos 5 años de sobrevivencia	Neurinomas Meningeomas Adenomas pituitarios Craniofaringeomas	Gangliocitomas (temporo-basales) Ependimomas de los ventrículos Papiloma de los plexos Espongioblastomas Angioblastomas (LINDAU)
Grado II semibenigno	Sobrevivencia post-operatoria entre 3—5 años	Adenomas pituitarios polimorfos	Gangliocitomas con distinta localización Ependimomas (cerebrales) Astrocitomas isomorfos Oligodendrogliomas isomorfos Pinealomas anisomorfos
Grado III semimaligno	Sobrevivencia post-operatoria entre 2—3 años	Meningeomas polimitóticos Neurinomas polimitóticos	Gangliocitomas polimorfos Ependimomas polimorfos Papilomas de los plexos polimorfos Astrocitomas polimorfos Oligodendrogliomas polimorfos Pinealomas polimorfos
Grado IV maligno	Sobrevivencia post-operatoria entre 6—15 meses	Sarcomas	Glioblastomas Méduloblastomas (Retinoblastomas) Sarcomas primitivos

los grados de los tumores son comparables entre sí.

Ahora todos los grupos tienen *una correlación de prognóstico para un tumor cerebral* siendo tomados estes datos por un morfólogo basándose en el examen microscópico.

Malignidad morfologica y clínica

Es necesario decir brevemente que las previsiones sobre el proceso del crecimiento puede en gran parte modificarse a través de la «malignidad clínica» de un tumor, como lo prueba el siguiente esquema.

Esquema III. *Malignidad «clínica» de un tumor intracraneal = Malignidad biológica (histológica) más*

---

1. Volumen total
2. Expansión tumoral con hernia
   temporal, cerebelar } presión del bulbo
3. Acción sobre circuito del liquido céfalorraguídeo: hidrocéfalo por oclusión
4. Acción sobre los vasos (infarto)
5. Acción sobre centros vitales: hipotálamo mesencéfalo, médula oblongata, etc.

La «malignidad clínica» sólo puede ser definida en casos aislados por el propio clínico llevando en cuenta su experiencia.

El morfólogo sólo puede dar ideas sobre el «crecimiento intrinseco» de un tumor e indicar a través de su clasificación morfólogica la experiencia de generaciones anteriores y también sobre el procedimiento biológico de determinados grupos.

Espero que este Atlas de clasificación de tumores intracraneanos puede ser de utilidad para el *trabajo cotidiano,* también tengo la esperanza de que nos ayude a todos nosotros en la unificación de la nomenclatura de dichos tumores y así permitir una mejor comprensión entre morfólogos y clínicos de todo el mundo.

Solamente entonces se conseguirá trabajar *de forma estadística correcta* en los problemas terapéuticos comparar los posibles resultados entre si.

Primero los términos precisan ser correlacionados, comprensibles y fáciles de ser traducidos en los términos de otra clasificación. En segundo lugar, es necesario que en la clasificación entren las variantes conocidas de un tumor; en tercer lugar, estas variantes tienen que poder ser analizadas con los métodos correspondientes de tinción o impregnación; esto se muestra en el presente Atlas.

La clasificación de los tumores intracraneanos no es siempre fácil porque ella frecuentemente no tiene una constitución celular pura. Aquí vale el viejo principio de «patologia clasica»: «a potiori fit denominatio», la clasificación depende del elemento celular que *más frecuentemente* aparece.

Para el morfólogo es difícil clasificar correctamente si dispone sólo de *partículas mínimas de tejido* para el examen.

Los resultados de la clasificación morfológica se van perfeccionando a medida que el neurocirujano envía *partes mayores de tejido* para el examen; esta es nuestra súplica al operador.

Al Atlas acompaña la esperanza de que él permita una clasificación morfológica y biológica de los tumores intracraneanos y ayude a los neurocirujanos en su trabajo.

Bibliografia p. 258

ВВЕДЕНИЕ

Удаленная опухоль подвергается микроскопическому исследованию для получения прогностических данных. При таком исследовании важное место принадлежит гистологической классификации. Поэтому морфологи в течение столетия совершенствуют классификацию опухолей различных органов по их микроскопическому строению. Таким образом устанавливается корреляция между послеоперационным выживанием и видом опухоли. На основании этого определяется «рост» опухоли. Кроме того имеются и другие признаки медленного и ускоренного роста опухоли.

В результате почти 50-летней работы над классификацией внутричерепных опухолей мы сейчас можем очень подробно дифференцировать отдельные группы этих опухолей. Нам известны наиболее часто встречающиеся структуры, клеточные типы и их варианты. Данные последних 30 лет свидетельствуют, что для опухолей специфичными являются также регрессивные процессы. На основании одного лишь анализа регрессивно измененной опухолевой ткани можно нередко поставить точный диагноз.

К истории вопроса

Свое начало классификация опухолей мозга берет с Вирхова (1846), открывшего глию. Чисто описательное деление Вирхова нашло дальнейшее развитие у Борста (1902) в его атласе опухолей. Со времени Мюллера (1838) основополагающий принцип классификации заключался в сопоставлении отдельных форм опухолей со стадиями развития клеток. Впервые по отношению к опухолям мозга этот принцип был применен Пиком и Бильшовским (1911), а также Рибертом (1918), но вершины от достиг лишь в подробнейших исследованиях Бейли и Кушинга (1926—1930). Они изучали клетки этих опухолей с помощью современных методов серебрения и сравнивали их с нормальными клетками на различных стадиях развития в процессе их созревания, основываясь на данных, полученных к тому времени школами немецких и испанских анатомов. Существовавшее ранее весьма сложное деление было постепенно упрощено. В настоящее время после различных изменений, внесенных Пенфилдом и Бергстрандом, а также на основе собственных данных, появилась обновленная схема, в которой классификации подлежат всего лишь каких нибудь 25 типов всех встречающихся в нейрохирургии опухолевых форм. Для опухолевых групп этой классификационной схемы стало хорошо известно среднее послеоперационное выживание, установленное по данным крупных американских и европейских клиник (Кушинг, Оливекруна, Тённис, клиника Мейо).

Наряду с этой схемой в мире применяются и другие, построенные на этом же принципе, классификационные схемы. Так, в странах Латинской Америки предпочитают классификацию Дель Рио Ортега, которая недавно была вновь изложена Полаком.

Лишь небольшое отклонение можно найти в атласе Расселл и Рубинстейна, где, правда, о послеоперационном диагнозе сказано только вскользь. На тех же принципах построен атлас Русси-Оберлена. И в этом атласе не освещены вопросы прогноза.

Наряду с делением Бейли и Кушинга, важнейшее значение приобрела классификация Керногена. В ней уже приводятся сведения о злокачественности. Керноген сочетает гистологическое деление по типу клеток с биологическими степенями злокачественности и выделяет 4 степени последней. Классификация Керногена получила большое распространение в странах с английским языком.

Наша собственная классификация (1951, 1956, 1965), насчитывающая 25 подвидов внутричерепных опухолей, возникла на основе тесного сотрудничества с нейрохирургами и поэтому отображает насущные практические потребности. Эта классификация нашла свое отражение в немецком и английском изданиях «Hirngeschwülste» была подробно освещена в «Handbuch der Neurochirurgie, Bd. III, Springer, Heidelberg (1956), в «Farbatlas der Hirntumoren» и, наконец, в «Lehrbuch der pathologischen Anatomie», Кауфмана (1958).

В нашей классификации преобладало стремление настолько просто описать внутричерепные опухоли, чтобы диагноз можно было уже поставить по парафиновым срезам при окраске анилином, то есть технике, применяемой в общих патоморфологических и нейроморфологических лабораториях. Действительно, в большом количестве случаев таким путем удается сделать правильное патоморфологическое заключение.

Однако, это было бы явным преуменьшением имеющихся еще трудностей, ибо в 10—20% случаев классифицирование внутричерепных опухолей является и сегодня большим искусством, которое приходит лишь с годами. Для этого нужно досконально знать все варианты клеточных форм и структуру каждой опухоли, а также многочисленные видоизменения, возникшие на почве регрессивных процессов. Эти варианты были в свое время подробно описаны и проиллюстрированы в книге «Handbuch der Neurochirurgie», которая была задумана как научное руководство, и поэтому оно несколько обширно для каждодневных практических целей. Кроме того, недостаточное знание немецкого языка затрудняет многим использование этого руководства. С другой стороны, в нашей второй книге «Hirngeschwülste» слишком мало иллюстраций, чтобы стать диагностическим справочником.

Поэтому целью настоящего издания является дополнение подробной текстовой части книги «Hirngeschwülste» бо́льшим количеством иллюстраций типичных опухолей и их вариантов. Сами же рисунки снабжены краткими подписями. Желающих получить более подробные сведения мы отсылаем к таким руководствам, как «Handbuch der Neurochirurgie» или «Hirngeschwülste». Большинство рисунков взято из «Handbuch der Neurochirurgie», что позволило сократить расходы на издание атласа и тем не менее включить в него большой иллюстративный материал.

Трудности терминологии

Опыт последних 10 лет показал, что отдельные школы не смогли прийти к единому мнению по вопросу терминологии внутричерепных опухолей. Это окончательно выяснилось на Международном симпозиуме по опухолям, состоявшемся в 1961 году в Кёльне. «Языковая путаница» и отсутствие согласованности по вопросам терминологии не устранены и до настоящего времени. Это в известной степени затрудняет статистическую обработку материала клиницистами и оценку различных методов лечения (хирургия, радио- и химиотерапия).

Вот почему мы обратились к классификации «Международного Противоракового Союза» («Unio Internationali Contra Cancrum») и взяли ее за основу нашей настоящей работы.

Международный Противораковый Союз исходил из представления о возможности полной унификации терминологии, если наиболее часто применяемые термины и дефиниции помещать рядом в виде синонимов. Все должно иллюстрироваться рисунками из крупных атласов, имеющихся в мировой литературе. Согласно рекомендации Международного Противоракового Союза, не следует отдавать предпочтения какой-либо одной школе, а лучше ориентироваться на наиболее употребительные, всем известные термины, даже если они в научном отношении уже не совсем состоятельны. При прочих равных условиях должны быть выделены более рациональные синонимы.

В частности, это можно проиллюстрировать на примере «гипернефромы».

Так, каждому общему патологу и клиницисту известно, что подразумевается под этим термином, хотя он с научной точки зрения неудачен и его следовало бы заменить. Поэтому в атласе Международного Противоракового Союза даются наряду с этим более современные термины.

В классификационной схеме Международного Противоракового Союза (1965) приведены почти все опухоли человека, однако их морфология едва лишь упомянута. Представлены там также встречающиеся в нейрохирургии опухоли, каждая из которых иллюстрируется одним рисунком. Такой атлас поэтому недостаточен для выявления природы внутричерепных опухолей. Его значение заключается только в попытке унификации номенклатуры. Поэтому вполне логично дополнить этот обзорный труд Международного Противоракового Союза работами по опухолям отдельных органов и систем.

Такая попытка освещения внутричерепных опухолей и предпринята нами в настоящей работе. Пришлось ориентироваться на предложения Международного Противоракового Союза даже в тех случаях, когда мы лично с научной точки зрения придерживались другого взгляда и иной группировки материала. В этом смысле отдельные разделы нами дополнены, хотя они, как спорные, еще и не были включены в схему Международного Противоракового Союза. В таких случаях, согласно положения Международного Противоракового Союза, приводятся известные синонимы. Это можно проследить на примере «уродливоклеточной саркомы».

Прогноз

Для клинициста значение морфологической классификации невелико, если в ней не содержится прогностических данных о послеоперационной выживаемости. Такие данные разрабатывались в течение 30 лет для каждой из групп классификационной схемы Бейли-Кушинга и в них хирург надеется найти более или менее точные сведения. В этом заключается секрет успеха предложений Керногена о выделении 4 степеней злокачественности. Здесь можно провести параллель с точкой зрения старых патологов, которые выражали понятия добро- и злокачественности опухоли таким определениями как «доброкачественная», «полудоброкачественная», «полузлокачественная» и «злокачественная», то есть тоже выделяли 4 степени. Однако эта классификационная схема Керногеном подробно разработана не была. Для ежедневных практических целей она нуждалась в модификации в соответствии с дальнейшим развитием нашей специальности. Общие сведения об отдельных опухолевых группах были детализированы и установлено, что не каждая опухолевая группа имеет 4 степени злокачественности, а обычно только 2 или по крайней мере 3.

Для практических целей представлялось особенно важным унифицировать степени злокачественности с целью возможности их сравнения. Например, олигодендроглиома II степени злокачественности по своим биологическим особенностям соответствует плексус-папилломе этой же II стадии злокачественности.

Такую попытку «выделения степеней» злокачественности мы в 1961 году представили на обсуждение Международного симпозиума по опухолям в Кёльне. В результате дальнейшей работы и практической проверки была создана схема, нашедшая также и электронно-микроскопическое обоснование в недавно опубликованной совместно с Векслером обзорной статье.

Мы считаем важным указать на наличие «переходных» степеней злокачественности, вроде тех, которые уже давно обнаружены в астроцитоме. Известно, что в 10% астроцитом либо есть злокачественные участки, либо обнаруживается склонность к злокачественному перерождению (Цюльх и Телчаров, 1948). Нами также установлено, что наряду с группной «изоморфных»,

Схема I. **Модификация степеней злокачественности внутричерепных опухолей**

Опухоли	I степень доброкачественные	II степень полудоброкачественные	III степень полузлокачественные	IV степень злокачественные
Ганглиоцитома				
изоморфная	+	+		
полиморфная			+	
Эпендимома				
изоморфная	+	+		
полиморфная			+	
Плексуспапиллома				
изоморфная	+			
полиморфная			+	
Астроцитома				
изоморфная		+		
полиморфная			+	
Олигодендроглиома				
изоморфная		+		
полиморфная			+	
Глиобластома				+
Спонгиобластома				
изоморфная	+			
полиморфная			+	
Медуллобластома				+
Пинеалома				
изоморфная	+			
неизоморфная		+		
полиморфная			+	
Невринома				
амитотическая	+			
полимитотическая			+	
Менингеома				
амитотическая				
(олигомитотическая)	+			
полимитотическая)			+	
Ангиобластома (Линдау)	+			
Саркома				+
Аденома гипофиза				
изоморфная	+			
полиморфная		+		
Краниофарингеома	+			

имеются еще и «полиморфные олигодендроглиомы» (1955), характеризующиеся бóльшей злокачественностью. Нами были также выявлены и изучены злокачественные формы спонгиобластом (1968—1969), плексус-папиллом, неврином, пинеалом и ганглиоцитом. Эти переходные степени злокачественности нашли свое отражение в классификационной схеме. Теперь оказалось возможным сравнение между собой опухолей всех степеней злокачественности. *Одинаковый прогноз* устанавливается *для опухолей одной*

Схема II. **Классификация опухолей мозга и их различные степени злокачественноти**

Степень злокачественности	Прогноз после «тотального» удаления	Опухоли	
		экстрацеребральные	интрацеребральные
I степень доброкачественные	Излечение или выживание в течение 5 и более лет	Невриномы Менингеомы Аденомы гипофиза Краниофарингеомы	Ганглиоцитомы (височнобазальные) Эпендимомы желудочков Плексуспапилломы Спонгиобластомы Ангиобластомы (Линдау)
II степень Полудоброкачественные	Послеоперационное выживание 3—5 лет	Аденомы гипофиза полиморфные	Ганглиоцитомы других локализаций Эпендимомы (церебральные) Астроцитомы, изоморфные Олигодендроглиомы, изоморфные Пинеаломы неизоморфные
III степень Полузлокачественные	Послеоперационное выживание 2—3 года	Менингеомы, полимитотические Невриномы, полимитотические	Ганглиоцитомы полиморфные Эпендимомы полиморфные Плексуспапилломы полиморфные Астроцитомы, полиморфные Олигодендроглиомы, полиморфные Пинеаломы, полиморфные
IV степень Злокачественные	Послеоперационное выживание 6—15 месяцев	Саркомы	Глиобластомы Медуллобластомы Первичные саркомы

и той же группы, правда, в пределах тех возможностей, которые дает морфологу микроскопическое исследование.

Морфологическая и клиническая злокачественность

Следует указать и на то, что предсказания о характере роста опухоли модифицируются в значительной степени «клинической злокачественностью» опухоли, что явствует из следующей схемы.

Схема III. **«Клиническая» злокачественность внутричерепных опухолей = биологической (гистологической) злокачественности плюс**

1. Увеличение объема
2. Смещения и вклинения
3. Воздействие на ликворные пути: гидроцефалия
4. Воздействие на артерии (инфаркты!) фаркты!)
5. Воздействие на витальные центры: гипоталамус и т. д.

Клиницист определяет «клиническую злокачественность», опираясь на свой опыт изучения конкретных случаев, а морфолог получает представление об «истинном росте» опухоли и, основываясь на разработанной морфологической классификации, может судить о биологических качествах определенных групп опухолей.

Я надеюсь, что настоящий атлас внутричерепных опухолей окажется полезным для повседневых практических целей. Я также выражаю надежду, что он поможет в унификации номенклатуры внутричерепных опухолей и будет тем самым способствовать установлению лучшего взаимопонимания между морфологами и клиницистами во всем мире. Только в этом случае можно будет получать безупречные статистические данные о лечении внутричерепных опухолей и сравнивать результат этого лечения. Для этого, во-первых, употребляемые термины должны быть понятными и легко переводимыми в понятия другой классификации; во-вторых, классификация должна отразить все известные варианты опухоли; в-третьих, материал должен окрашиваться и импрегнироваться соответствующими доступными методами. Все это нашло отражение в данном атласе.

Классификация внутричерепных опухолей не всегда проста, потому что не так уж часто приходится наблюдать «чистую» клеточную популяцию. Здесь действует старый принцип «классической патологии» — «e potiori fit denominatio», иными словами, классификация зависит от наиболее часто встречающихся клеточных элементов.

Морфологу трудно сделать правильное заключение, имея в своем распоряжении лишь очень мелкие кусочки ткани. Результаты морфологического исследования будут тем лучше, чем большими будут образцы тканей, направляемых нейрохирургом. В этом и состоит одна из наших просьб к нейрохирургу.

Еще раз питаем надежду, что настоящий атлас обеспечит морфологическую и биологическую классификацию внутричерепных опухолей и станет подспорьем в практической работе нейрохирурга.

Литература стр. 258

諸　言

患者の予後を正しく推定するためには，手術で剔出された腫瘍を顕微鏡的に検索し，かつ組織学的に分類することがまず必要である。それゆえ，この一世紀来，各種器官の腫瘍を，その組織像にしたがって分類する形態学が試みられてきた。その結果，患者の術後生存期間は腫瘍の種類に相関することが明らかとなった。このような理由から，特に腫瘍の発育度が問題にされた。腫瘍の発育度については，増殖が緩徐であるか，急速であるかを決める顕微鏡的な指標がある。

われわれが個々の腫瘍群をきわめて正確に鑑別出来るのは，この50年間の頭蓋内腫瘍の分類に関する研究の成果におうところが大きい。われわれはひん発する腫瘍の構造と細胞形態を知っているとともに，腫瘍の基本構造，細胞要素には多くの異型のあることも知っている。腫瘍の退行性変化の過程が，個々の腫瘍に特異的なものであることも，この30年間にわかった知見である。そこで退行性変化を示す腫瘍からも更に正確な診断をつけることが出来る。

歴史的展望：脳腫瘍の分類は，神経膠細胞の発見者である Virchow (1846) にはじまる。彼の分類は，記述的であったので，Borst (1902) によって改定された。Johannes Müller (1838) 以来，分類の基本的原則は，個々の腫瘍形態を細胞の発生段階と比較することであった。この原則は，Pick と Bielschowsky (1911)，更に Ribbert (1918) らにより，初めて脳腫瘍にも適用された。しかしこの試みは Bailey & Cushing (1926／30) の正確な研究によってその頂点に達した。彼らは，腫瘍細胞を新しい鍍銀法によって検索し，腫瘍細胞を正常の細胞と，また正常細胞が成熟するにいたるまでの各段階と比較した。このような成果は，ドイツおよびスペインの解剖学の知見によって裏付けられた。その後，しだいに複雑な分類が行われるようになってきた。今日では，Penfield と Bergstrand によって種々修正され，さらにそれをもとに得られた経験から改定された分類表が用いられている。この分類表では，脳外科でみられる腫瘍を25型に分類している。分類された腫瘍群については，欧米の臨床経験例 (Cushing, Olivecrona, Tönnis, Mayo-Clinic) から術後の平均生存期間が確実に推定される。

上記の分類表のほかに，世界中で各種の分類表—上述の原則に従ってはいるものの—が用いられている。たとえば Del Rio Hortega によって作られた分類表は，ラテンアメリカで好んで使われている。最近さらに Polak によっても作られた。Russel & Rubinstein の図譜には多少の相違がある。それは手術の予後について，ほとんど記載のないことである。Roussy-Oberling の分類表も同様で，予後についての記述がない。

Bailey & Cushing の分類とともに，Kernohan の分類は，もっとも重要なものである。この分類には腫瘍の悪性度についての説明が加えられている。Kernohan は細胞の形態を指標とした組織学的分類に，悪性度の生物学的段階区分を組み合せ，その結果，腫瘍の悪性度を4段階にわけた。この Kernohan の分類は，英語を使う国々で広く使われている。

頭蓋内腫瘍を25型に分類（1951，1956，1965）出来たのは神経外科医との共同研究に基づいている。すなわち，毎日の診療の経験から出来たものである。この分類は，ドイツ語版並びに英語版の「脳腫瘍」の基礎であるとともに，神経外科学叢書3巻 (Springer/Heidelberg 1956) に詳述された脳腫瘍とその異型の基礎になったものである。さらに又 Agfa および Leitz の援助で出来た「脳腫瘍のカラー図譜」と，Kaufmann の「病理解剖学」(1958) のなかの記載にもこの分類がとり入れられている。

頭蓋内腫瘍の分類をわれわれがここに供覧する目的は，腫瘍を簡潔に記載出来るようにすることである。腫瘍は Anilin 系の色素で染色したパラフィン切片で診断がつくようになったので，この方法は一般病理学および神経病理学教室に適うものである。事実，多数例の頭蓋内腫瘍の診断がこの方法でうまく行われている。

しかしながら，まだまだ軽んじえない困難な問題がある。それは頭蓋内腫瘍のうち，10～20％の症例を分類するためには，今日まで熟練した技術を必要とすることである。この技術は，ただ長年の経験から取得出来るものである。特に，細胞の形態と構築上，腫瘍には多種多様な異型のあること，またこれと同時に，退行性変化の過程で生ずる変形をも正確に知らねばならない。これらの変形については，神経外科学叢書に詳細な記載がある。この綜説は，この方面の科学的便覧にあたると考える。それゆえ，診療にたづさわる際には詳細すぎる。利用者の中には，ドイツ語に関する知識不足から，叢書内のわれわれの綜説の利用が困難な人もいる。「脳腫瘍」というわれわれの小さな本は，独習で診断がつけられるようになれるほど，多くの写真は掲載されていない。

この図譜出版の目的は，すでに出版した縮小型の教科書の説明を多数の定型的な腫瘍およびその異型を写真によって補うことである。しかし，写真にはただ簡単な説明のみをつけるべきであると思う。詳細な記載は叢書，「脳腫瘍」にあるので充分である。この図譜の写真の多くは，神経外科学叢書3巻からとったものである。したがって複写のための費用をはぶけ，しかも多くの写真を掲載することが出来た。

術語の混乱について：この10年間，われわれは頭蓋内腫瘍に関する術語が，それぞれの学派で異なることを経験して来たが，1961年に行われたKöln 国際脳腫瘍シンポジュームで，さらにはっきりと実証された。いまだに〝用語の混乱〟すなわち，術語についての理解不足がある。このことが，治療法(手術，放射線療法，化学療法)の効果について統計学的な検討を臨床医にさせることを困難にしている。

われわれは，国際対癌連合(Unio Internationalis Contra Cancrum)の分類に立ち帰って，その翻案を基礎とした。UICCは，研究者のしばしば用いる学名と定義を比べ，それぞれの同意語を判然とさせた時に，各種の学名を統一することが可能であると述べている。この場合には，世界中で既に出版されている腫瘍の図譜のなかの写真を用いて定義ならびに説明がなされねばならない。その際UICCの意図にもとづいて，特定の学派に特典を与えてはならない。事務的に仕事をすすめ，ひん繁に用いられている名称を利用すべきである。しかし，その名称がもはや科学的に根拠のないものになった時は，各研究者の良く知っているほかの名称を用いるべきである。ここでよく適合した同意語について述べることにする。

例として「副腎腫」について説明したい。副腎腫という名称が，科学的には妥当ではなく，改称すべきではあるが，この名称の腫瘍がどの様なものであるかは，一般病理学者および臨床家には周知のことである。副腎腫のような使い方をしたものと，新しい用語とがUICCの図譜には見だされる。

UICCの分類法(Springer-Verlag, Berlin-Göttingen-Heidelberg, 1965)には，人体にみられるほとんどすべての腫瘍が記載されてはいるが，腫瘍の形態学についての最初の手掛りを与えたにとどまる。さらに神経外科学の領域でみられる腫瘍についても写真をもちいて説明がなされている。しかしこの図譜は頭蓋内腫瘍の診断を学ぶためには，まだ不充分である。この図譜のもっている意義は，学名を統一化しようとするところにある。それゆえに，各種器官系の腫瘍についての研究成果を公表することでUICCの概括的な報告を補わねばならない。

この図譜を作ることは，頭蓋内腫瘍について上記の課題を実現させるための試みと云える。われわれは，腫瘍の分類を行う際にはUICCの提案を守ることにしているが，この図譜の一部には，いささか異なる見解と分類を用いたところがある。さらに，UICCが分類の中に取り入れていない二三のものについても補った。この種の腫瘍がUICCの分類に引用されていないのは，それら腫瘍に関して，まだ議論の余地があるからである。この場合に，われわれはUICCの取り扱い方に合致するようによく知られた同意語を用いた。それによって，UICCの仕事が更に発展すると思われたからである。それはわれわれの“Monstrozelluläres Sarkom”と云う記載に例をみる。

予後：形態学的分類のなかに腫瘍剔出後の患者の生存期間について記載のない場合，その分類は臨床家にとってそれほど大きな利用価値はない。このことは30年間を要して作られたBailey-Cushingの分類についても，さらにそれぞれの学派の分類についてもいえることである(1965)。外科医は出来るかぎり，正確かつ概括的な報告をもとめている。このことが動機となって，Kernohanは腫瘍の悪性度を4段階に区分するという偉大な成果を収めた。彼の分類は古くからの病理学の方法を用いて，腫瘍の悪性度を〝良性〟，〝亜良性〟，〝亜悪性〟，〝悪性〟の4段階にわけた。しかし，彼は個々の腫瘍についてこの分類規準をあてはめるところまではいかなかった。彼の分類が日常利用されるためには，さらに修正の必要がある。そこで，われわれの得た新しい結果をこの分類表にあてはめてみた。二三の腫瘍群については簡単な説明を加え，次に経験を考慮に入れて，個々の腫瘍群を4段階にわけずに，2ないし3段階に区分してみた。

実際的な活用には，悪性度を統一してそれぞれを比較することが可能なところに，特別な意義がある。たとえば，希突起膠腫の悪性度Ⅲは生物学的尺度を用いた場合，脉絡叢乳頭腫の悪性度Ⅲに一致しなければならない。

われわれは，1961年Kölnで行われた国際脳腫瘍シンポジュームの際の討論を通じて悪性度の段階区分の試みをさらに修正した。その後，実際的な仕事を通じて利用出来る分類表が作られた。この分類表はW. Wechslerと共著で出した総括的な論文のなかに，電顕所見をも含めて，簡潔にまとめられている。

われわれは，悪性度の移行段階を明らかにすることに重点をおいている。たとえば星膠細胞腫では移行段階のあることが古くから知られている。すなわち，星膠細胞腫のうち，約10%は局部的に悪性であるか，悪性型に移行しつつあるものである(Zülch u. Teltscharow 1948)。またわれわれは，稀突起膠腫には同形性を示すもののほかに，悪性度の高い多形性のものがあることを見つけた(1955)。更に，われわれは，海綿芽細胞腫(1968/69)，脉絡叢乳頭腫，神経鞘腫，松果体腫そして神経細胞腫の悪性型についての観察結果をもとり入れた。悪性度の移行段階は分類表のなかにとり入れてある。そしてすべての腫瘍を互いに比較出来るようにした。今ここに，ひとつのグループの脳腫瘍は，すべて同一の予後を示すグループであることが判る。形態学者のみによって作られたこ

表Ⅰ 神経外胚葉性脳腫瘍の悪性度（Grading）

腫　瘍	Ⅰ度 良性	Ⅱ度 亜良性	Ⅲ度 亜悪性	Ⅳ度 悪性
神経細胞腫 同　形　性	＋	＋		
多　形　性			＋	
上衣細胞腫 同　形　性	＋	＋		
多　形　性			＋	
脈絡叢乳頭腫 同　形　性	＋			
多　形　性			＋	
星膠細胞腫 同　形　性		＋		
多　形　性			＋	
稀突起膠腫 同　形　性		＋		
多　形　性			＋	
膠　芽　腫				＋
海綿芽細胞腫 同　形　性	＋			
多　形　性			＋	＋
髄　芽　腫				
松果体腫 同　形　性	＋			
不同形性		＋		
多　形　性			＋	
神経鞘腫 無分裂性	＋			
多分裂性			＋	
脳　膜　腫 無分裂性／希分裂性	＋			
多分裂性			＋	
血管芽細胞腫 (Lindau)	＋			
肉　　腫				＋
下垂体腺腫 同　形　性	＋			
多　形　性		＋		
頭蓋咽頭腫	＋			

表Ⅱ 脳腫瘍の分類とその悪性度の関係

悪性度	予　後	腫瘍 脳　外	 脳　内
Ⅰ　度 良　性	治癒又は ５年以上 生存可能	神経鞘腫 脳膜腫 下垂体腺腫 頭蓋咽頭腫	神経細胞腫（側頭一基底部） 上衣細胞腫（脳室） 脈絡叢乳頭腫 海綿芽細胞腫 血管芽細胞腫
Ⅱ　度 亜良性	術後生存 期間３－５年		星膠細胞腫（同形性） 稀突起膠腫（同形性） 上衣細胞腫（大脳・旁脳室） 神経細胞腫（一般）
Ⅲ　度 亜悪性	術後生存 期間１－３年	脳膜腫 （多分裂性） 神経鞘腫 （多分裂性）	神経細胞腫（多形性） 上衣細胞腫（多形性） 脈絡叢乳頭腫（多形性） 星膠細胞腫（多形性） 稀突起膠腫（多形性）
Ⅳ　度 悪　性	術後生存 期間６－12ケ月	肉腫（クモ膜，硬膜，硬膜外）	膠芽腫 髄芽腫（網膜芽細胞腫）

の種の分類は，顕微鏡的な検索のみに頼りすぎるきらいがある。

形態学的，臨床的悪性度：腫瘍の発育態度についての予想は，臨床的悪性度によって，さらに修正されることを指摘せねばならない。下表を参照されたい。

表Ⅲ　頭蓋内腫瘍の臨床的悪性度

生物学的（組織学的）悪性度と
1）脳容積の増大
2）ヘルニアを作った脳の移動＜側頭部／小脳部＞ヘルニア
3）脳脊髄液循環への影響：閉塞性脳水腫
4）血管への影響（梗塞）
5）脳幹部への影響：視床下部，延髄等

臨床的な悪性度は，臨床医自身が自験例を考察することによって決めることが出来る。形態学者は腫瘍の発育についての概念，更に過去の経験にのっとった形態学的分類を通して，各腫瘍群の生物学的態度を明らかにし得るにとどまる。

私は，この頭蓋内腫瘍の分類図譜が，日常利用されることを希望する。更にこの図譜が頭蓋内腫瘍の学名を統一するための助けとなり，それによって，形態学者と臨床医の協調が更にきん密になることを希望する。そうなれば，治療上の問題点を検討する際，統計学的にも正しく処理出来るようになり，結果も比較し得るようになる。そのためには，まず意味の明瞭な学名を用いるようにし，ほかの分類にもあてはめられるようにすべきである。第２に，分類に際して，その学名がすべて周知の腫瘍の異形についても該当せねばならない。第３に，この異形はそれに適した染色法又は鍍銀法で検索が可能でなければならない。それらの条件に合うようにこの図譜は作られている。

頭蓋内腫瘍の分類は，理解しやすいものではない。それはこの腫瘍が単一の細胞群からなることが少いからである。それゆえ分類は多数を占める細胞要素に負うという古典病理学の原則が重きをなす。

形態学者が検索のために小さな組織片のみしか得られない場合には，正しい分類をすることはむずかしい。脳外科医が検索のために，より大きな組織塊を形態学者に送る時のみ形態学的分類の正確さが増す。そこで常に大きな組織塊を送られるよう手術医にわれわれはお願いする。

この図譜が頭蓋内腫瘍の形態学的，生物学的分類を可能にし，それによって脳外科医を仕事の面で援助出来るように私の希望を本書に託する。

258頁の文献参照

Gangliocytomas

Ganglioneuroma, gangliogIioma, true neuroma, ganglioma, glioneuroblastoma, neuroastrocytoma, neurocytoma, neuroblastoma, Purkinjeoma etc.

Fig. 1 — Gangliocytomas

a)—d) Various patterns of the tumor cells in a gangliocytoma. Many cells have typical Nissl bodies and in between them lie the spindle or lymphoid cells of the interstitial tissue. In others the Nissl substance is present only as a fine powder. In the last two microphotographs one recognizes "ganglioid" nuclei only, while the true nature of the cells can only be determined with assurance from other positions of the tumor. In the literature these cells are designated as "neuroblasts".

a)—d) Verschiedene Bilder der Geschwulstzellen in einem Gangliocytom. Manche Zellen haben typische Nissl-Schollen und zwischen ihnen liegen die spindeligen oder lymphoiden Zellen des Zwischengewebes. Bei anderen ist die Nissl-Substanz nur feinstäubig vorhanden. Bei den letzten beiden Aufnahmen erkennt man nur noch „ganglioide" Kerne, während man auf die wahre Natur der Zellen mit Sicherheit nur aus anderen Stellen der Geschwulst schließen kann. Im Schrifttum werden diese Zellen als „Neuroblasten" bezeichnet.

a)—d) Différents aspects des cellules tumorales dans un gangliocytome. Beaucoup de cellules contiennent des blocs de Nissl typiques et sont mêlées à des cellules fusiformes ou lymphoïdes du tissu interstitiel. D'autres cellules ne contiennent plus qu'une substance de Nissl finement poussiéreuse. Dans les deux dernières images, on ne voit plus que les noyaux «ganglioïdes» et l'on ne peut reconnaître avec certitude la nature exacte de ces cellules que par l'examen d'autres endroits de la tumeur. Dans la littérature, on donne à ces cellules le nom de «neuroblastes».

a)—d) Diferentes imágenes de las células tumorales en un gangliocitoma. Algunas células tienen típicos grumos de Nissl; entre ellas se encuentran células fusiformes o linfoideas del conectivo. En otras la substancia de Nissl se encuentra en finas granulaciones. En las dos últimas fotos sólo se reconocen núcleos redondos mientras que la verdadera naturaleza de las células tumorales solo puede asegurarse en otras partes del tumor. En la literatura a estas células se las designa como neuroblastos.

a)—d) Различные картины опухолевых клеток ганглиоцитомы. В одних клетках имеются типичные зерна Ниссля, а между ними находятся веретенообразные или лимфоидные клетки межуточной ткани, в других вещество Ниссля представлено в виде мелкой пыли. В этих местах видны лишь «ганглиоидные» ядра; об истинной же природе опухоли можно судить только по другим участкам. В литературе эти клетки описываются как «нейробласты».

a)—d) 神経細胞腫における､多様な腫瘍細胞所見。多くの細胞は定型的な Nissl 顆粒を有し、間質には紡錘形あるいはリンパ球様細胞が存在している。図 c)— d) には「神経細胞様」核がみらるのみで、他の部分を参照して始めて確実な診断が下される。文献には、この細胞は「神経芽細胞」と記載されている。

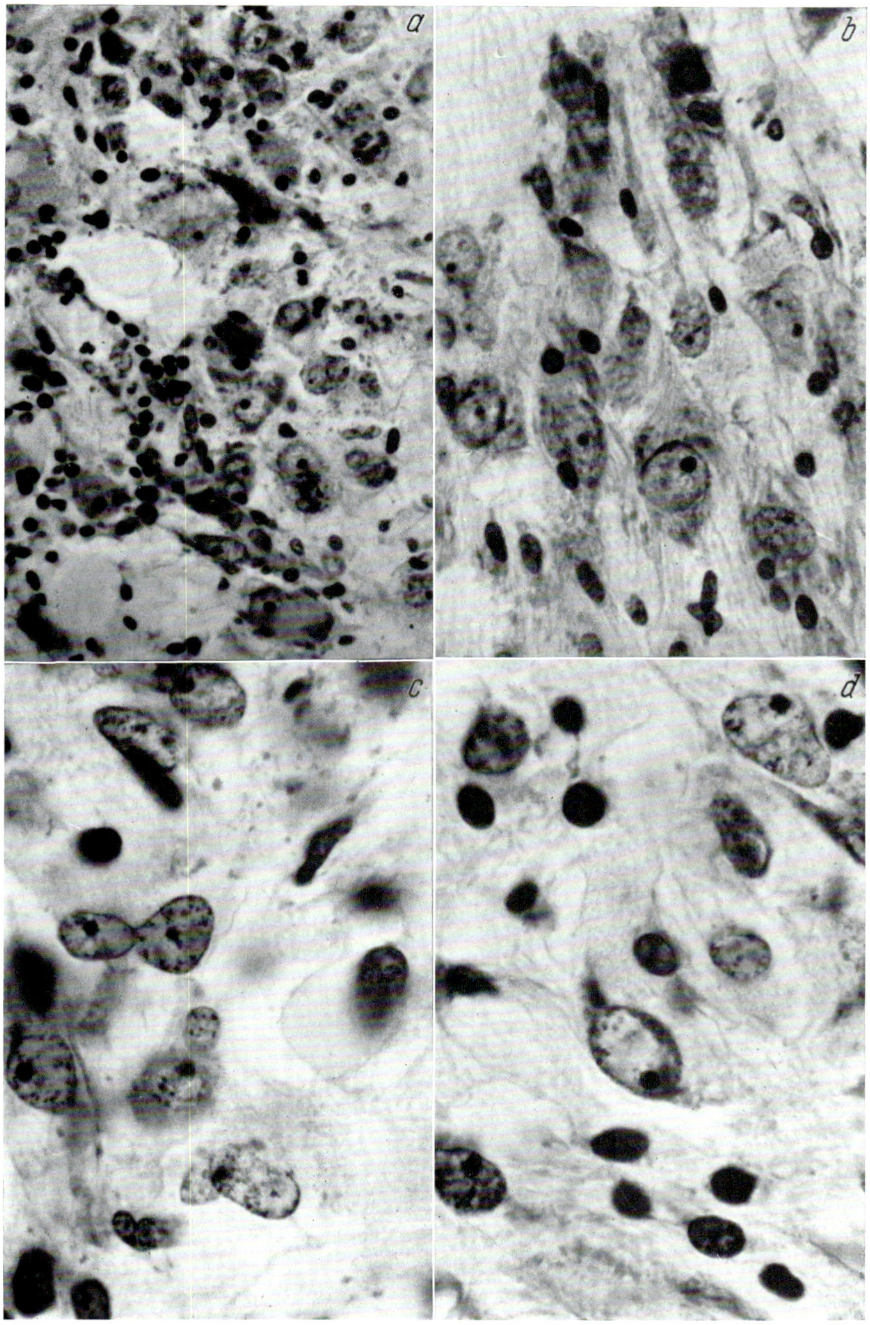

Fig. 1a—d: a ×218, b ×780, c and d ×1,040
Cresyl violet stain

Fig. 2 — Gangliocytomas

The cells of the gangliocytoma:

a) "Matured", partly binucleated ganglion cells in a small gangliocytoma of the head of the caudate nucleus.

b) Large ganglion cells with Nissl granules.

c) and d) Typical cells of a gangliocytoma of a sympathetic ganglion.

Die Zellen des Gangliocytoms:

a) „Ausgereifte", z.T. doppelkernige Ganglienzellen in einem kleinen Gangliocytom des Schweifkernkopfes.

b) Große Ganglienzellen mit Nissl-Schollen.

c) und d) Typische Zellen eines Gangliocytoms des Sympathicus.

Les cellules du gangliocytome.

a) Cellules nerveuses arrivées à « maturité » et parfois binucléées, dans un petit gangliocytome de la tête du noyau caudé.

b) Volumineuses cellules ganglionnaires contenant des blocs de Nissl.

c) et d) Cellules typiques d'un gangliocytome du sympathique.

Células en los gangliocitomas:

a) Células ganglionares «maduras» en parte binucleadas en un pequeño gangliocitoma del núcleo caudal.

b) Grandes células ganglionares con grumos de Nissl.

c) y d) Típicas células de un gangliocitoma del simpático.

Клетки ганглиоцитомы:

a) «Зрелые», частично двуядерные ганглиозные клетки в малой ганглиоцитоме головки хвостатого ядра,

b) Крупные ганглиозные клетки с субстанцией Ниссля.

c) и d) Типичные клетки ганглиоцитомы симпатического нерва.

神経細胞腫の腫瘍細胞。

a) 二核性細胞を混じた「成熟」神経細胞。尾状核頭部の小腫瘍にみられたもの。

b) Nissl 顆粒をもった大型の神経細胞。

c) および d) 交感神経節細胞腫の定型的な腫瘍細胞。

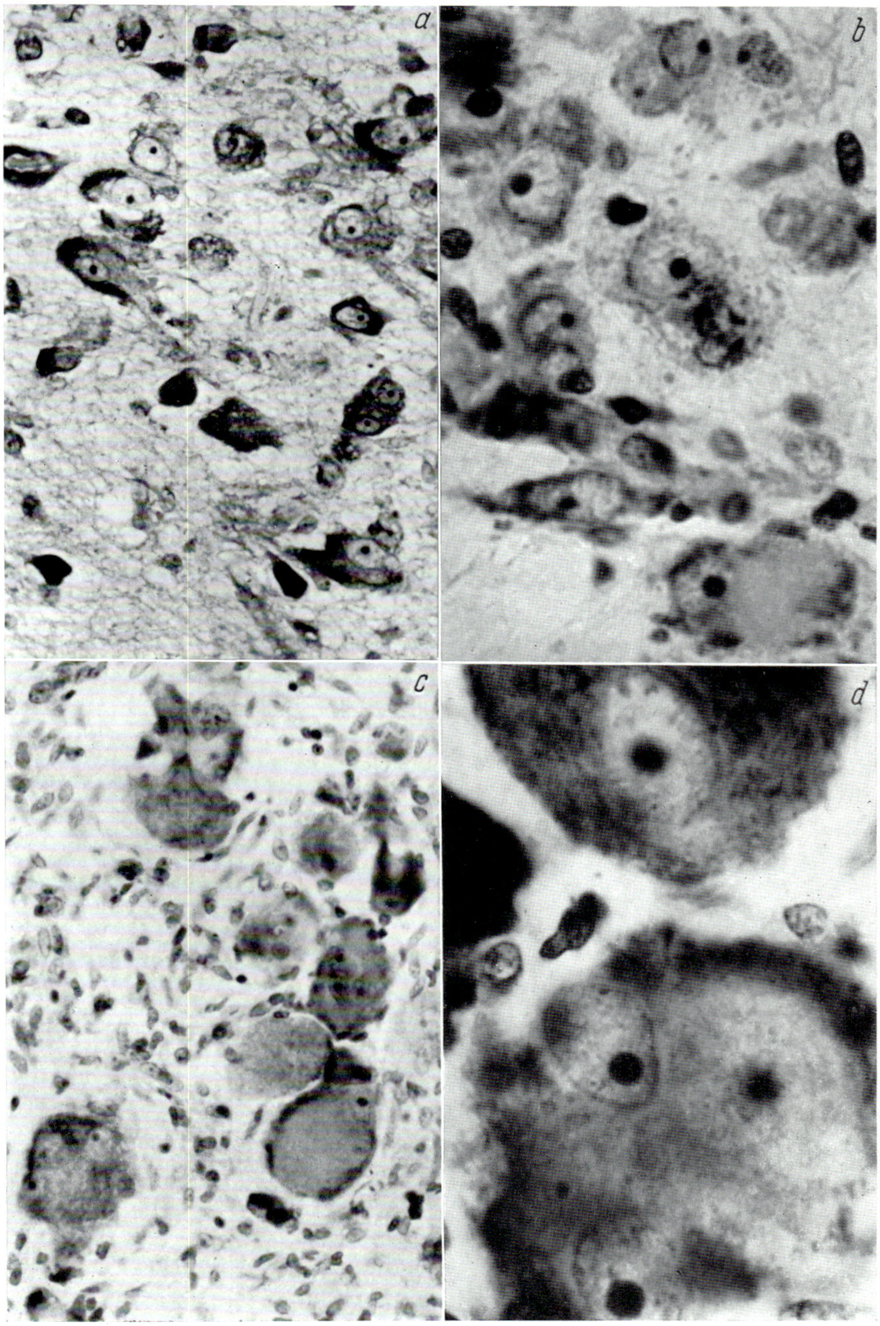

Fig. 2a—d: a ×272 b ×548, c ×120, d ×1,040
Cresyl violet stain

Fig. 3 — Gangliocytomas

Concerning the architecture of the gangliocytoma:

a) and b) The extensive connective tissue with blood vessels leaves individual islands free, in which the ganglion cells are located.

c) The pia (*top*), extensively infiltrated by tumor cells, is sharply delineated from the brain (*bottom*). In the outer layers of the brain one sees a reactive macrogliosis.

d) The pia is infiltrated by a gangliocytoma (*right*). Marked increase of the adventitia of the blood vessels, which extend from the leptomeninges into the brain. The adventitial spaces are filled with "round cells".

Zur Architektur des Gangliocytoms:

a) und b) Das reichliche Bindegewebe mit Gefäßen läßt einzelne Inseln frei, in denen die Ganglienzellen liegen.

c) Die von den Geschwulstzellen reichlich infiltrierten weichen Häute (oben) sind vom Hirn scharf abgetrennt (unten). In den obersten Schichten des Hirns sieht man eine reaktive Makrogliose.

d) Die weichen Häute sind von einem Gangliocytom infiltriert (rechts). Deutliche Vermehrung der Adventitia an den Gefäßen, die von der Leptomeninx in das Hirn einstrahlen. Die adventitiellen Räume sind mit „Rundzellen" gefüllt.

L'architecture du gangliocytome.

a) et b) Des travées riches en tissu conjonctif et en vaisseaux séparent des îlots de cellules ganglionnaires.

c) Les cellules tumorales infiltrent abondamment la leptoméninge (au-dessus) sans envahir le cerveau (au-dessous), dont les couches superficielles présentent une macrogliose réactionnelle.

d) La leptoméninge (à droite) est infiltrée par un gangliocytome. Epaississement important de l'adventice des vaisseaux leptoméningés, qui pénètrent dans le cerveau. Les espaces adventitiels sont bourrés de «cellules rondes».

Arquitectura del gangliocitoma:

a) y b) El abundante tejido conectivo, con sus vasos, deja islas libres, en las que se disponen las células ganglionares.

c) Las leptomeninges, intensamente invadidas por las células tumorales (arriba) están vigorosamente separadas del cerebro (abajo). En las capas más superiores de éste se observa una macrogliosis reactiva.

d) Las leptomeninges están infiltradas por un gangliocitoma (derecha). Evidente crecimiento de la adventicia en los vasos que penetran en el cerebro a partir de las leptomeninges. Los espacios adventiciales están llenos de células redondas.

К строению ганглиоцитомы:

a) и b) В обильной соединительной ткани с сосудами имеются отдельные островки ганглиозных клеток.

c) Обильно проросшие опухолевыми клетками мягкие мозговые оболочки (вверху) четко отграничены от мозговой ткани (внизу). В наиболее верхних слоях мозга виден реактивный макроглиоз.

d) Инфильтрированные ганглиоцитомой мягкие мозговые оболочки (справа). Четкое размножение адвентиции сосудов, проникнущие из лептоменинкса в мозг. Адвентициальные полости полны «круглыми клетками».

神経細胞腫の組織像:

a) および b) 血管をともなった豊富な結合組織が、いくつかの神経細胞集団（島）をつゝんでいる。

c) 多数の腫瘍細胞が浸潤している軟膜（図上）と、境界の明瞭である脳の最表層に、反応性マクログリヤの増殖がおこっている。

d) 軟膜は神経細胞によって浸潤されている（図右)。軟膜から脳実質内に入る血管の外膜は高度の増殖を示す。外膜腔に「円形細胞」が存在している。

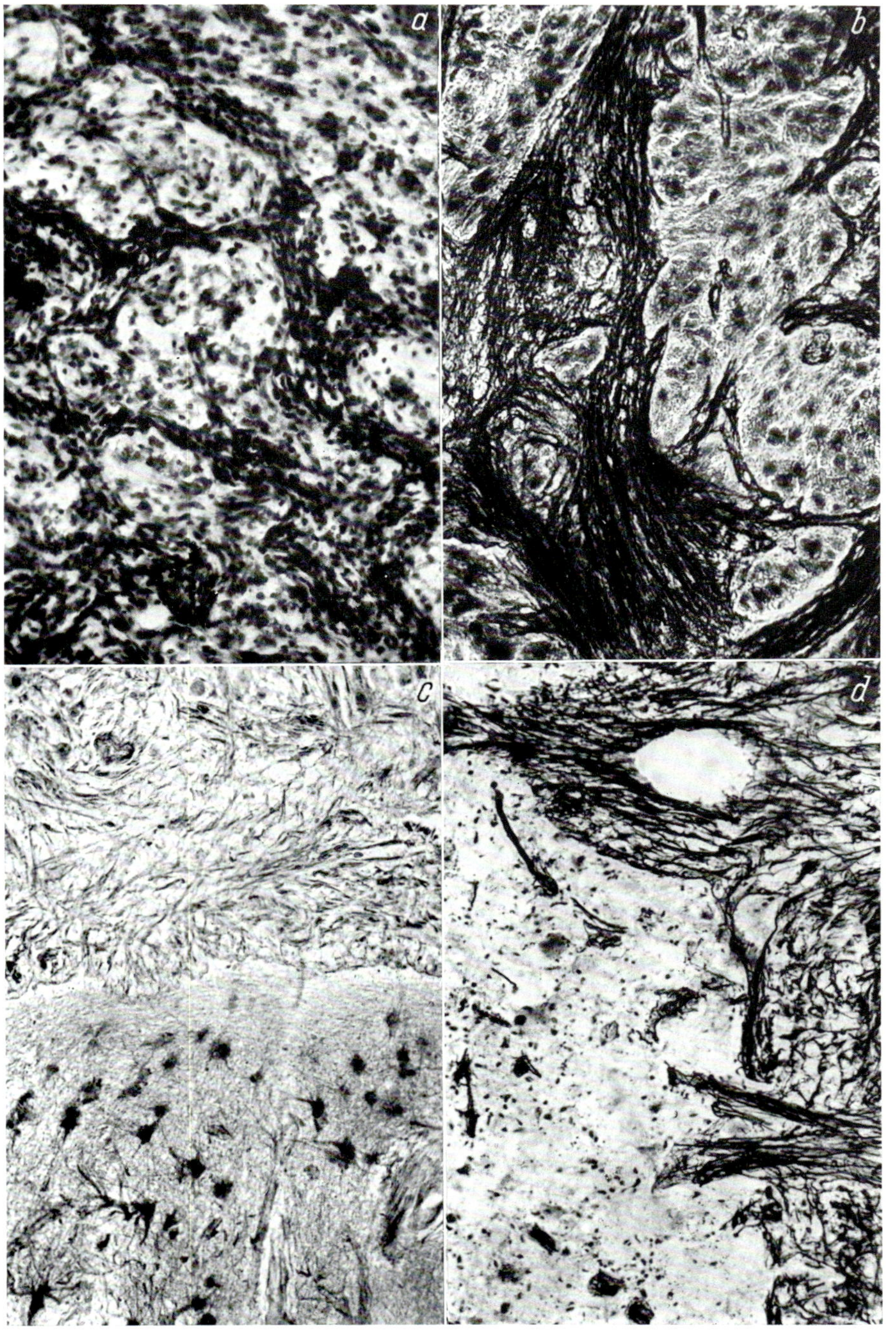

Fig. 3a—d: a ×120. Cresyl violet stain
b ×104. Tannin silver method
c ×75. Gold sublimate method
d ×96. PERDRAU's method

Fig. 4 — Gangliocytomas

a)—c) Multinucleated ganglion cells from a malignant gangliocytoma. All the cells are "mature". Biologically, the tumor behaved like a glioblastoma.

d) *Bottom:* A binucleated ganglion cell with only a few Nissl granules. *Top:* A large ganglion cell containing finely powdered calcification. The dark spindle-shaped nuclei belong to connective tissue cells.

a)—c) Mehrkernige Ganglienzellen aus einem malignen Gangliocytom. Die Zellen tragen sämtlich die Zeichen höchster ,,Reife". Biologisch verhielt sich die Geschwulst wie ein Glioblastom.

d) Unten liegt eine doppelkernige Ganglienzelle mit nur wenig Nissl-Schollen, oben eine große mit feinstäubiger Verkalkung. Die dunklen spindeligen Kerne gehören zu Bindegewebszellen.

a)—c) Cellules nerveuses multinucléées dans un gangliocytome malin. Les cellules présentent tous les signes d'une «maturité» complète. Au point de vue biologique, la tumeur a évolué comme un glioblastome.

d) A la partie inférieure, on note une cellule nerveuse binucléée et contenant peu de blocs de Nissl. A la partie supérieure, une grande cellule nerveuse est chargée de calcifications finement poussiéreuses. Les noyaux foncés et allongés appartiennent aux cellules du tissu conjonctif.

a)—c) Células ganglionares multinucleadas de un gangliocitoma maligno. La totalidad de las células muestra signos de máxima «maduración». Biológicamente el tumor se comporta como un glioblastoma.

d) Abajo se ve una célula ganglionar binucleada con solo unos pocos grumos de Nissl; arriba una célula grande presenta una fina granulación calcárea. Los núcleos obscuros, fusiformes, pertenecen a células del conectivo.

a)—c) Многоядерные ганглиозные клетки злокачественной ганглиоцитомы. Все келтки обладают признаками высшей «зрелости». Биологически опухоль ведет себя как глиобластома.

d) Внизу видна двуядерная ганглиозная клетка с небольшим количеством субстанции Ниссля; вверху крупная ганглиозная клетка с обызвествлением в виде мелкой пыли. Темные веретенообразные ядра принадлежат соединительно-тканным клеткам.

a)—c) 悪性神経細胞腫の多核神経細胞。これらの細胞は、全体として高度に成熟した所見をそなえている。この腫瘍の生物学的態度は、膠芽腫のそれに相当する。

d) 図の下に僅少の Nissl 顆粒をもつ２核性神経細胞、上部に微細な石灰化を示す神経細胞がある。濃染した紡錘形核は結合組織細胞のもの。

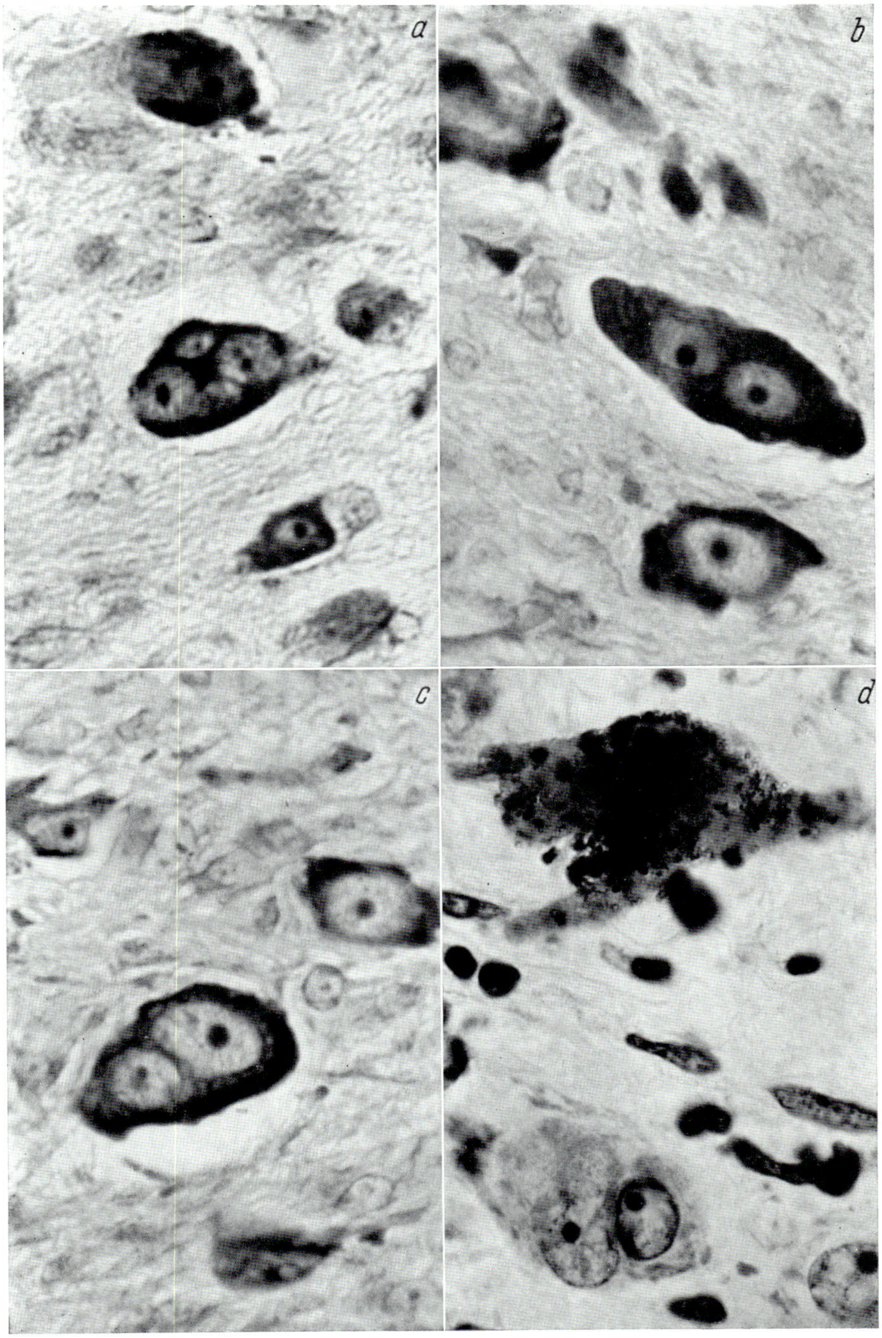

Fig. 4a—d: a—c ×648, d ×1,040
Cresyl violet stain

Fig. 5 — Gangliocytomas

Characteristic of the peripheral gangliocytoma are:

a) Small lymphocyte-like (or medulloblast-like) cells, b) neuroblastic cell types, the ganglion-cell nature of which is apparent, and c) large mature often multinucleated ganglion cells. The mitotic figures indicate the rapid rate of growth, although mature ganglion cells are produced.
b) Some portions of these tumors are composed entirely of mature ganglion cells with abundant Nissl substance.
c) These cells are frequently dysplastic and multinucleated. There are, in addition, multinucleated cells with undifferentiated nuclei and without Nissl substance. The nature of these cells is not clear.
d) Also characteristic of peripheral gangliocytoma (sympathetic, adrenal) is an admixture of undifferentiated cells of unknown origin, neuroblasts and ganglion cells in various stages of maturity.

a) Beim peripheren Gangliocytom ist das Nebeneinander von kleinen „lymphoiden“ (oder medulloblastomartigen) Zellen, von neuroblastenartigen Typen, denen man die Ganglienzellnatur schon ansieht und von großen ausgereiften, oft mehrkernigen Ganglienzellen charakteristisch. Mitosen weisen auf die rasche Proliferation hin, obwohl auch ausgereifte Ganglienzellen gebildet werden.
b) Einzelne Partien dieser Tumoren bestehen fast ausschließlich aus ausgereiften Zellen mit reichlichem Besatz an Nisslkörpern.
c) Diese Zellen sind oft mehrkernig und dysplastisch. Man sieht außerdem mehrkernige Zellen mit undifferenzierten Kernen und ohne Nisslsubstanz, deren Natur nicht klar ist.
d) Ein Gemisch von undifferenzierten Zellen, deren Natur nicht identifizierbar ist, von Neuroblasten und von Ganglienzellen aller Reifungsstufen ist für die „peripheren“ Gangliocytome (Sympathicus, Nebennieren) charakteristisch.

a) Dans le gangliocytome périphérique, il est caractéristique de trouver des cellules lymphoïdes (ou «médulloblastiques») parmi des cellules de type neuroblastique, dont la nature ganglionnaire peut déjà se reconnaître, et de grandes cellules nerveuses différenciées et souvent multinucléées. Les mitoses témoignent d'une prolifération rapide, quoique des cellules ganglionnaires différenciées soient formées.
b) Dans certaines zones de cette tumeur, il existe presque uniquement des cellules ganglionnaires différenciées, riches en blocs de Nissl.
c) Souvent, ces cellules contiennent plusieurs noyaux et ont une allure dysplasique. On voit entre autres des cellules multinucléées, à noyaux indifférenciés et sans substance de Nissl, dont la nature n'est pas élucidée.
d) Le mélange de cellules indifférenciées, dont la nature n'est pas identifiable, de neuroblastes et de cellules ganglionnaires à tous les stades de la maturation est caractéristique du gangliocytome «périphérique» (sympathique, surrénale).

a) En los gangliocitomas periféricos aparecen otras células pequeñas «linfoides» (semejantes «méduloblastoma») de tipo neuroblástico, viéndose su naturaleza de célula ganglionar con varios núcleos caracteristicos de la misma.
Numerosas mitosis muestran la rapidez de la proliferación aunque lleguen a células ganglionares.
b) Fragmento de este mismo tumor constituido por gran cantidad de células com corposculos de Nissl.
c) Estas células son multinucleares y displásicas. Otras células poseen núcleo indiferenciado y sin substancia de Nissl, por lo que es difícil decir de que naturaleza son.
d) Mezcladas con células indiferenciadas cuya naturaleza no se puede identificar existe toda la gama, desde neuroblastos hasta células ganglionares de tipo gangliocitoma «periférico» (simpático, supra-renal).

Continued on page 42.

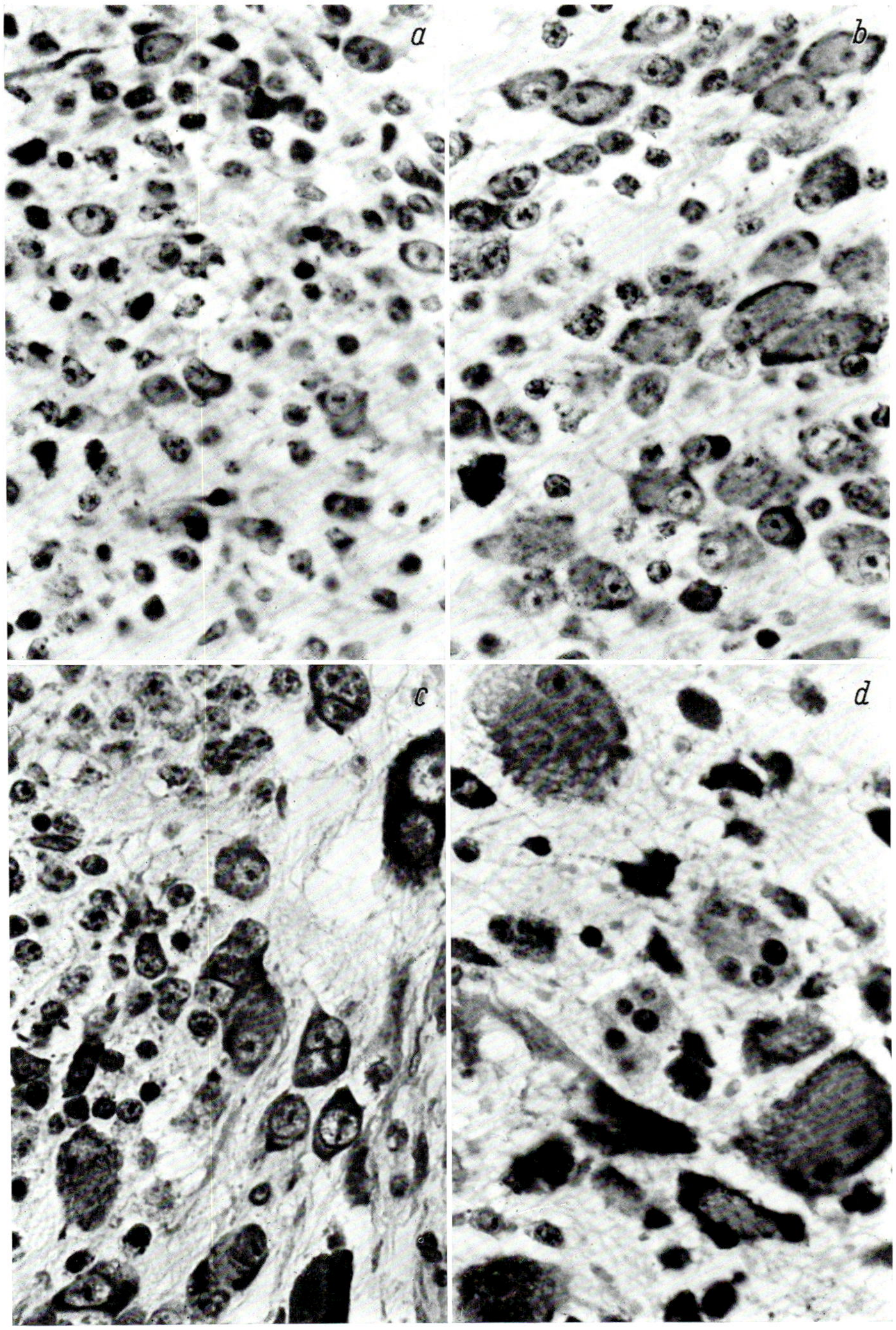

Fig. 5a—d: ×500. Cresyl violet stain

Fig. 5 — Gangliocytomas (continued)

a) Характерное для периферической ганглиоцитомы сосуществование мелких «лимфоидных» (или «медуллобластомоподобных») клеток, нейробластоподобных клеток, в которых уже прослеживается ганглиозноклеточная природа и крупных зрелых, нередко многоядерных ганглиозных клеток. Митозы свидетельствуют о быстрой пролиферации, хотя идет и образование зрелых ганглиозных клеток.

b) Отдельные участки этих опухолей состоят почти исключительно из зрелых клеток с обилием телец Ниссля.

c) Эти клетки чаще всего многоядерны и диспластичны. Видны еще и неясной природы многоядерные клетки с недифференцированными ядрами и без субстанции Ниссля.

d) Характерное для «периферической» ганглиоцитомы (симпатикус, надпочечники) смешение недифференцированных клеток неясной природы, нейробластов и ганглиозных клеток всех стадий созревания.

a) 末梢の神経細胞腫の特色は、小リンパ球様(または髄芽細胞腫様)細胞、神経芽細胞様ではあるが神経細胞の構造をもつ細胞、成熟ししばしば多核性である大きな神経細胞が共存することである。分裂像は急速な腫瘍増殖を示すが、他方成熟した神経細胞もできている。

b) 二三の腫瘍部は Nissl 顆粒に富む成熟型細胞からなる。

c) この腫瘍細胞はしばしば多核で異型的である。さらに未分化核を有し、しかも Nissl 顆粒をもたない多核細胞をみとめることがあるが、この細胞の由来は不明である。

d) 性質を同定出来ない未分化細胞、神経芽細胞、さらにすべての成熟段階を示す神経細胞が混在することは末梢性神経細胞腫(交感神経、副腎)の特色である。

Ependymomas

Fig. 6—14

Ependymoblastoma, adenoglioma, glioependymoma, ependymoepithelioma, ependymoglioma, ependymocytoma, "Pfeilerzellgliom", blastoma ependymale, subependymoma, "neuroepithelioma", occasionally they were also described as "angiosarcomas"

Ependymal Tumors in Tuberous Sclerosis

Fig. 15

Spongioneuroblastoma, subependymal glioma, subependymal (glomerate) astrocytoma, subependymal giant-cell astrocytoma

Fig. 6 — Ependymomas

Typical architecture of an ependymoma. Numerous blood vessels with nucleus-free cuffs give the tumor its peculiar appearance (leopard skin). The expanding growth against the cerebral cortex is clearly discernible.

Typische Architektur eines Ependymoms. Zahlreiche Gefäße mit den kernfreien Manschetten geben der Geschwulst das eigenartige Aussehen („Jaguarfell"). Man erkennt deutlich das verdrängende Wachstum gegen die Hirnrinde.

Architecture typique de l'épendymome. Les nombreux vaisseaux entourés d'une manchette anucléée donnent à la tumeur son aspect particulier (peau de jaguar). La croissance tumorale refoule l'écorce cérébrale.

Arquitectura típica de un ependimoma. Numerosos vasos con sus manguitos perivasculares libres de núcleos prestan al tumor su característico aspecto (en piel de leopardo). Se ve claramente la tendencia invasiva hacia el cortex cerebral.

Типичное строение эпендимомы. Многочисленные сосуды с безъядерными поясами придают опухоли характерный вид тигровой шкуры. Четко виден экспансивный рост по отношению к коре мозга.

上衣細胞腫の定型的な組織構造。まわりに無核の外套をもつ多くの血管が特有な模様を作っている（ジャガー毛皮様)。脳皮質を圧迫して増殖する様子が明らかに認められる。

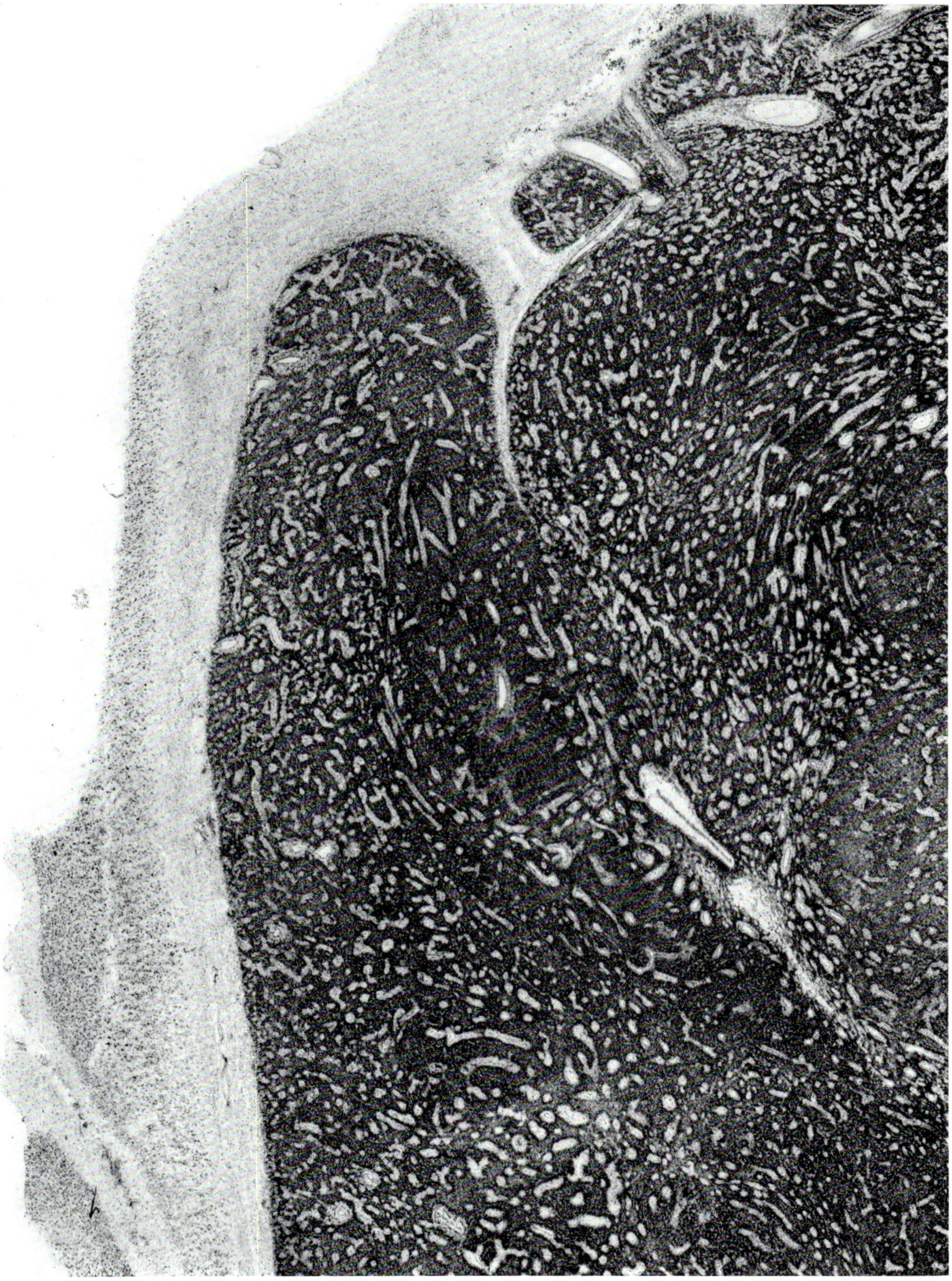

Fig. 6: ×14.5. Nissl stain

Fig. 7 — Ependymomas

Typical architecture of an ependymoma at higher magnification:

a) Highly cellular tumor, partitioned by regularly placed blood vessels. Around the vessels lie nucleus-free cuffs.
b) The same architecture at higher magnification.
c) Magnification of a). One sees chromatin-rich nuclei as well as a mitosis.
d) Ependymal canals in an ependymoma of the fourth ventricle.

Typische Architektur eines Ependymoms bei höherer Vergrößerung:

a) Man sieht eine zellreiche Geschwulst, die durch regelmäßig gelagerte Gefäße unterteilt wird. Um die Gefäße liegen kernfreie Manschetten.
b) Die gleiche Architektur mit höherer Vergrößerung.
c) Vergrößerung von a). Man sieht chromatinreiche Kerne sowie eine Mitose.
d) Ependymschläuche in einem Ependymom des 4. Ventrikels.

Architecture typique de l'épendymome à un plus fort grossissement,

a) Tumeur très cellulaire, qui est cloisonnée par les vaisseaux disposés régulièrement. Autour des vaisseaux, on note les manchettes anucléées.
b) La même architecture à un grossissement plus fort.
c) Agrandissement d'un morceau de a). Parmi les noyaux riches en chromatine, on voit une mitose.
d) Canal épendymaire dans un épendymome du 4e ventricule.

Arquitectura típica de un ependimoma a mayor aumento:

a) Se ve un tumor muy celular estructurado por vasos uniformemente colocados. Alrededor de los vasos se ven zonas libres de núcleos.
b) La misma arquitectura a mayor aumento.
c) Aumento de a). Se ven núcleos ricos en cromatima, y una mitosis.
d) Tubo ependimario en un ependimoma del cuarto ventrículo.

Типичное строение эпендимомы под большим увеличением:

a) Богатоклеточная опухоль с равномерно распределенными кровеносными сосудами. Безъядерные пояса в окружности кровеносных сосудов.
b) Та же структура опухоли под бóльшим увеличением.
c) Снимок a) под бóльшим увеличением. Видны гиперхромные ядра и митоз.
d) Канальцы в эпендимоме 4-го желудочка.

より強拡大でみた上衣細胞腫の定型的な組織構造。

a) 腫瘍組織は細胞に富み、整然とならぶ血管によって区画されている。腔が血管を外套状にとりまいている。
b) a)とおなじ構造の強拡大。
c) a)の強拡大像。核はクロマチンに富む。核分裂が1個みとめられる。
d) 第4脳室の上衣細胞腫にみられた腺腔様構造。

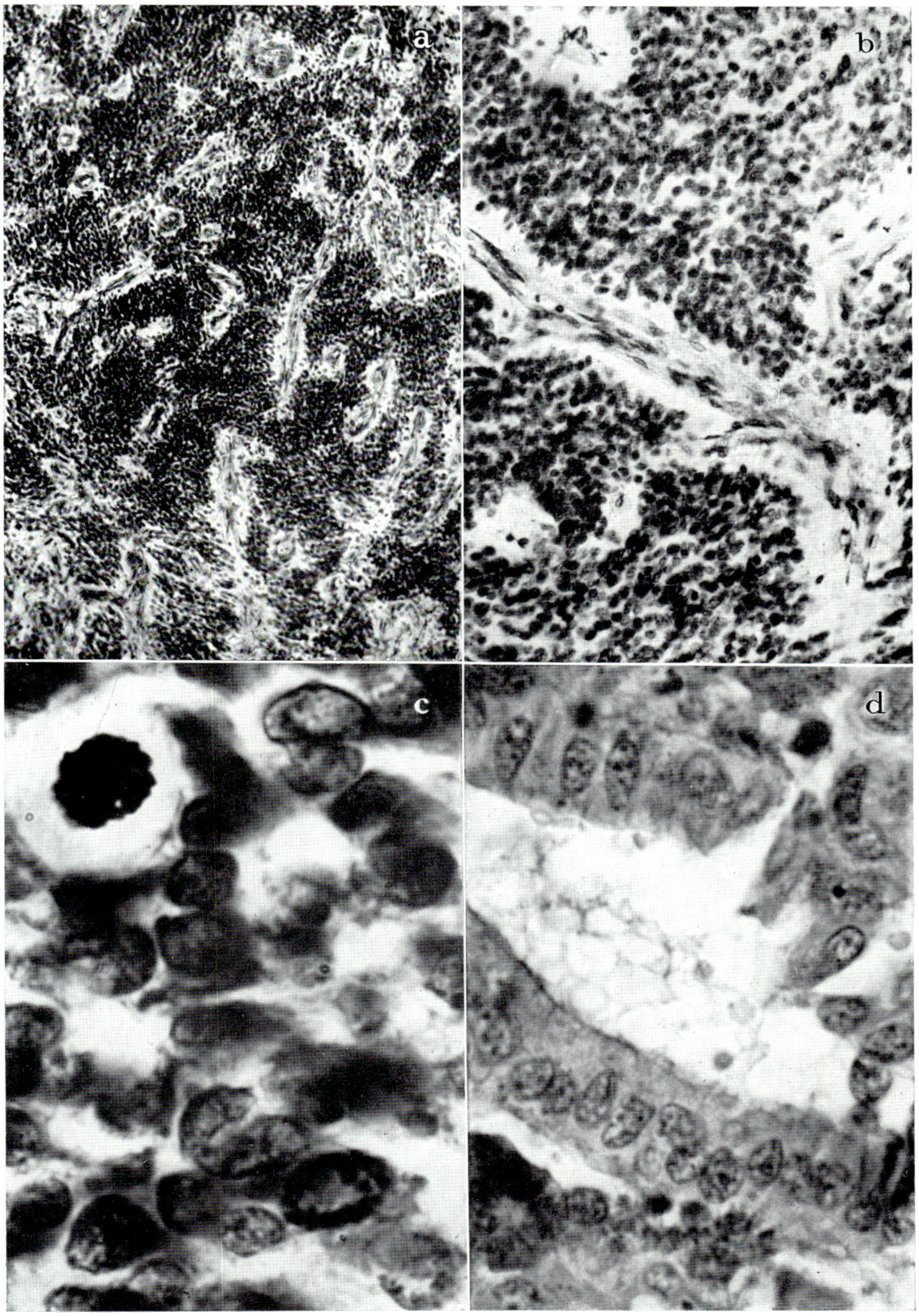

Fig. 7a—d: a ×64, b ×380, c ×1,400. Cresyl violet stain
d ×920. H. & E. stain

Fig. 8 — Ependymomas

Architecture of the perivascular zone in an ependymoma:

a) Perivascular "halo", in which the vascular feet in the nucleus-free zones are well demonstrated.
b) Magnification of the cell processes in the nucleus-free zones.
c) Vascular feet in the nucleus-free perivascular space.
d) Often the vascular processes of the cells are well demonstrated with gold sublimate.

Architektur der perivasculären Zone im Ependymom:

a) Perivasculärer „Strahlenkranz", wobei die Gefäßfüße in den kernfreien Zonen sich gut darstellen.
b) Vergrößerung der Zellfortsätze in den kernfreien Zonen.
c) Gefäßfüße im kernfreien perivasculären Raum.
d) Oft stellen sich die Gefäßfortsätze der Zellen auch mit Goldsublimat gut dar.

Architecture des zones périvasculaires de l'épendymome.

a) «Couronne radiaire» périvasculaire, où l'on reconnaît bien les pieds vasculaires dans la zone anucléée.
b) Vue à un plus fort grossissement des prolongements cellulaires dans la zone anucléée.
c) Pieds vasculaires dans la zone périvasculaire anucléée.
d) Les prolongements vasculaires des cellules sont souvent bien mis en évidence par l'imprégnation à l'or sublimé.

Arquitectura de la zona perivascular de un ependimoma.

a) Corona radiada perivascular; en las zonas anucleadas se ven muy bien los pies vasculares.
b) Aumento de las prolongaciones celulares en las zonas anucleadas.
c) Algunos pies vasculares en zonas perivasculares anucleadas.
d) Frecuentemente, tambien con el oro sublimado, se ponen bien de manifiesto los pies celulares de las células.

Строение периваскулярной зоны в эпендимоме:

a) Периваскулярная «лучистая корона». Хорошо видны сосудистые ножки в безъядерных зонах.
b) Отростки клеток в безъядерных зонах. Большое увеличение.
c) Сосудистые ножки в безъядерной периваскулярной зоне.
d) Сосудистые ножки клеток видны при импрегнации золото-сулемовым методом.

上衣細胞腫における、血管周囲の組織構造。

a) 血管周囲の「放射冠」。細胞の血管足が無核帯に明瞭に染色されている。
b) 血管周囲無核帯にみとめる細胞突起の強拡大像。
c) 無核帯の血管足。
d) 上衣細胞腫の血管足は、金昇汞法によってもしばしばよく染る。

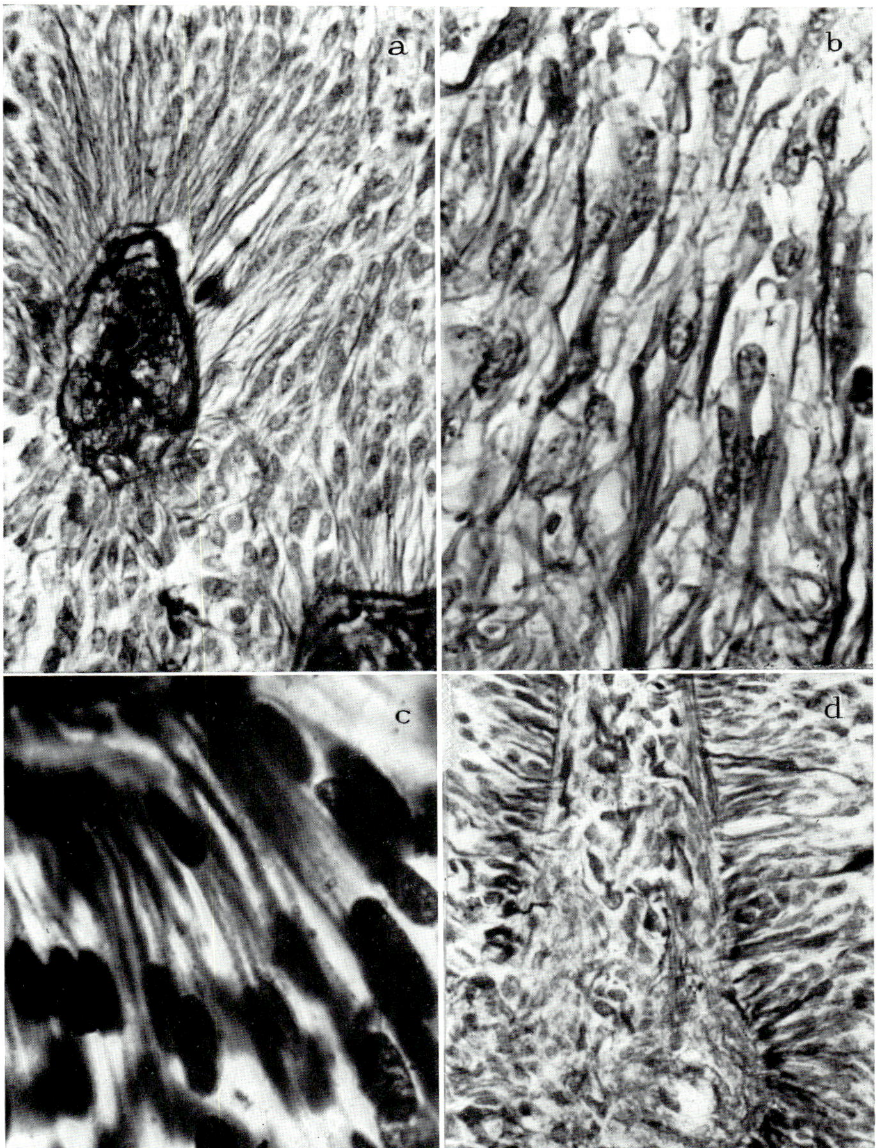

Fig. 8a—d: a ×312, b ×920, c ×1,400. Mallory's stain
d ×312. Gold sublimate method

Fig. 9 — Ependymomas

Ependymoma with a true ependymal canals. Quite frequently, these occur caudal to the midbrain.

a) and b) A true "corona radialis".

c) Higher magnification showing ependymal canals lined by a single layer of uniform ependymal cells. No mitotic figures.

Ependymom mit echten Ependymkanälen. Sie kommen besonders häufig caudal vom Mittelhirn vor.

a) u. b) Man sieht noch echte „Strahlenkronen".

c) Vergrößerung eines Ependymschlauches, einzeiliges, einschichtiges Ependym. Keine Mitosen.

Ependymome contenant de vrais canaux épendymaires, tels qu'on en trouve avec une fréquence particulière caudalement par rapport au mésencéphale.

a) et b) On voit encore de véritables «couronnes radiaires».

c) Vue au fort grossissement d'un canal épendymaire, dont la paroi est constituée d'une seule rangée de cellules. Pas de mitoses.

Ependimoma con canales ependimarios verdaderos.
Encuentranse frecuentemente en las partes posterior del cerebro medio.

a) y b) Se ven tambien «rosetas» verdaderas.

c) Aumento de un canal ependimaria con sus celulas constitutivos unilineares. Ninguna mitosís.

Эпендимома с истинными эпендимарными канальцами, особенно часто встречающимися каудальнее среднего мозга.

a) и b) Еще видны истинные «лучистые короны».

c) Увеличение эпендимарной полости. Однорядная, однослойная эпендима. Митозы отсутствуют.

上衣管をともなった上衣細胞腫。上衣細胞腫は多く中脳尾部に発生する。

a) および b) 放射冠をみとめる。

c) 上衣管および一層の上衣細胞の強拡大像。分裂像はみとめられない。

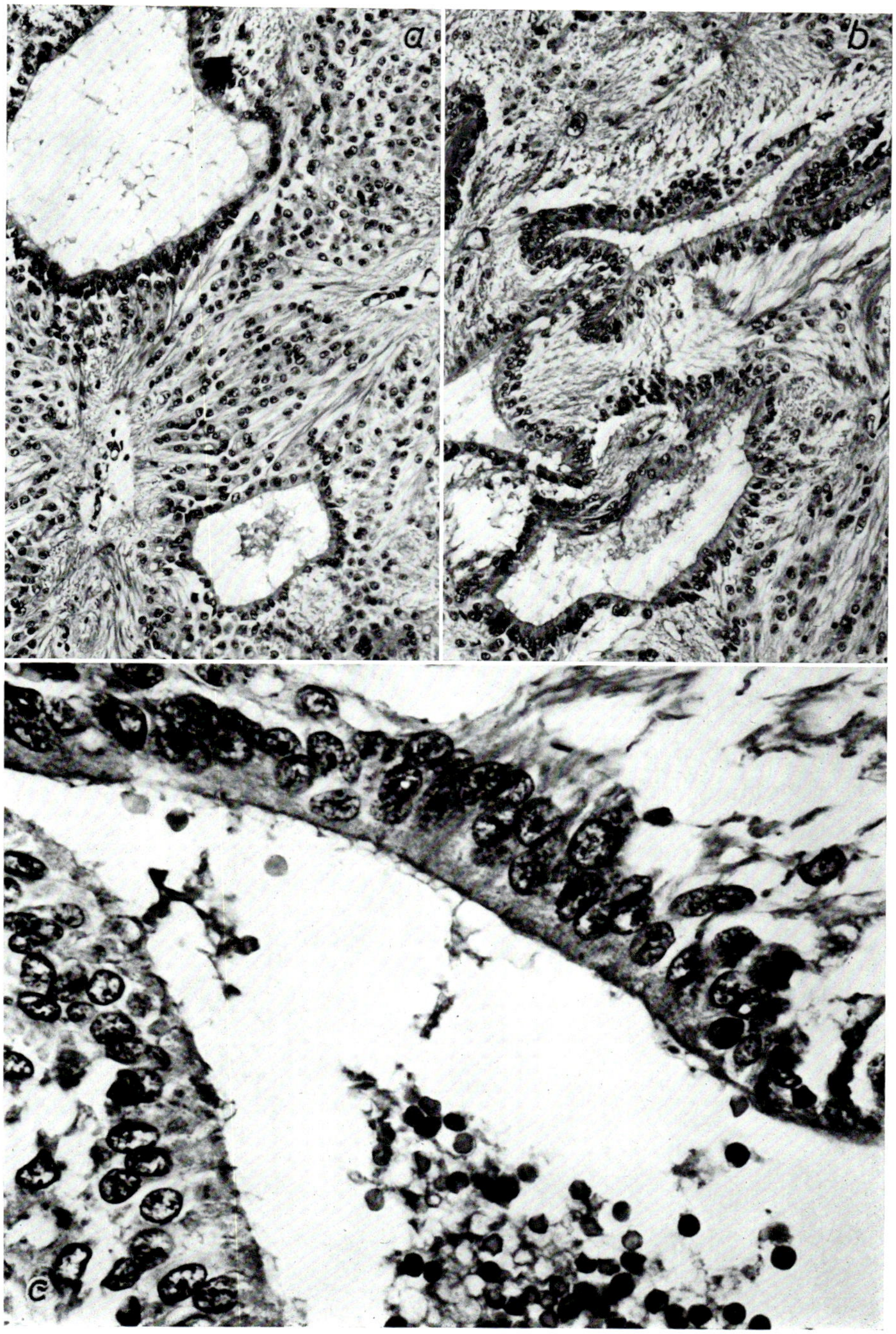

Fig. 9a—c: a and b ×125, c ×500
H. & E. stain

Fig. 10 — Ependymomas

Variants of the ependymoma:

a) A typical "true rosette" formed by the arrangement of the cells around a small cavity in an ependymoma of the fourth ventricle.

b) Numerous ependymal canals and rosettes in an ependymoma of the fourth ventricle.

c) Papillary ependymoma of the filum terminale with marked regressive changes due to mucoid degeneration and hyalinization. The tumor cells are preserved only in a few bands around the mucoid capsules.

d) Sections showing even more markedly regressive changes in the same case as in c).

Varianten im Ependymom:

a) Typische „echte Rosette" in einem Ependymom des 4. Ventrikels durch Lagerung der Zellen um einen kleinen Hohlraum.

b) Zahlreiche Ependymschläuche und Rosetten in einem Ependymom des 4. Ventrikels.

c) Papilläres Ependymom der Conus/Cauda-Gegend (Filum terminale) mit starken regressiven Veränderungen durch Verschleimung und Hyalinisierung. Die Geschwulstzellen sind nur noch in wenigen Bändern um die verschleimten Kapseln erhalten.

d) Noch stärker regressiv veränderte Partien im gleichen Falle wie c).

Variantes de l'épendymome.

a) Dans un épendymome du 4e ventricule, une «rosette vraie» typique s'est formée par la disposition des cellules autour d'un petit espace vide.

b) Formation de nombreux tubes épendymaires et de rosettes dans un épendymome du 4e ventricule.

c) Ependymome papillaire du filum terminale, dans la région du cône terminal et de la queue de cheval. D'importantes transformations régressives sont la conséquence d'un gonflement et d'une hyalinisation. Quelques cordons de cellules tumorales persistent encore autour des travées œdématiées.

d) En d'autres endroits de la tumeur précédente, les transformations régressives sont encore plus prononcées, comme c).

Variantes en los ependimomas.

a) Típicas «rosetas verdaderas» en un ependimoma del cuarto ventrículo, por disposición de las células alrededor de un pequeño espacio vacío.

b) Abundantes tubos ependimarios y rosetas en un ependimoma del cuarto ventrículo.

c) Ependimoma papilar de la región del cono (filum terminale) con intensos procesos regresivos del tipo de la degeneración mucosa y de la hialinización. Las células tumorales se conservan sólo en pequeñas bandas alrededor de la cápsula.

d) Zonas tumorales con procesos regresivos más intensos en el mismo caso que c).

Варианты эпендимомы:

a) Эпендимома 4-го желудочка с типичными «истинными розетками», образованными вследствие расположения клеток вокруг маленькой полости.

b) Эпендимома 4-го желудочка с множественными канальцами и розетками.

c) Папиллярная эпендимома области конуса и конского хвоста (конечной нити) с выраженными регрессивными изменениями, вызванными мукоидным перерождением и гиалинозом. Опухолевые клетки сохранились лишь в отдельных тяжах в окружности слизистоперерожденных участков опухоли.

d) Тот же случай. Еще более выраженные регрессивные изменения отдельных участков опухоли.

上衣細胞腫の変異像。

a) 定型的な「真正ロゼッテ」。小管腔をかこむ細胞配列。第4脳室の上衣細胞腫にみられたもの。

b) 第4脳室上衣細胞腫にみる多数の腺腔とロゼッテ。

c) 粘液様、硝子様変性をともない、高度な退行変化を示す脊髄円錐、馬尾（脊髄終末線維）部の乳頭状上衣細胞腫。腫瘍細胞は、粘液性被膜をかこみ、少数の索をなして存在しているのみ。

d) c)図と同一例の、さらに変性の強い部分。

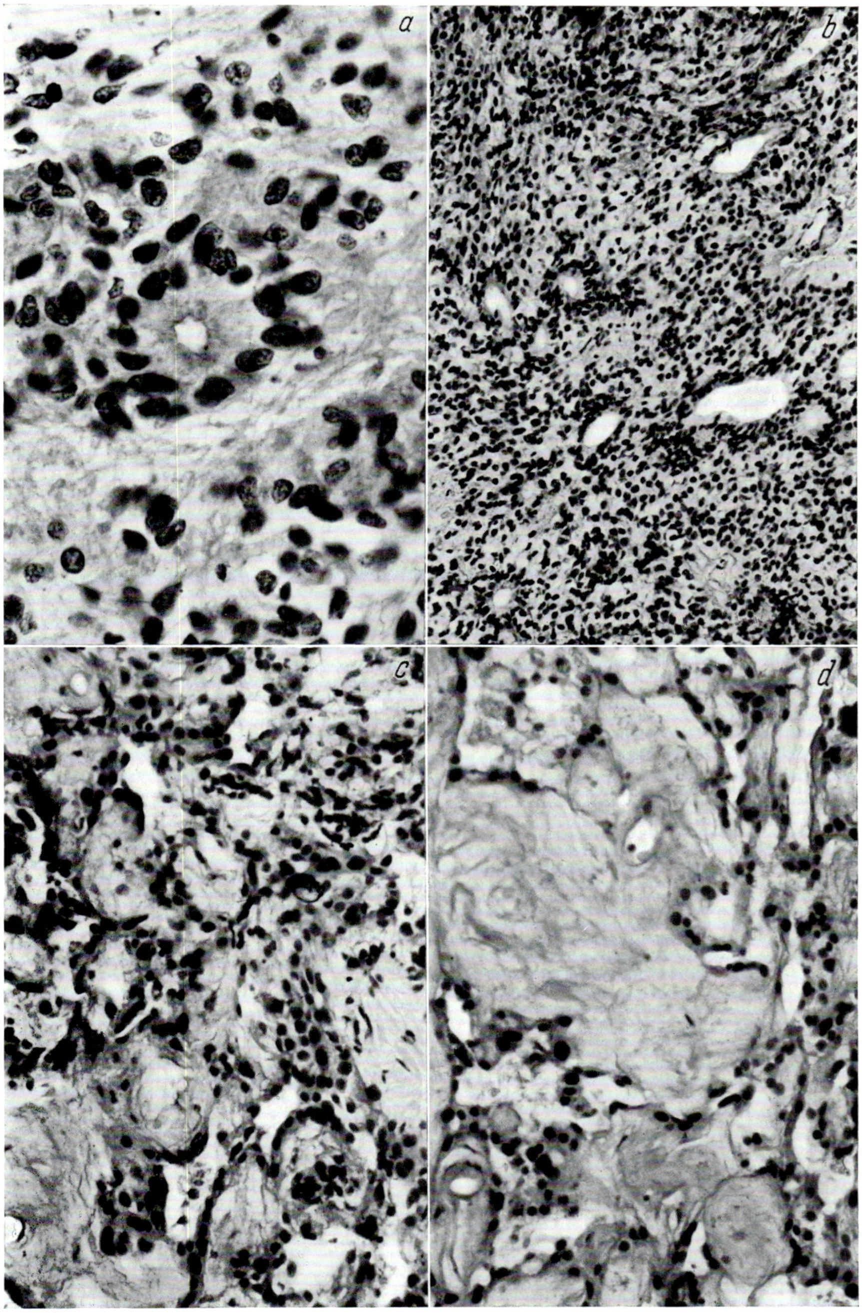

Fig. 10a—d: a ×272, b ×96, c and d ×136
H. & E. stain

Fig. 11 — Ependymomas

Various stages of "atrophic" changes in an ependymoma:
a) Distinct enlargement of the nucleus-free, perivascular zones. A "cylindroma-like" pattern occurs.
b) The typical architecture of the ependymoma is hardly recognizable, because the tumor parenchyma is limited to a few bands and the nucleus-free spaces have expanded further.
c) Cell impoverishment has progressed in individualized parts, the architecture is just recognizable as a "halo" (*top left.*)
d) Extreme cell impoverishment in the intraspinal tumor cones of an ependymoma of the fourth ventricle. Only isolated clusters of bands of tumor cells still appear.

Verschiedene Stadien „atrophischer" Veränderungen im Ependymom:
a) Deutliche Vergrößerung der kernfreien, perivasculären Zonen. Es entsteht ein „cylindromartiges" Bild.
b) Die typische Architektur des Ependymoms ist kaum mehr zu erkennen, weil das Geschwulstparenchym auf einige Bänder beschränkt ist und sich die kernfreien Räume weiter verbreitert haben.
c) Die Zellverarmung ist in einzelnen Teilen fortgeschritten, die Architektur nur noch links oben als „Strahlenkrone" eben erkennbar.
d) Hochgradige Zellverarmung im intraspinalen Geschwulstzapfen eines Ependymoms des 4. Ventrikels. Es erscheinen nur noch einzelne Grüppchen oder Bänder von Geschwulstzellen.

Différents stades de transformations «atrophiques» de l'épendymome.
a) Elargissement important des zones anucléées périvasculaires, ce qui donne une image ressemblant au cylindrome.
b) On ne reconnaît presque plus l'architecture typique de l'épendymome, car le parenchyme tumoral est réduit à quelques cordons cellulaires et les zones anucléées se sont davantage élargies.
c) Dans certaines régions, l'appauvrissement cellulaire s'est accentué, mais l'architecture peut encore se reconnaître dans la partie supérieure gauche de la figure, sous forme de «couronne radiaire».
d) Important appauvrissement cellulaire dans le prolongement intra-spinal d'un épendymome du 4e ventricule. Il ne persiste plus que quelques groupes ou cordons de cellules tumorales.

Diferentes estadíos de modificaciones atróficas en un ependimoma.
a) Claro aumento de las zonas anucleadas perivasculares. Se constituye un cuadro de tipo cilindromatoso.
b) La típica arquitectura de un ependimoma ya casi no se reconoce. El parénquima tumoral ha quedado reducido a algunas bandas y las zonas avasculares han continuado ampliándose.
c) El empobrecimiento celular ha progresado en algunas zonas. La arquitectura en corona radiada sólo es reconocible arriba, a la izquierda.
d) Pronunciado empobrecimiento celular en las prolongaciones intraespinales de un ependimoma del cuarto ventrículo. Aparecen solo algunos grupos o bandas de células tumorales.

Различные стадии «атрофических» изменений в эпендимоме:
a) Отчетливое увеличение безъядерных периваскулярных зон. Возникает «цилиндромоподобная» картина.
b) С трудом различается типичное строение эпендимомы, так как паренхима опухоли представлена отдельными тяжами, а безъядерные зоны еще больше расширились.
c) Еще большее обеднение отдельных участков опухолевыми клетками. Лишь слева вверху различима характерная для эпендимомы «лучистая корона».
d) Выраженное обеднение клетками в центре интраспинального выроста эпендимомы 4-го желудочка. Видны лишь отдельные группы или тяжи опухолевых клеток.

上衣細胞腫の「萎縮性」変化の諸段階。
a) 無核の血管周囲腔の著明な拡大。この場合､「円柱上皮腫」様の像を呈する。
b) 腫瘍実質が索状に凝縮し、無核性部分が拡大したために、上衣細胞腫の定型的所見はほとんどみとめられない。
c) 細胞密度は、ところどころ、さらに減少し、上衣細胞腫構造は、図左上の「放射冠」によって、かろうじて示されるのみである。
d) 第4脳室上衣細胞腫の脊椎腔内進入栓にみられた、きわめて細胞の少ない部分。わずかに腫瘍細胞の小群ないし索がみられるのみである。染色性も低下している。

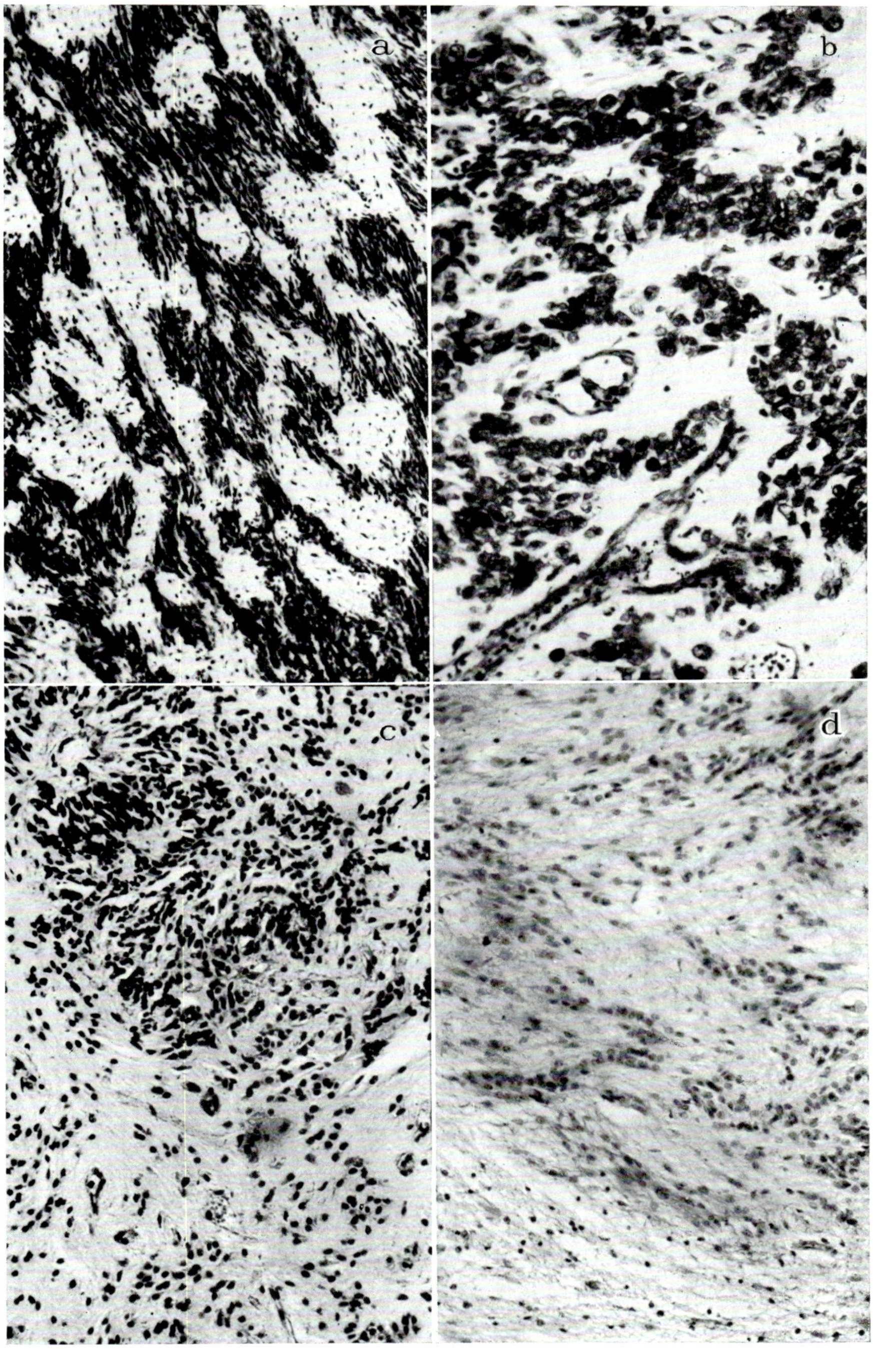

Fig. 11a—d: a ×120, Nissl stain
b ×200, c and d ×154. Cresyl violet stain

Fig. 12 — Ependymomas

a) Ependymoma of the aqueduct. The architecture is typical; the nuclei, however, are lying almost against the vessel walls. The cells are oriented radially to the vessels.
b) Ependymoma of the fourth ventricle. In the dense areas there is a tendency to form pseudo-rosettes which are considered characteristic for the medulloblastoma.
c) A type of palisading of cells in a cerebral ependymoma.
d) Ribbons of cells which at first glance resemble the classical description of the "medulloepithelioma"

a) Ependymom des Aquädukts. Die Architektur ist typisch, doch reichen die Kerne bis fast an die Gefäßwände heran. Die Zellen sind radiär um die Gefäße gelagert.
b) Ependymom des 4. Ventrikels. In den kompakten Partien sieht man eine auffällige Neigung zur Lagerung in Pseudorosetten, die sonst als typisch für das Medulloblastom gilt.
c) Eigenartig reihenförmige Lagerung der Zellen in einem Großhirnependymom.
d) Lagerung in Zellbändern, die auf ersten Blick an das „Medulloepitheliom" der klassischen Beschreibung erinnern.

a) Ependymome de l'aqueduc. L'architecture est typique; cependant les noyaux touchent presque les parois vasculaires. Les cellules sont disposées de façon radiaire autour des vaisseaux.
b) Ependymome du IVe ventricule. Dans les régions denses, on note une tendance marquée à la disposition en pseudo-rosettes, qui sont par ailleurs considérées comme étant typiques du médullo-blastome.
c) Disposition particulière des cellules en palissades dans un épendymome d'un hémisphère cérébral.
d) Disposition en cordons, qui rappellent au premier coup d'oeil la description classique du «médullo-épithéliome».

a) Ependimoma del acueduto. La arquitetura es típica, los núcleos alcanzan cerca de la pared del vaso. Las células estan colocadas radialmente en torno de los vasos.
b) Ependimoma del 4° ventrículo. En zonas compactas pueden verse formaciones en pseudorosetas como las que se consideran típicas del meduloblastoma.
c) Modo particular de agruparse las células en forma alargada en un ependimoma del cerebro.
d) Agrupamiento en yuxtaposición que recuerda a primera vista el «meduloepitelioma» de la descripción clasica.

a) Эпендимома сильвиева водопровода типичного строения, хотя ядра почти достигают стенок сосудов. Клетки располагаются радиарно вокруг сосудов.
b) Эпендимома 4-го желудочка. В компактных участках видна типичная для медуллобластомы склонность к образованию псевдорозеток.
c) Своеобразное расположение клеток рядами в эпендимоме больших полушарий головного мозга.
d) Тяжи клеток, сходные на первый взгляд с классическим описанием «медуллоэпителиомы».

a) 中脳水道部の上衣細胞腫。定型的な構造であるが、腫瘍細胞は血管壁に接している。細胞は血管を中心に放射状に並んでいる。
b) 第4脳室部の上衣細胞腫。細胞の密集部に髄芽細胞腫に特徴的な偽ロゼッテ形成の傾向をみとめる。
c) 大脳上衣細胞腫に認めた腫瘍細胞の列状配列。
d) 細胞索をみとめる。これは古くから髄上皮細胞腫と記載された腫瘍に相当する。

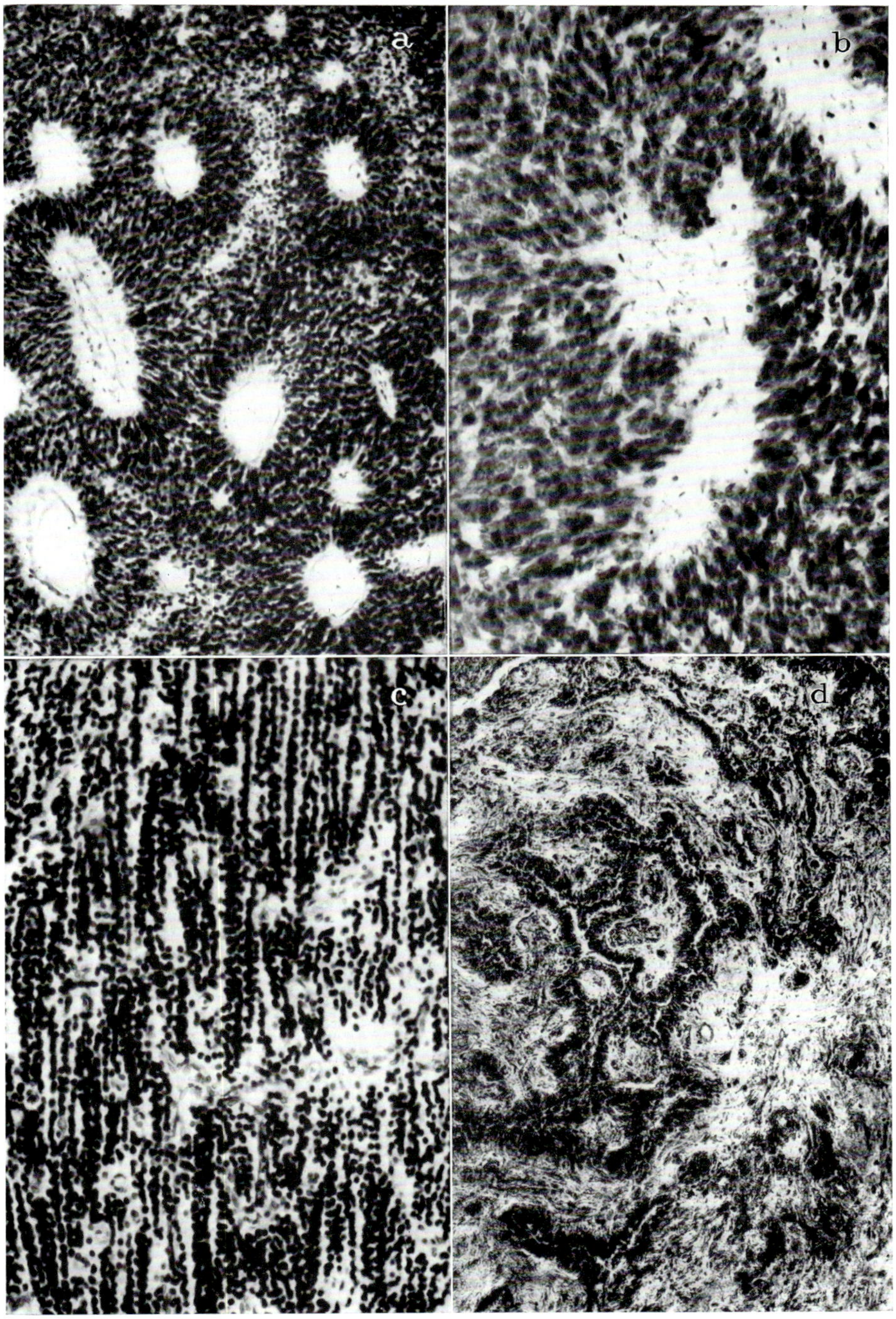

Fig. 12a—d: a ×112, c ×128. Nissl stain
b ×180, d ×86. Cresyl violet stain

Fig. 13 — Ependymomas

a) Unusually compact layer (epithelial sheet) of cells in a recurring cerebral ependymoma. Rare giant cells.
b) Sagittal section through the medulla oblongata: ependymoma of the floor of the fourth ventricle. In some places the tumor has penetrated the ependyma.
c) Increased anaplasia in a recurring cerebral ependymoma. The distribution of the vessels is quite irregular.
d) Metastasis of a cerebral ependymoma to the leptomeninges.

a) Eigenartig solide kompakte (plattenepithelartige) Lagerung der Zellen im Rezidiv eines Großhirnependymoms. Einzelne Riesenzellen.
b) Sagittalschnitt durch die Medulla oblongata: auf dem Boden des 4. Ventrikels sitzt ein Ependymom, das aber an einzelnen Stellen das Ependym durchbrochen hat.
c) Starke Verwilderung im Rezidiv eines Großhirnependymoms. Die Lagerung der Gefäße ist besonders unruhig.
d) Metastase eines Großhirnependymoms in die weichen Häute.

a) Disposition particulièrement compacte des cellules (comme un épithélium pavimenteux) dans une récidive d'un épendymome cérébral. Rares cellules géantes.
b) Coupe sagittale du bulbe: l'épendymome a son siège sur le plancher du IVe ventricule, mais il traverse l'épendyme par endroits.
c) Anarchie importante au niveau d'une récidive d'un épendymome cérébral. La disposition des vaisseaux est particulièrement désordonnée.
d) Métastase d'un épendymome cérébral dans la leptoméninge.

a) Particular agrupamiento celular (de tipo epitelio plano) en una recidiva de un ependimoma del cerebro. Células grandes.
b) Corte sagital del bulbo raquídeo. Ependimoma del 4° ventrículo que parte de una zona bien localizada del epéndimo.
c) Marcada atipia en una recidiva de un ependimoma del cerebro. El aglomerado vascular es intranquilo.
d) Metástasis de un ependimoma del cerebro en la meninge.

a) Своеобразное плотное компактное (подобно плоскому эпителию) расположение клеток в рецидивирующей эпендимоме больших полушарий головного мозга. Единичные гигантские клетки.
b) Сагиттальный разрез через продолговатый мозг: на дне 4-го желудочка находится эпендимома, прорвавшая в отдельных местах эпендиму.
c) Густое беспорядочное разрастание опухолевых клеток в рецидивирующей эпендимоме больших полушарий головного мозга. Выделяется особенно беспорядочное разрастание сосудов.
d) Метастаз эпендимомы больших полушарий головного мозга в мягкие мозговые оболочки.

a) 大脳上衣細胞腫の再発部に認められた腫瘍細胞（扁平上皮様）の充実性配置。二三の巨細胞。
b) 延髄の矢状断。第4脳室の底部に上衣細胞腫をみとめ、この腫瘍は数個所で上衣層を貫通している。
c) 大脳上衣細胞腫の再発部に見られた高度の荒廃。血管走行に乱れがある。
d) 軟膜へ転移した大脳上衣細胞腫。

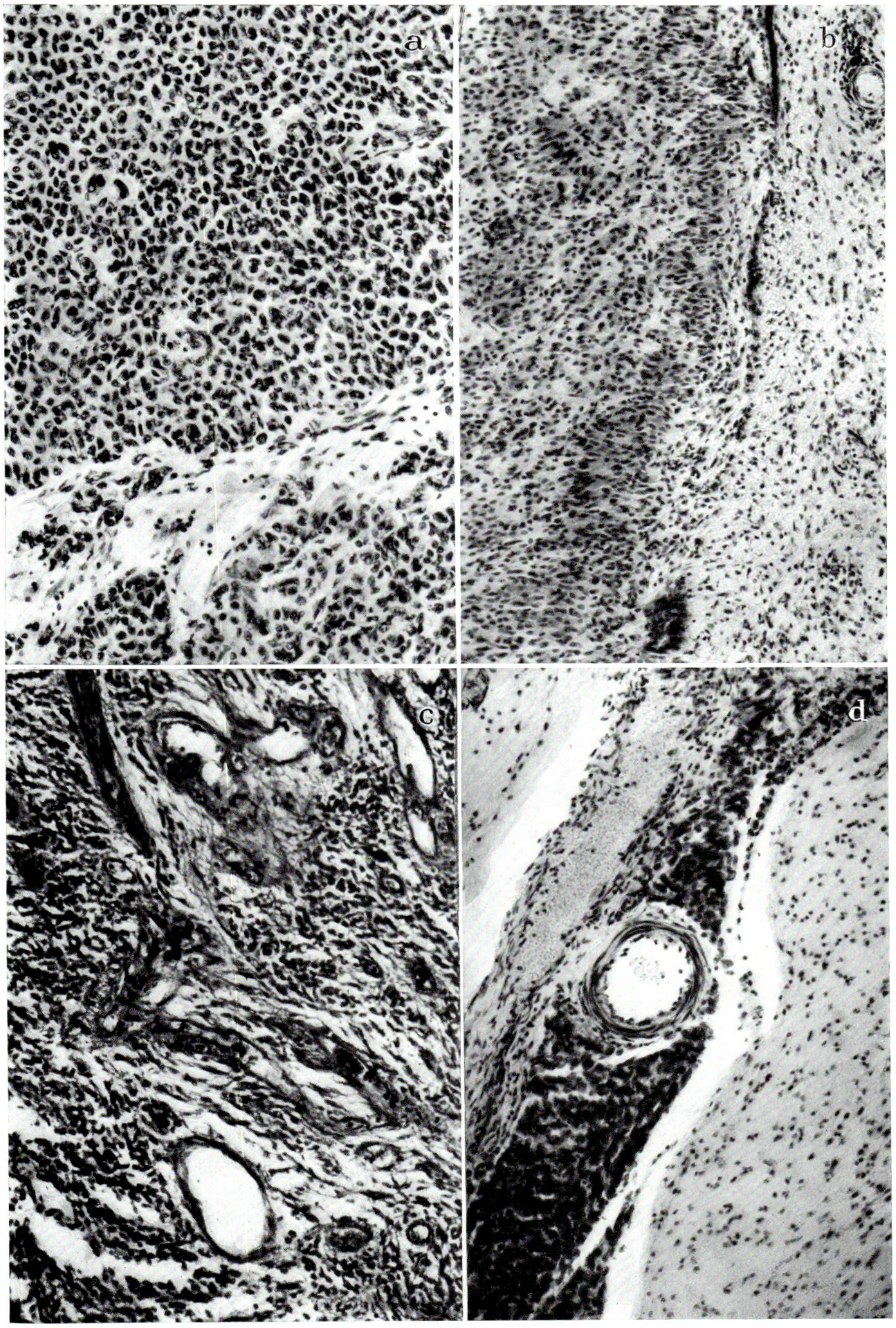

Fig. 13a—d: a ×288, d ×104. Nissl stain
b ×84. Cresyl violet stain
c ×112. H. & E. stain

Fig. 14 — Ependymomas

a) Papillary-trabecular variant of ependymoma which occurs only in the lateral recess of the cerebellar-pontine angle. The variation of this form from a true papilla of the plexus papilloma is noticeable by comparison with Fig. 16.
b) and c) In certain ependymoma-like tumors which undergo rapid growth (numerous mitoses), epithelial ribbons and hollow spaces develop. These ribbons of cells and spaces are similar to those seen in medulloepitheliomas (compare with Fig. 9a, 10b).

a) Papillär-trabekuläre Variante des Ependymoms, die nur im Recessus lat. des Kleinhirn-Brückenwinkels vorkommt. Der Unterschied von den echten Papillen des Plexuspapilloms wird durch Vergleich mit Abb. 16 sichtbar.
b) u. c) In manchen ependymomartigen Tumoren mit raschem Wachstum (zahlreiche Mitosen!) findet man epitheliale Bänder und Hohlräume, wie sie beim Medulloepitheliom vorkommen sollten (vgl. aber die andersartig geformten Hohlräume in Abb. 9a, 10b).

a) Variante papillo-trabéculaire de l'épendymome, qu'on retrouve uniquement dans le récessus latéral entre le cervelet et le pont. La différence avec les vraies papilles du papillome du plexus devient apparente lors de la comparaison avec la Fig. 16.
b) et c) Dans maintes tumeurs épendymaires à croissance rapide (mitoses nombreuses!), on trouve des cordons cellulaires épithéliaux et des cavités, comme c'est le cas dans le «médullo-épithéliome» (à comparer cependant avec les différentes cavités de la Fig. 9a, 10b).

a) Variante de ependimoma en forma de papilas y trabéculas en el receso lateralis del angulo pontino cerebelar. La diferencia con el verdadero papiloma de plexos coroideos se puede ver comparando con la Fig. 16.
b) y c) En varios tumores ependimarios com rápido crecimiento (numerosas mitosis) encuéntranse cordones y cavidades como si se tratase de «meduloepiteliomas» (comparar con la Fig. 9a, 10b).

a) Папиллярный трабекулярный вариант эпендимомы. Встречается только в боковом вывороте мосто-мозжечкового угла. Отличие от истинных сосочков плексус-папилломы можно проследить путем сравнения с рис. 16.
b) и c) В некоторых эпендимоподобных опухолях с быстром ростом (многочисленные митозы!) обнаруживают эпителиальные тяжи и полости, которые встречаются в «медуллоэпителиоме» (сравните, однако, по-разному образованные полости на рис. 9a, 10b).

a) 小脳－橋角部外側窩の乳頭状一梁状構造を示す上衣細胞腫の亜型。この乳頭と脉絡叢乳頭腫にみられる真正乳頭とのちがいは16図と比較すると明らかになる。
b) と c)急速な発育をする（多数の分裂像！）上衣細胞腫様の腫瘍には髄上皮細胞腫でみられるような上皮索と管腔が見られる。(図9a,10bにみられる種々な形をした管腔と比較せよ)。

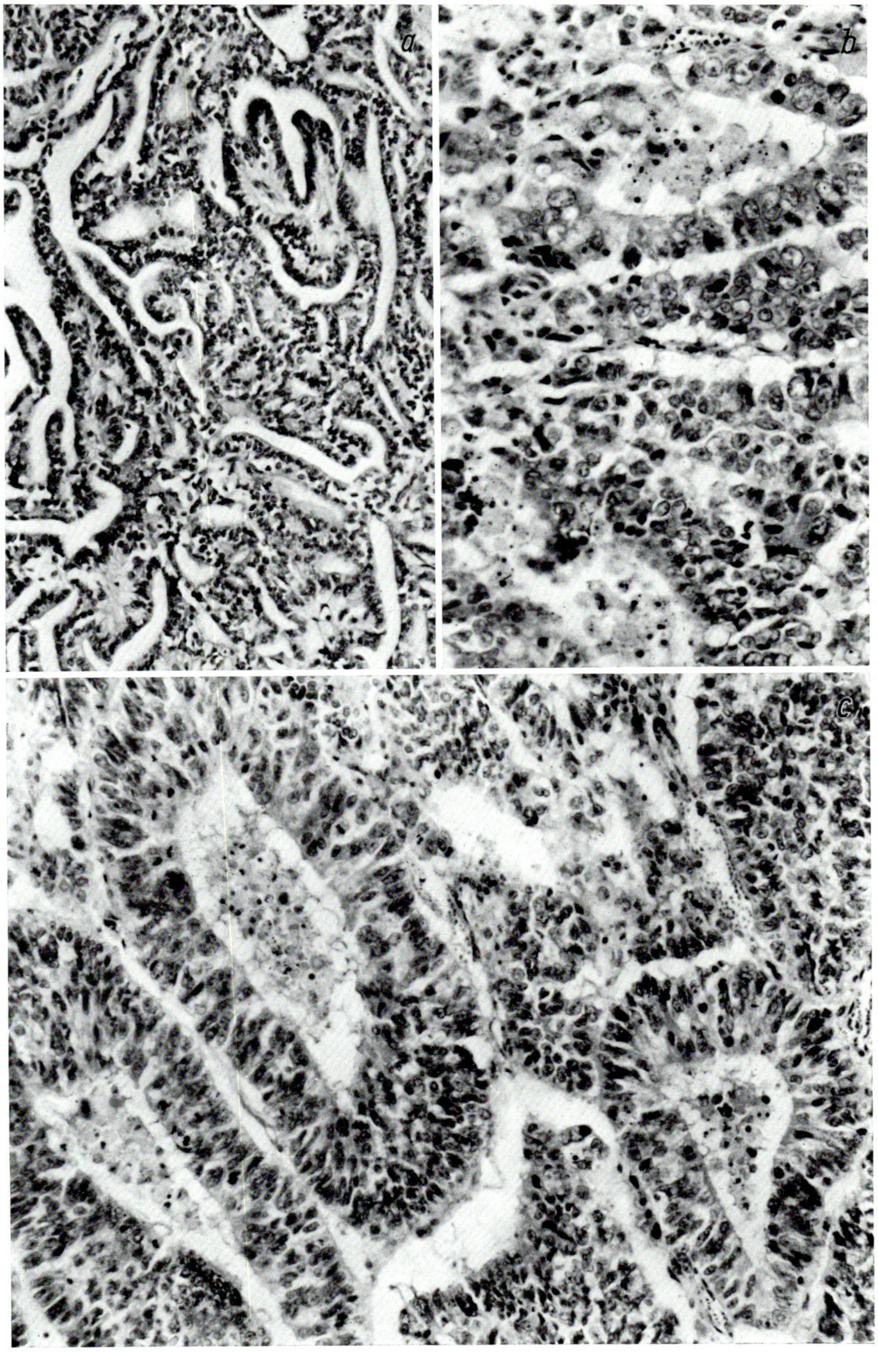

Fig. 14a—c: a × 84, b—c × 125. H. & E. stain

Fig. 15 — Ependymal Tumors in Tuberous Sclerosis

a) Typical arrangement of spindle shaped cells with abundant cytoplasm in lines interrupted by vessels. The vessels are surrounded by nucleus-free zones.
b) Very large cells with vesicular nuclei and large nucleoli are, in general, radially oriented to the vessels.
c) Demonstration of the conformation of cells and their processes with gold sublimate.
d) Blepharoplasts as demonstrated with HEIDENHAIN's hematoxylin.

a) Typische Anordnung der spindeligen cytoplasmareichen Zellen in Zügen, unterbrochen von einzelnen Gefäßen mit kernfreien Räumen.
b) Sehr großleibige Zellen mit bläschenförmigen Kernen und großem Nucleolus, die meist radiär zu den Gefäßen angeordnet sind.
c) Gute Abbildung der Außenform der Zellen und ihrer Fortsätze durch Goldsublimat.
d) Darstellung der Blepharoblasten mit HEIDENHAINs Hämatoxylin.

a) Agencement typique en bancs de poissons des cellules fusiformes riches en cytoplasme. Présence de quelques vaisseaux entourés d'une zone anucléée.
b) Volumineuses cellules à noyau vésiculaire et à gros nucléole, disposées le plus souvent radiairement autour d'un vaisseau.
c) Mise en évidence des contours cellulaires et de leurs prologements par l'or sublimé.
d) Mise en évidence des blépharoblastes par l'hématoxyline d'HEIDENHAIN.

a) Típica disposición en hilera de las células ricas en citoplasma y de forma alargada, alternando con vasos y zonas libres de núcleos.
b) Células grandes con núcleo vesiculoso y nucleolo grande, la mayoría dispuesta radialmente en torno de los vasos.
c) Buena imagen de la forma celular con sus prolongamientos evidenciados por el oro sublimado.
d) Presencia de bléfaroblastos puestos de manifiesto por la Hematoxilina de HEIDENHAIN.

a) Типичное расположение богатых цитоплазмой клеток в виде тяжей, прерываемых единичными сосудами. Видны безъядерные участки.
b) Клетки с очень большим телом, с пузырькоподобными ядрами и большим ядрышком. Радиарное расположение клеток по отношению к сосудам.
c) Четкое изображение внешнего вида клеток и их отростков при обработке золотосулемовым методом.
d) Блефаробласты, окрашенные по ГАЙДЕНГАЙНУ.

a) 紡錘形の胞体に富む細胞が列状に並ぶ定型像。この構造は無核の周囲腔を伴った血管によってつらぬかれている。
b) 胞状核と大型の核小体を伴った胞体に富む細胞が、主として血管に向って放射状にならぶ。
c) 鍍金によって、細胞の外形と突起が染出される。
d) Heidenhain ヘマトキシリン染色で Blepharoplast が染出される。

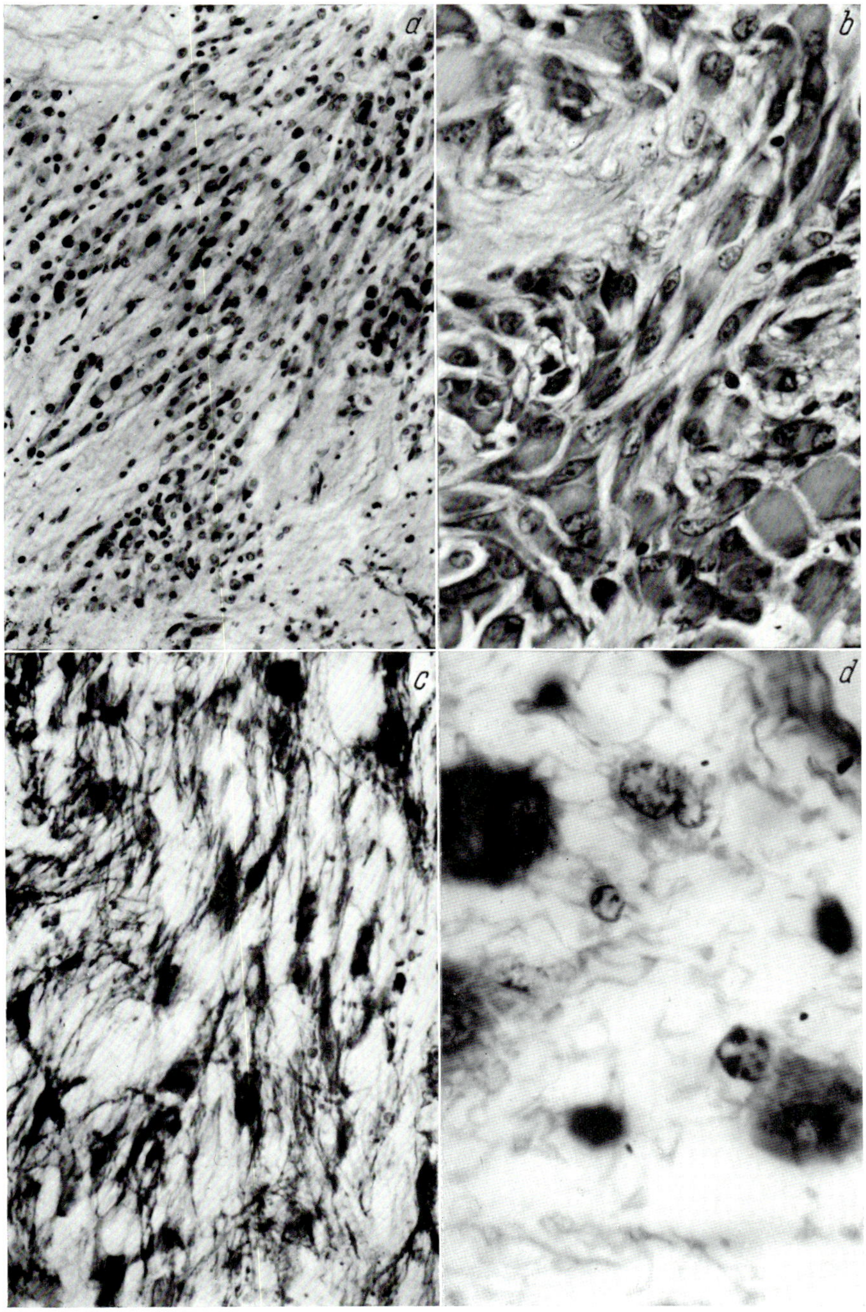

Fig. 15a—d: a ×160. Nissl stain
b ×160. Cresyl violet stain
c ×280. Gold sublimate impregnation
d ×1,152. Heidenhains hematoxylin

Plexus Papillomas

Choroid plexus papilloma, epithelioma, carcinoma or adenoma of the choroid plexus, choroid, epithelioma, choroid papilloma

Neuroepitheliomas

Fig. 17c

Fig. 16 — Plexus Papillomas

General view of a plexus papilloma:

a) Distinct formation of papillae with a central stroma. Around the papillae lie the parietal cells, regularly located.
b) In higher magnification one can discern the papillae better. In most of them there is a capillary vessel. The epithelial cells are pavement-shaped or cylindrical.
c) Magnification of a). One can discern here the thionin estained granules in the outer zone of the cells.
d) The stroma is especially well demonstrated in this illustration of the elastic fibers in the vascular wall.

Übersichtsbild eines Plexuspapilloms:

a) Klare Ausbildung von Papillen mit zentralem Stroma. Um die Papillen liegen die Belegzellen regelmäßig gelagert.
b) In der Vergrößerung erkennt man die Papillen noch besser. In der Mehrzahl von ihnen liegt ein capilläres Gefäß. Die Epithelien sind pflasterförmig oder zylindrisch.
c) Vergrößerung von a). Man erkennt hier die Thionin-färbbaren Granula in der Außenzone der Zellen.
d) Das Stroma wird besonders gut durch die Abbildung der Elasticafasern im Gefäß dargestellt.

Vue d'ensemble d'un papillome du plexus.

a) Formation de papilles caractéristiques, munies de leur stroma axial et bordées par une couche régulière de cellules.
b) A un plus fort grossissement, on reconnaît encore mieux les papilles, dont la majorité contiennent un capillaire. L'épithélium prend un aspect pavimenteux ou cylindrique.
c) Grossissement de a). Dans la portion externe des cellules, on reconnaît les granules colorés par la thionine.
d) Par la coloration des fibres élastiques des vaisseaux, on met bien le stroma en évidence.

Visión de conjunto de un papiloma del plexo coroideo:

a) Clara formación de papilas con estroma central. Sobre ellas descansan las células de revestimiento, uniformemente situadas.
b) A más aumento se reconocen mejor las papilas. En la mayoría de ellas hay un vaso capilar. Los epitelios son de tipo estratiforme o cilíndrico.
c) Aumento de a). En la zona externa de las células se reconocen los gránulos tingibles por la tionina.
d) El estroma se pone especialmente de manifiesto por la imagen de las fibras elásticas en el vaso.

Обзорный снимок плексус-папилломы:

a) Четкое папиллярное строение. Строма в центре сосочка. Вокруг сосочков равномерно расположены выстилающие клетки.
b) Сосочки еще отчетливее видны под большим увеличением. В большинстве сосочков определяется капилляр. Наличие плоского или цилиндрического эпителия.
c) Рис. a) под большим увеличением. Видны окрашенные тионином гранулы на наружном конце клеток.
d) Особенно отчетливо видна строма при окраске на эластические волокна.

脈絡叢乳頭腫の概観像。

a) 中心に間質のある乳頭構造が明瞭に認められる。乳頭は、規則正しくならんだ細胞でおおわれている。
b) 中拡大像。乳頭の多くは間質に毛細血管を有し、上皮細胞は敷石あるいは円柱状である。
c) 図a)の強拡大。上皮細胞の表層に、チオニンに染まる顆粒をみとめる。
d) 弾性線維染色によって、乳頭の間質は明瞭となる。

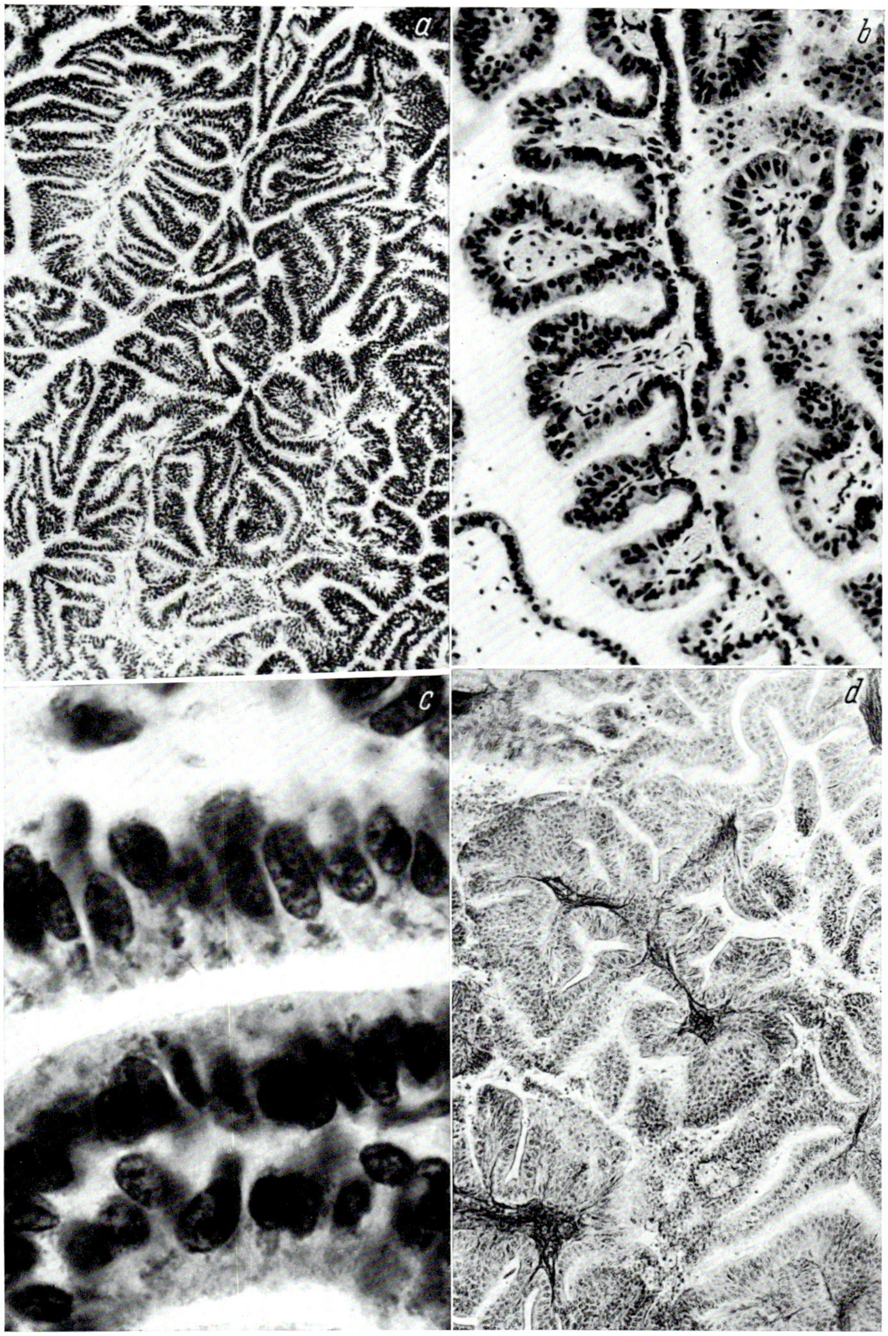

Fig. 16a—d: a ×62. Nissl stain
b ×240. Cresyl violet stain
c ×1,000 Nissl stain, d ×94
El. van Gieson-stain

Fig. 17 — Plexus Papillomas

a) The basic architecture is recognizable in the polymorphic plexus papilloma; in these cases one sees psammoma bodies. The epithelium is irregular and contains hyperchromatic and polymorphic cells.
b) The papillary type of basic architecture is also present in other locations of the same tumor. Psammoma bodies are visible. Here the epithelium is even more irregular and in places the papillary structure is not retained; the epithelial cells and polymorphic giant cells being interspersed.
c) "True rosettes" are seen in a highly cellular medulloblastoma type of tumor from the basilar portion of the frontal lobe. This tumor should be included in the neuroepithelioma group.
d) Grotesque, multinucleated, giant cells are found in the corona radialis of a "polymorphic" (malignant, dedifferentiated) ependymoma. The more dedifferentiated ependymomas lose part of the corona radialis architecture. The cells become epithelioid and hyperchromatic giant cells are scattered throughout the tumors. The mitotic index is high.

a) Beim polymorphen Plexuspapillom erkennt man noch die Grundstruktur dieser Tumorart, in diesem Falle erinnern daran einzelne Psammomkörner. Doch ist die Epithellinie bereits unruhig geworden und man erkennt einzelne hyperchromatische und polymorphe Zellen.
b) Im gleichen Falle sieht man an einer anderen Stelle auch noch eine papillenartige Grundstruktur. Auch sind Psammomkörner sichtbar. Doch wird hier die Unruhe des Epithels stärker. Man erkennt polymorphe Riesenzellen und die papilläre Struktur geht durch Zusammenwachsen dieser Gewebspartien verloren.
c) In einem sehr zellreichen, medulloblastomartigen Tumor des basalen Frontallappens finden sich „echte Rosetten". Dieser Tumor sollte in die Gruppe der Neuroepitheliome gerechnet werden.
d) Im Strahlenkranz eines „polymorphen" (maligne entdifferenzierten) Ependymoms finden sich groteske mehrkernige hyperchromatische Riesenzellen. Das weitgehend entdifferenzierte Ependymom hat z.T. die Architekturen der „Strahlenkronen" verloren, die Zellen sind epitheloid geworden und werden überall von hyperchromatischen Riesenzellen durchsetzt. Die Zahl der Mitosen ist groß.

a) Dans le papillome polymorphe des plexus, on reconnaît encore la structure fondamentale de ce type de tumeur; dans le cas présent, des calcosphérites (psammomes) y font penser. Cependant, l'alignement épithélial est devenu irrégulier et l'on reconnaît certaines cellules hyperchromatiques et polymorphes.
b) A un autre endroit de la même tumeur, on voit également une structure fondamentale papillomateuse ainsi que des grains psammomateux, mais l'irrégularité de l'assise épithéliale devient ici plus marquée. On reconnaît des cellules géantes polymorphes et la structure papillaire tend à s'estomper par suite de la croissance tumorale.
c) Dans une tumeur de type médulloblastique, riche en cellules et occupant la base du lobe frontal, on trouve de «vraies rosettes». Cette tumeur serait à classer dans le groupe des «neuroépithéliomes».
d) Dans la couronne radiaire d'un épendymome «polymorphe» (malin et indifférencié), on trouve des cellules géantes multinucléées à noyaux monstrueux et hyperchromatiques. Cet épendymome largement dédifférencié a perdu en partie son architecture en couronne radiaire. Les cellules ont pris un aspect «épithélioïde» et sont mêlées à de nombreuses cellules géantes hyperchromatiques. Le nombre de mitoses est élevé.

a) Esta estructura recuerda el papiloma polimorfo de plexos coroideos, incluso con cuerpos psamomatosos. Son células epiteliales intranquilas, pudiéndose ver células hipercromáticas y polimorfas.
b) En el mismo caso, en otro campo se ve todavía la estrutura papilar, cuerpos psamomatosos. Aquí la intranquilidad epitelial es más marcada. Aparecen células gigantes polimorfas y los vasos no llegan a acompañar su crecimiento.
c) En un tumor denominado meduloblastoma, rico en células, de la región frontal encuéntranse rosetas verdaderas. Este tumor debe colocarse en el grupo de los «neuroepiteliomas».
d) En una corona radiada de un ependimoma «polimorfo» (indiferenciación maligna) encuéntranse células con varios núcleos hipercromáticos y grotescos. En los ependimomas muy indiferenciados pueden perder la estrutura en «corona radiada». Las células son «epiteloides», muchas de ellas son hipercromáticas y grandes. La cantidad de mitosis es muy grande.

Continued on page 70

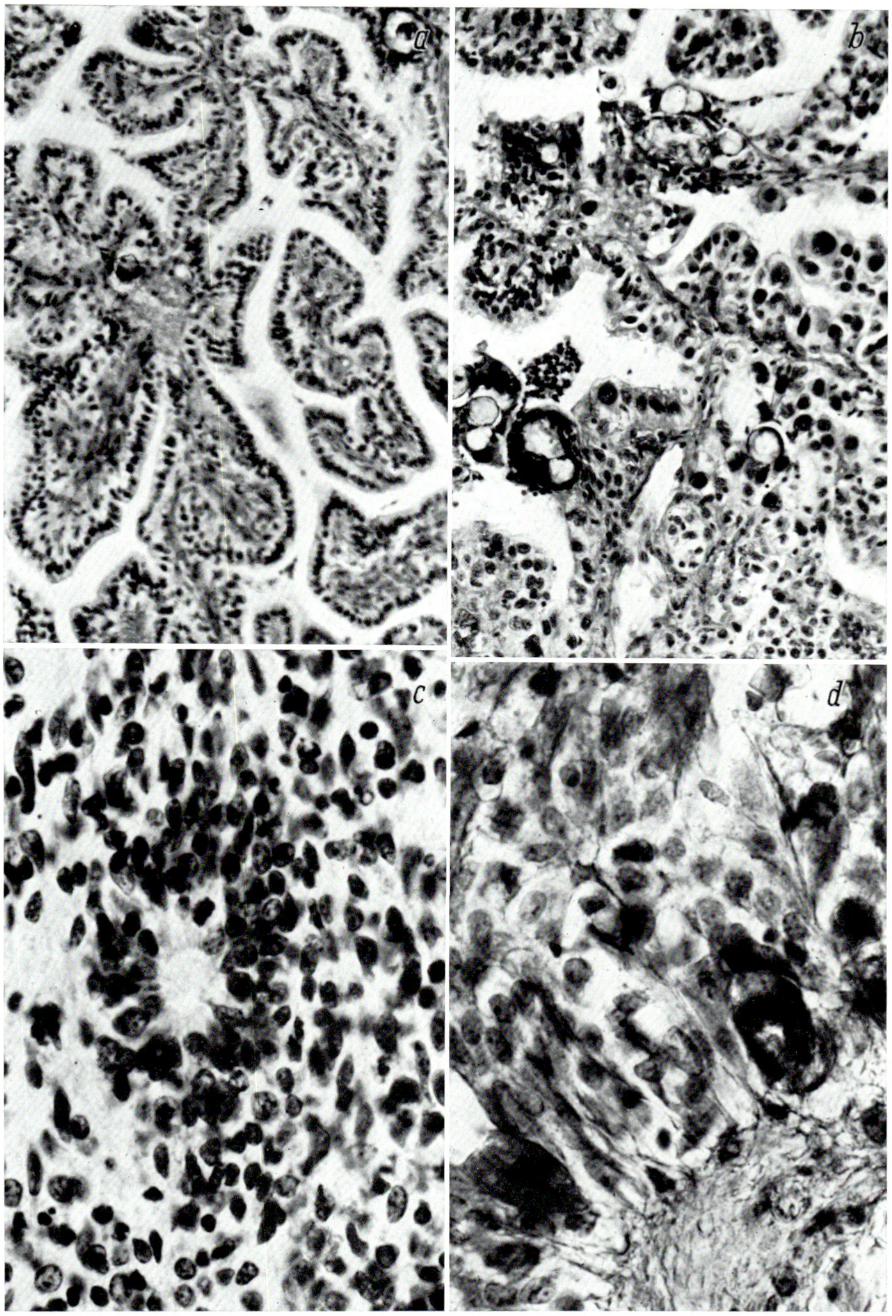

Fig. 17a—d: a ×125, b ×125, c and d ×500
a—c Cresyl violet stain
d H. & E. stain

Fig. 17 — Plexus Papillomas (continued)

a) В полиморфной плексус-папилломе еще прослеживается основная структура этого вида опухоли. В представленном случае об этом напоминают единичные псаммомные зёрна. Однако эпителиальные ряды потеряли свою упорядоченность и видны единичные гиперхромные и полиморфные клетки.

b) В этом же случае в другом участке еще видна характерная сосочковая структура. Имеются псаммомные зерна. Однако эпителиальные ряды стали еще более беспорядочны. Прослеживаются полиморфные гигантские клетки, а сосочковая структура исчезает вследствие сращения этих участков.

c) «Истинные розетки» в богатоклеточной медуллобластомоподобной опухоли базальных отделов лобной доли. Эту опухоль следовало бы отнести к группе «нейроэпителиом».

d) В лучистой короне «полиморфной» (злокачественной, недифференцированной) эпендимомы находятся причудливые многоядерные гиперхромные гигантские клетки.
Значительно дедифференцированная эпендимома частично утратила структуру «лучистых корон», клетки стали «эпителиоидными» и повсюду пронизаны гиперхромными гигантскими клетками. Велико количество митозов.

a) 多形性の脉絡叢乳頭腫でも、この腫瘍の基本構造を知ることが出来る。本例では Psammom 体をみる。上皮の配列はすでに乱れており、二三の濃染性、多形性の細胞をみとめる。

b) 同上例の他の部で、乳頭状の基本構造を見るときに、Psammon 体もみとめられる。上皮配列のみだれは、さらに増している。多形性の巨細胞があり、さらに乳頭状構造はこの組織の癒合によって失われる。

c) 前頭葉下部の、細胞に富む髄芽腫様腫瘍内に、真正ロゼットがみられる。この腫瘍は神経上皮腫に分類されるべきものである。

d) 多形性（悪性未分化型）上衣細胞腫の放射冠内に異様な形をした多核、濃染性の巨細胞をみる。さらに未熟な上衣腫は放線冠の構造を失い、腫瘍細胞は上衣細胞様になる。そして濃染性の巨細胞が混在する。分裂中の細胞が多い。

Retinoblastomas

Fig. 18

Neuroepithelioma of the retina with or without rosettes.

Astrocytomas

Fig. 19—27

Fibrillary/protoplasmic/gemistocytic astrocytoma, glioma durum, spider-cell glioma, "Pinselzellgliom", star-cell glioma, astroma, amoeboid-cell glioma, astrocytoma grade I—III, giant cell astrocytoma.

Fig. 18 — Retinoblastomas

a) In some retinoblastomas appear "true rosettes" in which a central empty space is noted.
b) Characteristic of the retinoblastoma *without* "true rosettes" is the aggregation of densely packed tumor cells around blood vessels, and areas of tissue necrosis between.

a) In manchen Retinoblastomen bilden sich „echte Rosetten", bei denen ein Hohlraum in der Mitte eines Zellkranzes liegt.
b) Für das Retinoblastom *ohne* echte Rosetten ist die Bildung dichter zelliger Mäntel von Geschwulstzellen um die Tumorgefäße charakteristisch, während zwischen diesen das Geschwulstgewebe durch Nekrose zerfällt.

a) Dans de nombreux rétinoblastomes, il se forme de «vraies rosettes» qui présentent une cavité à l'intérieur de la couronne cellulaire.
b) Lorsqu'il ne contient pas de véritables rosettes, le rétinoblastome est caractérisé par l'accumulation de nombreuses cellules tumorales autour des vaisseaux, tandis que le tissu néoplasique se nécrose entre ces cordons.

a) En algunos retinoblastomas aparecen «rosetas verdaderas» con una cavidad en el centro.
b) En el retinoblastoma *sin* rosetas verdaderas aparecen formaciones densas, con células hinchadas, con la vascularización característica, entremezcladas con tejido necrosado.

a) Образование «истинных розеток» в некоторых ретинобластомах с полостью в середине короны.
b) Характерное для ретинобластомы без истичных розеток образование плотных муфт из опухолевых клеток вокруг сосудов опухоли с некротическим распадом опухолевой ткани.

a) 真正ロゼットをともなわない網膜芽細胞腫では、腫瘍内血管の周囲に腫瘍細胞からなる鞘が形成されるのが特徴的である。この鞘の間にある腫瘍組織は、壊死におちいる。
b) 多くの網膜芽細胞腫には、真正ロゼットが形成される。この場合中央部に腔が存在する。

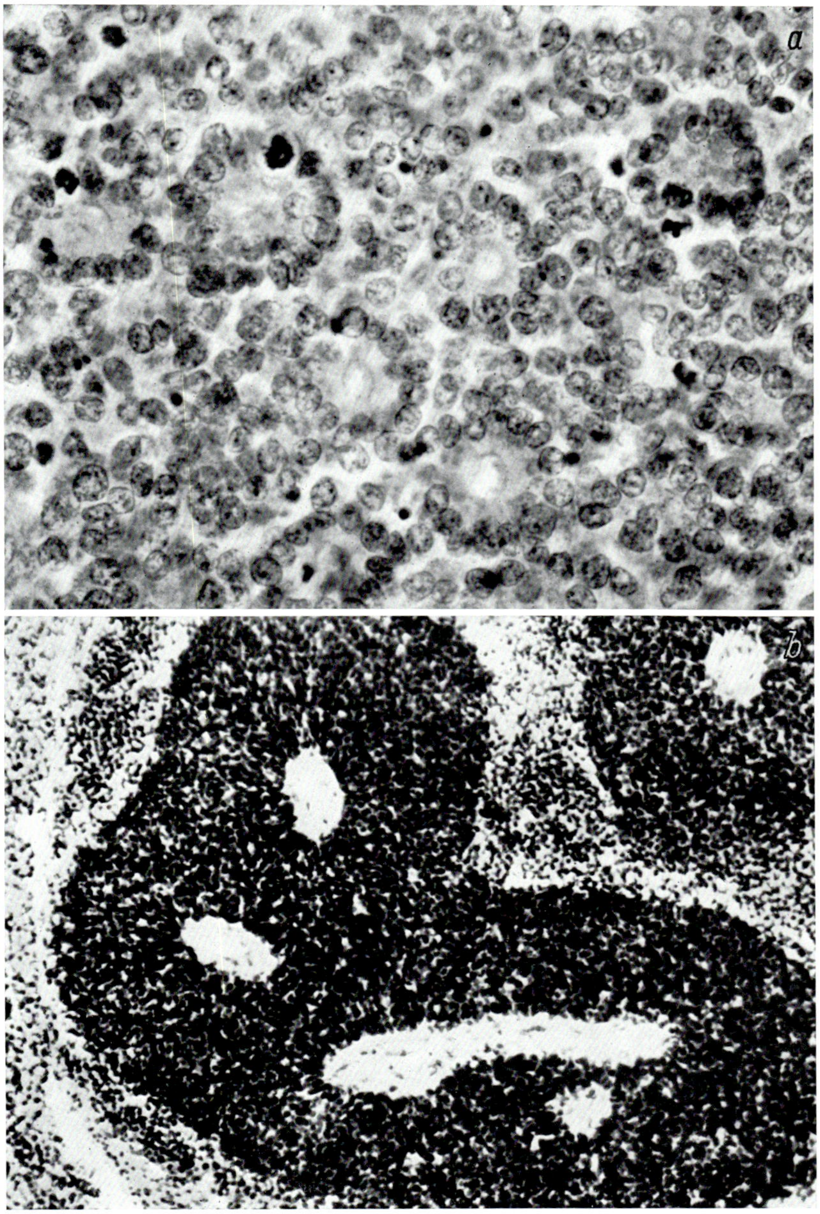

Fig. 18a and b: a ×500, b ×125
H. & E. stain

Fig. 19 — Astrocytomas

Fiber formation — impregnation with gold sublimate.

a) Unusually heavy fiber formation.
b) In comparison to a), only slight fiber formation.
c) Middle-grade fiber formation. The cells are seen at higher magnification.
d) A single fibrillary giant astrocyte among other large-bodied, but predominantly protoplasmic astrocytes.

Faserbildung bei Imprägnation mit Goldsublimat.

a) Außergewöhnlich starke Faserbildung.
b) Im Vergleich zu a) nur geringe Faserbildung.
c) Mittelgradige Faserbildung. Man sieht die Zellen in höherer Vergrößerung.
d) Einzelner fibrillärer Riesenastrocyt mit anderen, großleibigen, aber vorwiegend protoplasmatischen Astrocyten.

Mise en évidence des fibres gliales par l'imprégnation à l'or sublimé.

a) Formation exceptionnellement dense de fibres gliales.
b) Par rapport à la figure précédente, la production de fibres est discrète.
c) Réseau fibrillaire modéré. Les cellules apparaissent à un plus fort grossissement.
d) Astrocyte géant isolé, de type fibrillaire, parmi d'autres astrocytes volumineux de type protoplasmique.

Formación de fibras. Método del oro sublimado.

a) Intensa formación de fibras, mas de lo normal
b) En comparación con a) escasa formación de fibras.
c) Formación de fibras de mediana intensidad. Se ven las células a mayor aumento.
d) Astrocito fibrilar gigante, junto con otros grandes pero predominantemente protoplasmáticos.

Образование волокон при импрегнации золото-сулемовым методом.

a) Необычайно интенсивное образование волокон.
b) Слабое образование волокон в сравнении с a).
c) Умеренное образование волокон; клетки видны под большим увеличением.
d) Единичный фибриллярный гигантский астроцит и другие крупные, преимущественно протоплазматические астроциты.

金昇汞法でみた線維形成像。

a) きわめて高度な線維形成。
b) 図a)と比較し、ごく軽度な線維形成。
c) 中等度の線維形成。細胞の強拡大像が示されている。
d) 胞体の大きい形質性星膠細胞と、1個の線維性巨星膠細胞。

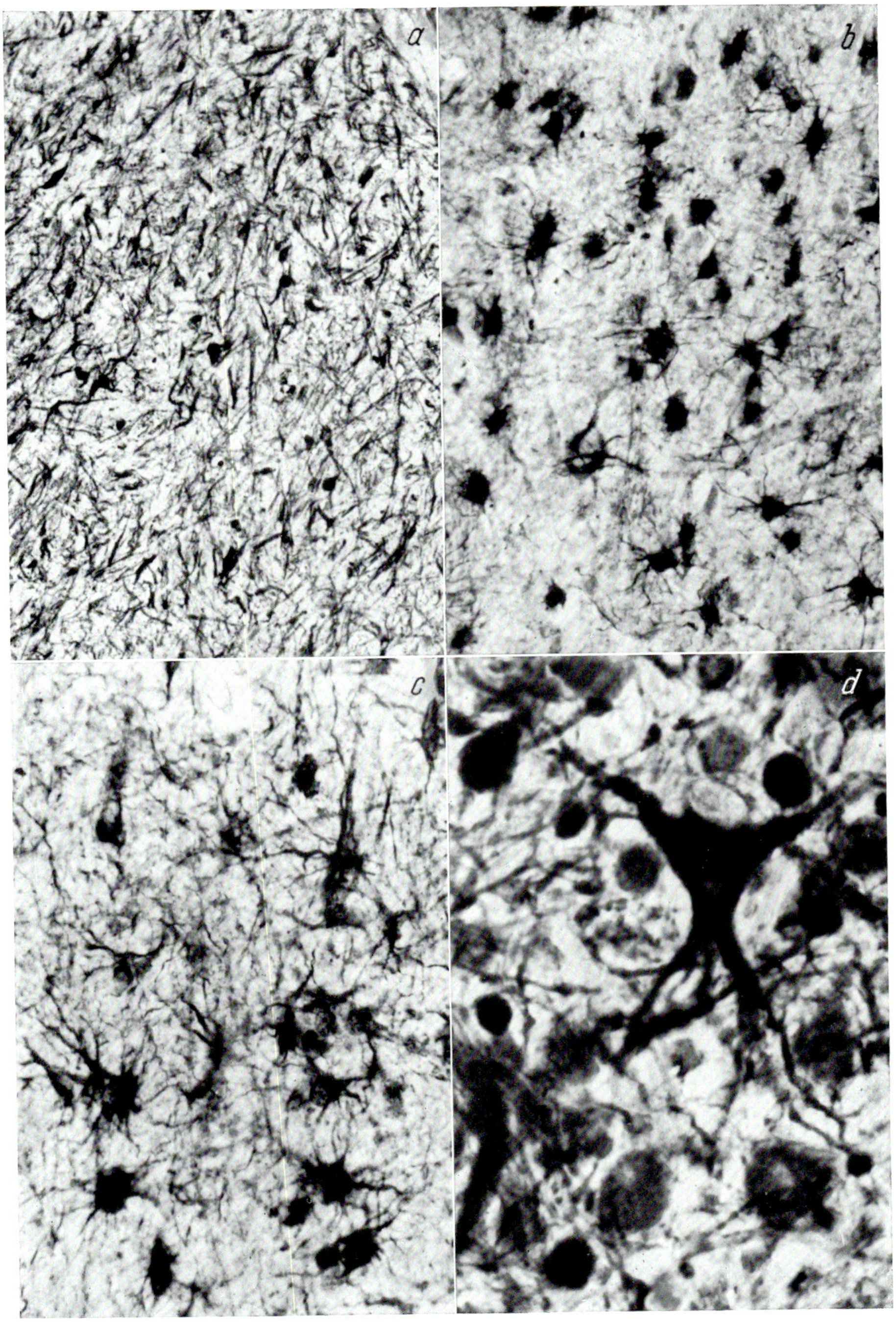

Fig. 19a—d: a ×72, b ×272, c ×336 and d ×580
Gold sublimate impregnation

Fig. 20 — Astrocytomas

a) Typical nuclear shapes in a fibrillary astrocytoma (aniline stain): roundish or oval nuclei with a prominent chromatin network. Occasionally the nucleus is somewhat vesicular and a nucleolus stands out clearly, particularly in the case of fibrillary forms.
b) Small, medium-sized and large nuclei in an astrocytoma around the aqueduct. *Top left:* An ependymal canal, a remnant of the former lining of the lumen.
c) Small, medium-sized and large nuclei in a predominantly fibrillary astrocytoma. In some elements one can also recognize the cell body, demonstrated with aniline staining. The nuclei lie in little clusters, two or three together. *Top:* A ganglion cell of the infiltrated region.
d) Often several nuclei fuse to form a symplasmatically connected and multinucleate-appearing cell-mass. Fibrillary astrocytoma.

a) Typische Kernformen in einem fibrillären Astrocytom bei Anilinfärbung: rundliche oder ovale Kerne mit kräftigem Chromatinnetz. Gelegentlich ist der Kern auch etwas blasiger und es hebt sich ein Nucleolus ab, besonders bei fibrillären Formen.
b) Kleine, mittelgroße und größere Kerne in einem Astrocytom des Aquädukts. Links oben ein Ependymschlauch als Rest der ehemaligen Auskleidung des Lumens.
c) Kleinere, mittelgroße und große Kerne in einem vorwiegend fibrillären Astrocytom. Bei einigen Elementen erkennt man auch den Zelleib mit Anilinfärbung dargestellt. Die Kerne liegen auch in Grüppchen zu 2—3 beieinander. Oben liegt eine Ganglienzelle des infiltrierten Gebietes.
d) Oft schließen sich mehrere Kerne zu einer symplasmatisch verbundenen und mehrkernig erscheinenden Zelle zusammen. Fibrilläres Astrocytom.

a) Dans l'astrocytome fibrillaire coloré par l'aniline, les noyaux sont caractérisés par leur forme arrondie ou ovale et leur réseau grossier de chromatine. Parfois, le noyau est légèrement gonflé et contient un nucléole, particulièrement dans les formes fibrillaires.
b) Noyaux petits, moyens et volumineux dans un astrocytome de l'aqueduc. En haut à gauche, on note un canal épendymaire, vestige de l'ancien recouvrement de la lumière.
c) Noyaux petits, moyens et volumineux dans un astrocytome à prédominance fibrillaire. Le colorant d'aniline met aussi en évidence le corps cellulaire de quelques éléments. Les noyaux se rassemblent parfois par petits groupes de deux ou trois. A la partie supérieure de la figure, on reconnaît une cellule nerveuse de la zone infiltrée.
d) Plusieurs noyaux s'accolent souvent pour constituer un symplasme et une cellule d'aspect multinucléé. Astrocytome fibrillaire.

a) Típica forma de los núcleos de un astrocitoma fibrilar, teñidos por la anilina: núcleos redondos y ovales con una densa red cromatínica. Ocasionalmente el núcleo es algo claro y se destaca en el un nucleolo, especialmente en las formas fibrilares.
b) Núcleos pequeños, medianos y grandes, en un astrocitoma del acueducto. Arriba y a la izquierda un tubo ependimario, resto del epitelio primitivo que recubría el lumen.
c) Núcleos pequeños, medianos y grandes en un astrocitoma predominantemente fibrilar. En algunos elementos se reconoce también el cuerpo celular teñido por la anilina. Los núcleos se reúnen en grupos de a dos y tres. Arriba hay una célula ganglionar del tejido invadido.
d) Frecuentemente varios núcleos se funden en una sola célula, multinucleada y de protoplasma único. Astrocitoma fibrilar.

a) Типичные формы ядер фибриллярной астроцитомы, окрашенной анилином: округлые или овальные ядра с обильной хроматиновой сетью; пузырькообразные ядра с четким ядрышком — особенность, характерная для фибриллярных астроцитом.
b) Мелкие, средние и крупной величины ядра в астроцитоме области сильвиева водопровода. Вверху слева остаток эпендимарной выстилки.
c) Преимущественно фибриллярная астроцитома с мелкими, средними и крупной величины ядрами. В некоторых элементах при окраске анилином видно также тело клетки. Ядра расположены группами по 2—3. Вверху инфильтрированного участка ганглиозная клетка.
d) Фибриллярная астроцитома. Часто несколько ядер образуют симпласт, сходный с многоядерной клеткой.

Continued on page 78

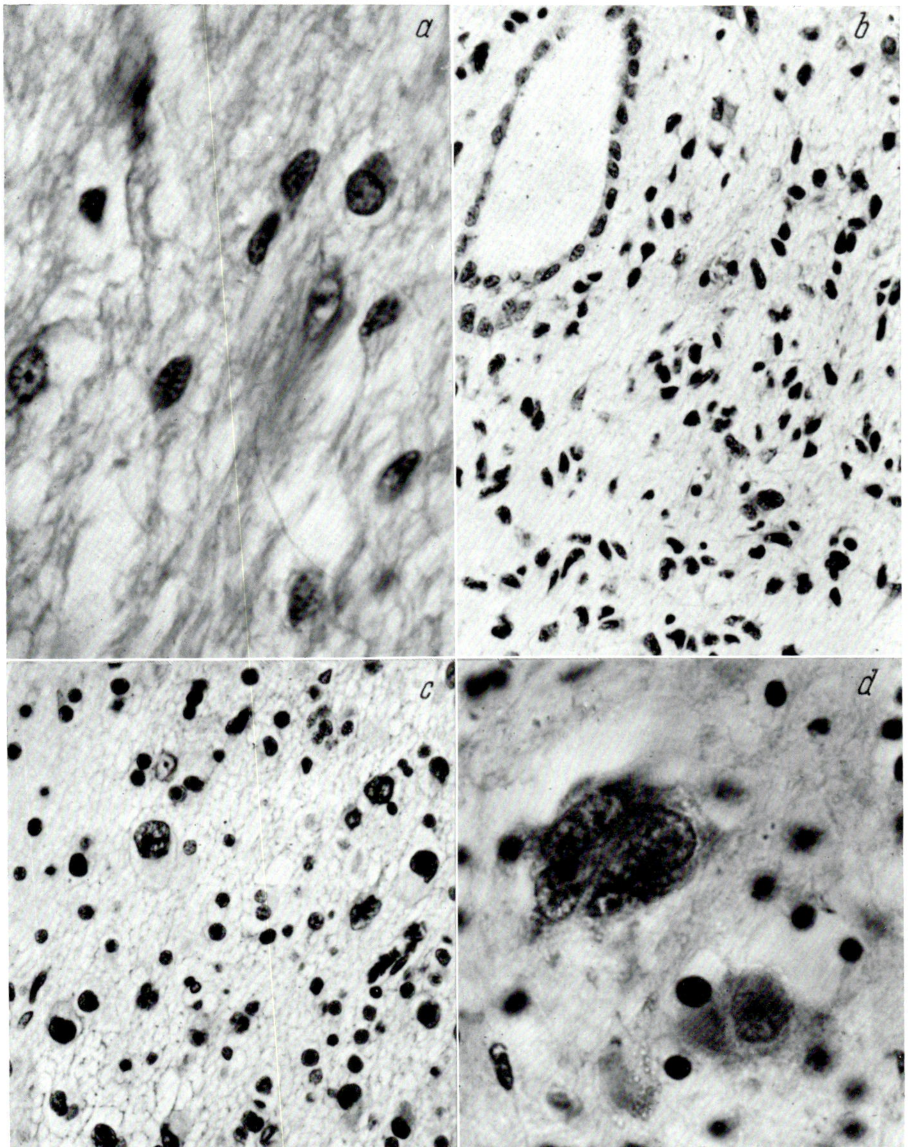

Fig. 20a—d: a ×648, b and c ×272, d ×576
Cresyl violet stain

Fig. 21 — Astrocytomas

a) and b) Gigantocellular, predominantly protoplasmic astrocytoma.
c) Protoplasmic astrocytoma with mucoid degeneration of the tissue. One sees numerous regressive changes.
d) Gigantocellular, predominantly protoplasmic astrocytoma, where, between the cells, glial fibers can still be discerned.

a) u. b) Gigantocelluläres, aber vorwiegend protoplasmatisches Astrocytom.
c) Protoplasmatisches Astrocytom mit schleimiger Entartung des Gewebes. Man sieht zahlreiche regressive Veränderungen.
d) Gigantocelluläres, vorwiegend protoplasmatisches Astrocytom, wo zwischen den Zellen noch deutliche Fasern zu erkennen sind.

a) et b) Astrocytome giganto-cellulaire, mais de type surtout protoplasmique.
c) Dans ce cas d'astrocytome protoplasmique, on voit une transformation muqueuse du tissu et de nombreuses altération régressives.
d) On peut encore voir nettement les fibres courant entre les cellules de cet astrocytome giganto-cellulaire à prédominance protoplasmique.

a) y b) Astrocitoma gigantocelular predominantemente protoplasmático.
c) Astrocitoma protoplasmático con degeneración mucoide del tejido. Se ven muchas modificaciones regresivas.
d) Astrocitoma gigantocelular, predominantemente protoplasmático en el que todavía se pueden reconocer claramente fibras entre las células.

a) и b) Гигантоклеточная, преимущественно протоплазматическая астроцитома.
c) Протоплазматическая астроцитома с мукоидной дегенерацией ткани. Многочисленные регрессивные изменения.
d) Гигантоклеточная, преимущественно протоплазматическая астроцитома. Между клетками еще четко прослеживаются волокна.

a) および b) 大細胞性、しかし大部分、形質性の星膠細胞腫。
c) 粘液様変性を伴った形質性星膠細胞腫。変性した細胞が多数みられる。
d) 大細胞性、形質性星膠細胞腫。細胞間に、グリヤ線維がまだ明らかに染出される。

Fig. 20 — Astrocytomas (continued)

a) Nissl 染色でみられる線維性星膠細胞腫の定形的な核。明瞭なクロマチン網をもつ、円形あるいは楕円形の核。特に線維性の細胞では核はやゝ明るく、核小体はときにきわだってみえる。
b) 中脳水道部星膠細胞腫にみられた、種々の大きさの核。図左上に細胞の遺残により形成された管をみとめる。
c) おもに線維性の星膠細胞腫における、種々の大きさの核。アニリン色素でも若干の細胞に細胞体が染出される。これらの核はまた、2〜3 個づつ小群をなしているものもある。図上に、浸潤巣に残存した神経細胞が 1 個みとめられる。
d) しばしば数個の細胞が集合して、多核細胞を形成する。線維性星膠細胞腫の 1 例。

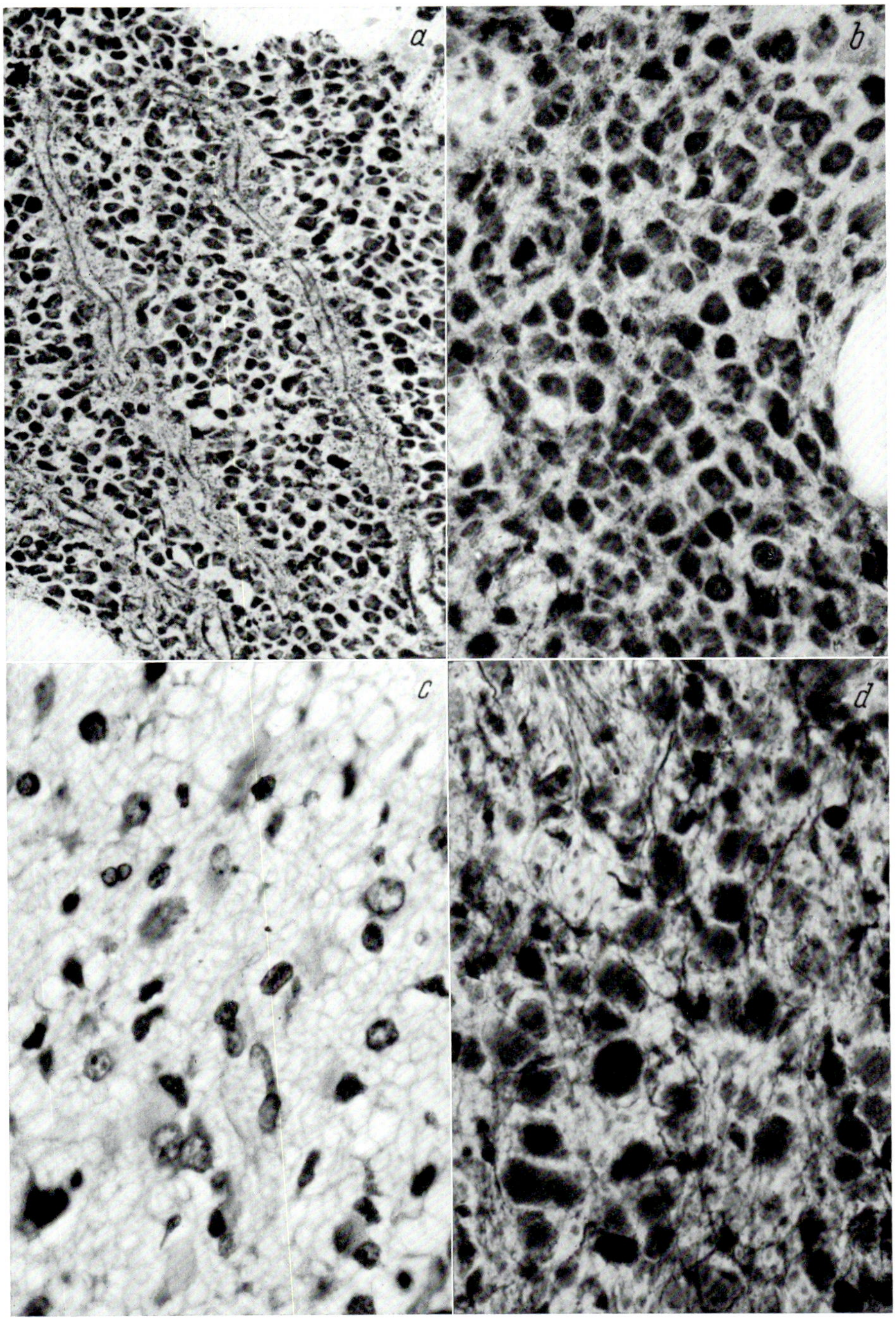

Fig. 21 a—d: a ×90, b ×180, d ×172. Gold sublimate method
c ×488. Cresyl violet stain

Fig. 22 — Astrocytomas

Predominantly gigantocellular astrocytoma: Coarse cells with pyknotic nuclei, usually located peripherally. Occasionally one finds multinucleated cells.

Vorwiegend gigantocelluläres Astrocytom, plumpe Zellen mit meist randständig gelegenen pyknotischen Kernen. Gelegentlich findet man auch mehrkernige Zellen.

Astrocytome à prédominance giganto-cellulaire, dont les cellules massives contiennent un noyau pycnotique et généralement refoulé à la périphérie. A certains endroits, on trouve également des cellules multinucléées.

Astrocitoma predominantemente gigantocelular; células tumefactas con núcleos picnóticos, la mayoría situados periféricamente. Ocasionalmente se encuentran células multinucleadas.

Преимущественно гигантоклеточная астроцитома; клетки уродливы, ядра гиперхромны и расположены по краям. Встречаются также многоядерные клетки.

主として、大細胞性の星膠細胞腫。細胞は大きく丸味を帯びていて、核は濃縮状、多くは辺在している。ときには多核細胞をみとめる。

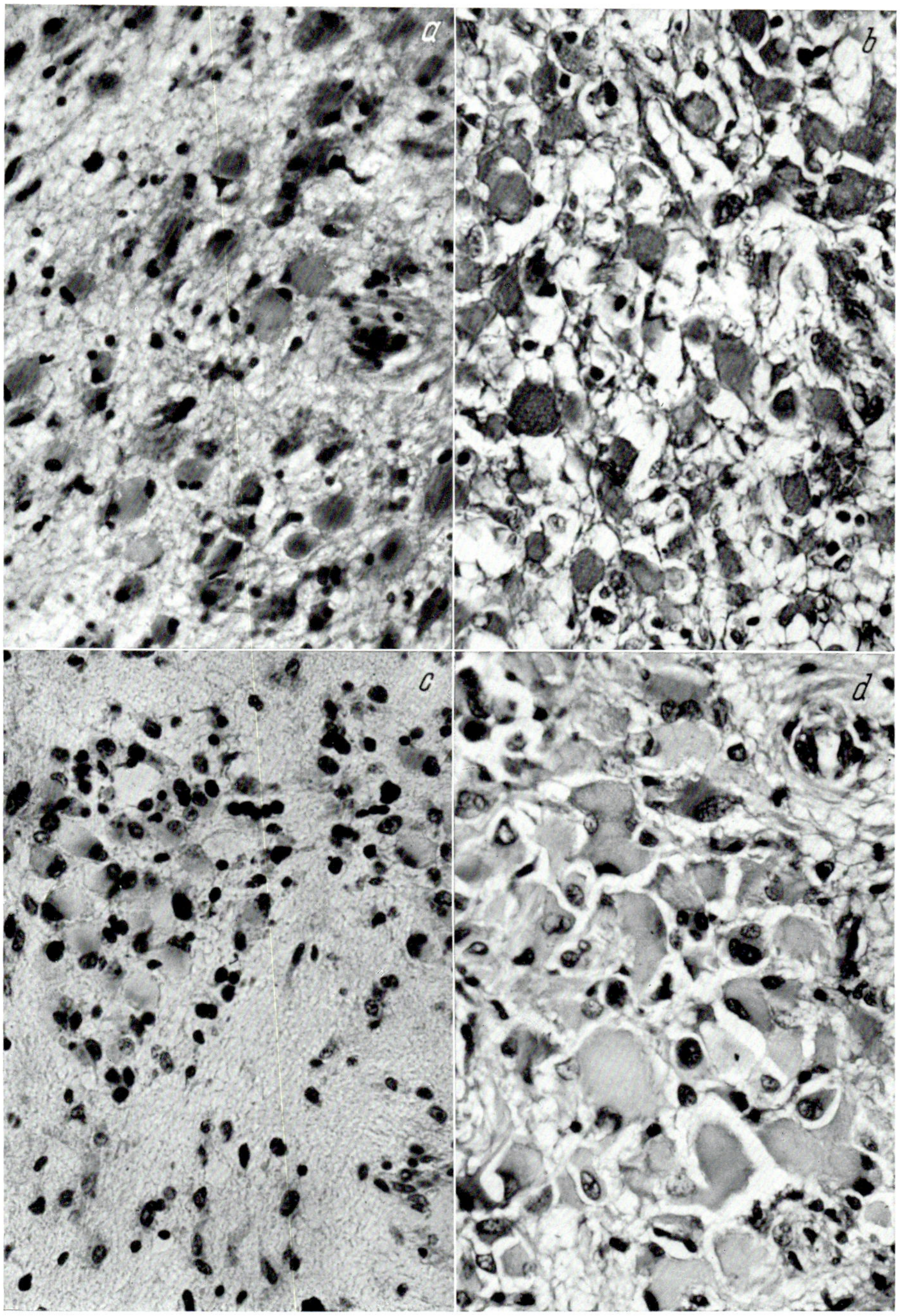

Fig. 22a—d: a ×112, b and d ×272. Cresyl violet stain
c ×112. H. & E. stain

Fig. 23 — Astrocytomas

a) Peculiar extension of an astroblastoma in the marginal zone: Vascular buds protrude like fingers into the healthy tissue and become sheated by a dense mantle of worm-shaped glial cells. From these buds the cells grow into the tissue and assume "mature" forms.
b) Blood vessel lying within a typical astroblastoma: Around the somewhat thickened adventitia, the coarse tumor cells are barely visible by impregnation and lie in a radial arrangement. The vascular connective tissue is specifically impregnated.
c) Astroblastoma with large, predominantly astrocyte-like cells.
d) Same case as b), stained with cresyl violet.

a) Eigenartige Ausbreitung eines Astroblastoms in der Randzone: Gefäßsprossen reichen wie Finger in das gesunde Gewebe und werden dabei von einem dichten Mantel wurmförmiger Gliazellen eingescheidet. Von dieser Knospe wachsen die Zellen ins Gewebe aus und nehmen dort reifere Formen an.
b) Gefäß im Inneren eines typischen Astroblastoms: Um den Adventitiamantel, der vielleicht etwas verbreitert ist, liegen in radiärer Anordnung die plumpen, durch Imprägnation eben sichtbaren Geschwulstzellen. Das Gefäßbindegewebe ist spezifisch imprägniert.
c) Astroblastom mit großen, hier vorwiegend astrocytenartigen Zellen.
d) Gleicher Fall wie b).

a) Extension caractéristique à la périphérie d'un astroblastome: des bourgeons vasculaires pénètrent dans le tissu comme des digitations et sont entourés par une gaine épaisse de cellules gliales vermiculaires. A partir de ces bourgeons, les cellules infiltrent le tissu environnant, où elles prennent une forme plus «mure».
b) Vaisseau au sein d'un astroblastome typique: les cellules tumorales, massives et bien mises en évidence par l'imprégnation métallique, se disposent de façon radiaire autour de la gaine adventitielle, qui est peut être un peu épaissie. Le tissu conjonctif du vaisseau est imprégné de façon spécifique.
c) Astroblastome à grandes cellules qui, dans ce cas, ressemblent à des astrocytes.
d) Même cas que dans b).

a) Crecimiento característico de un astroblastoma. En la periferia, proliferaciones vasculares alcanzan como dedos el tejido sano y se encuentran limitadas por un denso manto de células gliales alargadas. A partir de estos vasos las células crecen en el tejido tomando alli formas más maduras.
b) Vaso en el interior de un astroblastoma típico: alrededor de la adventicia, quizás algo engrosada, se colocan radialmente las células tumorales, visibles por la impregnación. El tejido conectivo vascular está específicamente impregnado.
c) Astroblastoma con células grandes, aquí predominantemente de tipo astrocítico.
d) El mismo caso que b).

a) Своеобразное расрастание клеток астробластомы в краевой зоне. Пальцевидное проникновение сосудистых ветвей в здоровую ткань. Эти сосуды заключены в оболочку, образованную густо расположенными вытянутыми клетками; отсюда эти клетки врастают в ткань, принимая там зрелые формы.
b) Сосуд внутри типичной астробластомы: вокруг несколько расширенной адвентиции радиарно расположены импрегнируемые уродливые опухолевые клетки. Сосудистая соединительная ткань импрегнируется специфически.
c) Астробластома с преимущественно крупными астроцитомоподобными клетками.
d) Случай b).

a) 星膠芽細胞腫の辺縁部における、独特な浸潤様式。神経膠細胞よりなる厚い鞘をともなって、血管芽があたかも指のように正常組織内に浸入する。神経膠芽細胞は、ここから組織内に増殖して行き、そこでより成熟した形になる。
b) 定型的星膠芽細胞腫のなかにみられる血管。おそらく、やゝ拡張した血管外膜の周囲に、丸味を帯びかろうじて鍍銀された腫瘍細胞が、放射状に存在している。血管結合組織は、特異的に染出されている。
c) ここでは、ほとんど大型の星膠細胞様の細胞からなる星膠芽細胞腫。
d) 図 b) と同一例

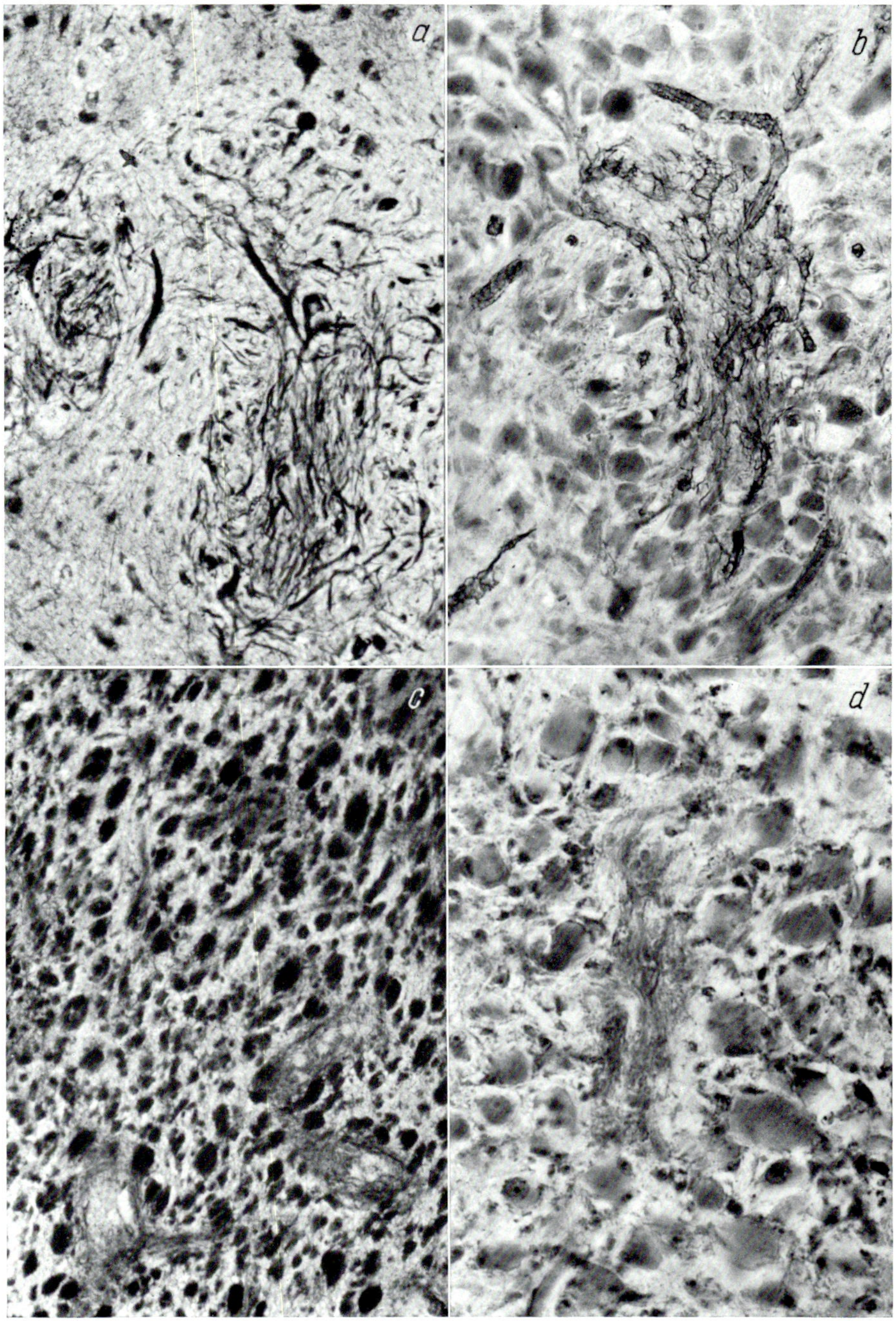

Fig. 23a—d: a ×108. Gold sublimate method
b ×112. Perdrau's impregnation
c ×96. H. & E. stain
d ×112. Cresyl violet stain

Fig. 24 — Astrocytomas

Typical patterns of an astroblastoma.

a) Coarse, large-bodied cells, usually with short processes, lie radially around the blood vessels.

b) Between the cells, mucoid disintegration of the tissue is beginning. Meanwhile, the fiber-forming tumor cells still lie radially around the vessels.

c) Typical "pseudopapillary" architecture in an astroblastoma. It arises by cystic degeneration of the tissue at a distance from the blood vessels, while the tumor cells close to the vessels are preserved.

d) See c).

Typische Bilder eines Astroblastoms.

a) Plumpe, großleibige Zellen, meist mit kurzen Fortsätzen, liegen radiär um die Gefäße.

b) Zwischen den Zellen beginnt der schleimige Zerfall des Gewebes. Vorläufig liegen um die Gefäße noch die faserbildenden Geschwulstzellen in radiärer Anordnung.

c) Typische ,,pseudopapilläre" Architektur in einem Astroblastom. Sie entsteht durch cystischen Zerfall des Gewebes fern von den Gefäßen, während die gefäßnahen Geschwulstzellen erhalten bleiben.

d) Siehe c).

Images typiques de l'astroblastome.

a) Cellules massives, riches en cytoplasme, généralement munies de courts prolongements et situées de façon radiaire autour des vaisseaux.

b) Début de la désintégration spongieuse du tissu entre les amas de cellules tumorales, qui persistent le long des vaisseaux entourés de fibres à disposition radiaire.

c) Architecture «pseudo-papillaire» typique dans un cas d'astroblastome. Elle est causée par la dégénérescence kystique du tissu à distance des vaisseaux, tandis que les cellules tumorales restent intactes à proximité des vaisseaux.

d) voir c)

Imágenes típicas de un astroblastoma.

a) Células groseras de protoplasma grande, la mayoría con pequeñas prolongaciones situadas radialmente a los vasos.

b) La degeneración mucosa del tejido se inicia entre las células. Alrededor de los vasos todavía quedan células tumorales formadoras de fibras, en disposición radiada.

c) Típica arquitectura «pseudopapilar» en un astroblastoma. Se constituye por la degeneración quística del tejido lejos de los vasos, mientras persisten las células cercanas a estos últimos.

d) Ver c).

Типичные картины астробластомы.

a) Крупные, уродливой формы клетки с преимущественно короткими отростками, радиарно расположенными вокруг сосудов.

b) Мукоидный распад ткани между клетками. Наличие вокруг сосудов радиарно расположенных волокнообразующих опухолевых клеток.

c) Типичное псевдопапиллярное строение астробластомы, обусловленное кистозным распадом тканей на отдалении от сосудов. Вблизи сосудов опухолевые клетки сохранены.

d) См. c).

星膠芽細胞腫の定型像。

a) 丸味をおびた、胞体の大きい細胞が、多くは短い突起をもって放射状に血管をかこんでいる。

b) 腫瘍組織の粘液様崩壊が起ってはいるが、血管周囲には、まだ線維形成細胞が放射状に残存している。

c) 星膠芽細胞腫の定型的な「偽乳頭」構造。この像は、血管に接する腫瘍細胞が残存し、血管から離れた部位が嚢胞状崩壊を起すことによって生ずる。

d) c)参照。

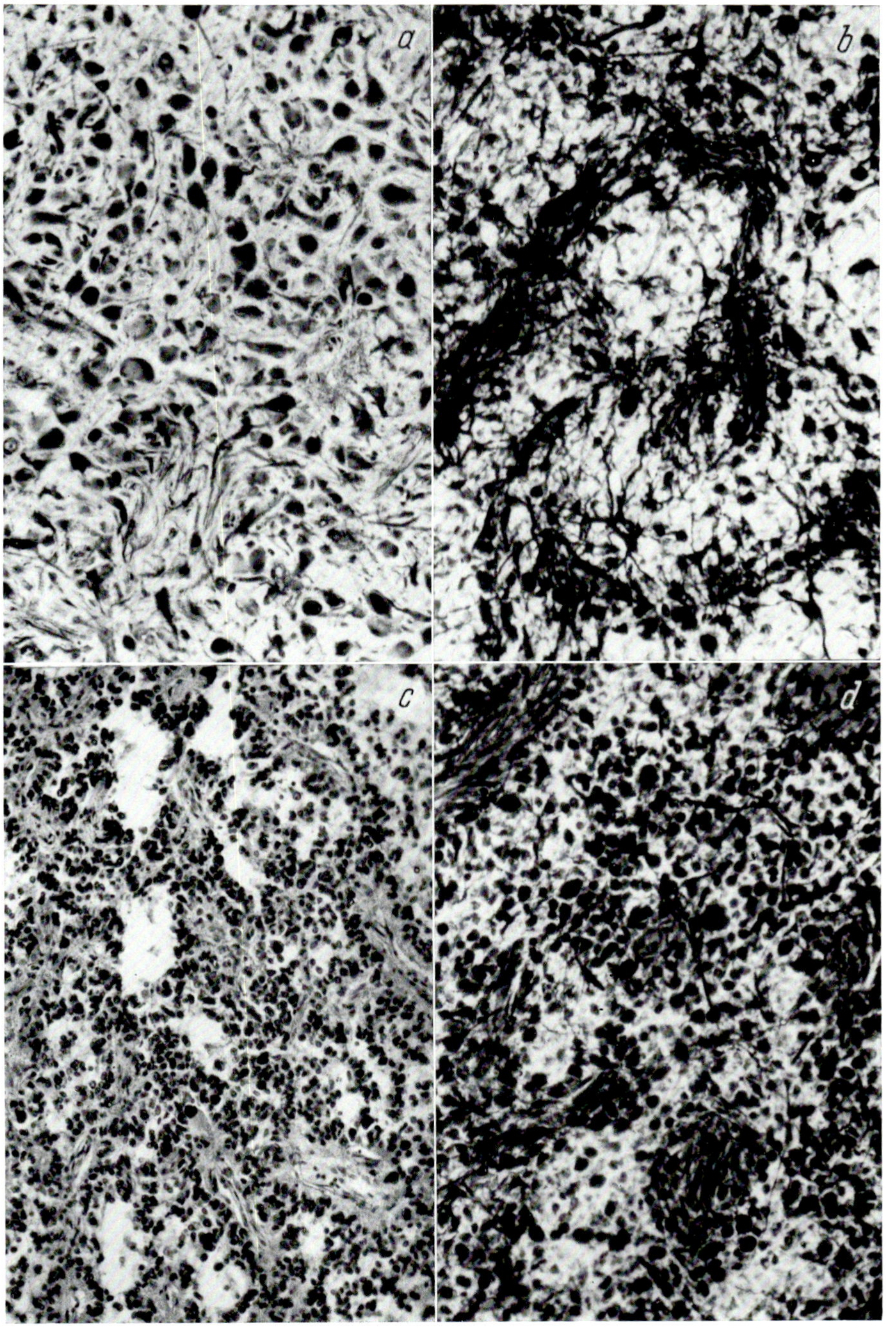

Fig. 24a—d: a ×84, b ×104. Gold sublimate method
c and d ×76. Cresyl violet stain

Fig. 25 — Astrocytomas

Various forms of regressive changes, in particular, mucoid transformation up to cyst formation in fibrillary and protoplasmic astrocytomas. Single, multinucleated cells can be recognized.

Verschiedene Formen der regressiven Veränderungen, insbesondere der schleimigen Umwandlung bis zur Cystenbildung in fibrillären und protoplasmatischen Astrocytomen. Man erkennt einzelne mehrkernige Zellen.

Différentes formes d'altération régressive dans des astrocytomes fibrillaires et protoplasmiques, notamment depuis la transformation muqueuse jusqu'à la formation de kystes. On observe quelques cellules multinucléées.

Diferentes formas de los procesos regresivos, en especial de la transformación mucosa hasta la formación de quistes, en astrocitomas fibrilares y protoplasmáticos. Se ven algunas células multinucleadas.

Фибриллярная и протоплазматическая астроцитомы. Различные формы регрессивных изменений, в особенности мукоидная дегенерация вплоть до кистообразования. Единичные многоядерные клетки.

線維性および形質性星膠細胞腫の、粘液様変性から嚢胞形成にいたる退行性変化。数個の多核巨細胞がある。

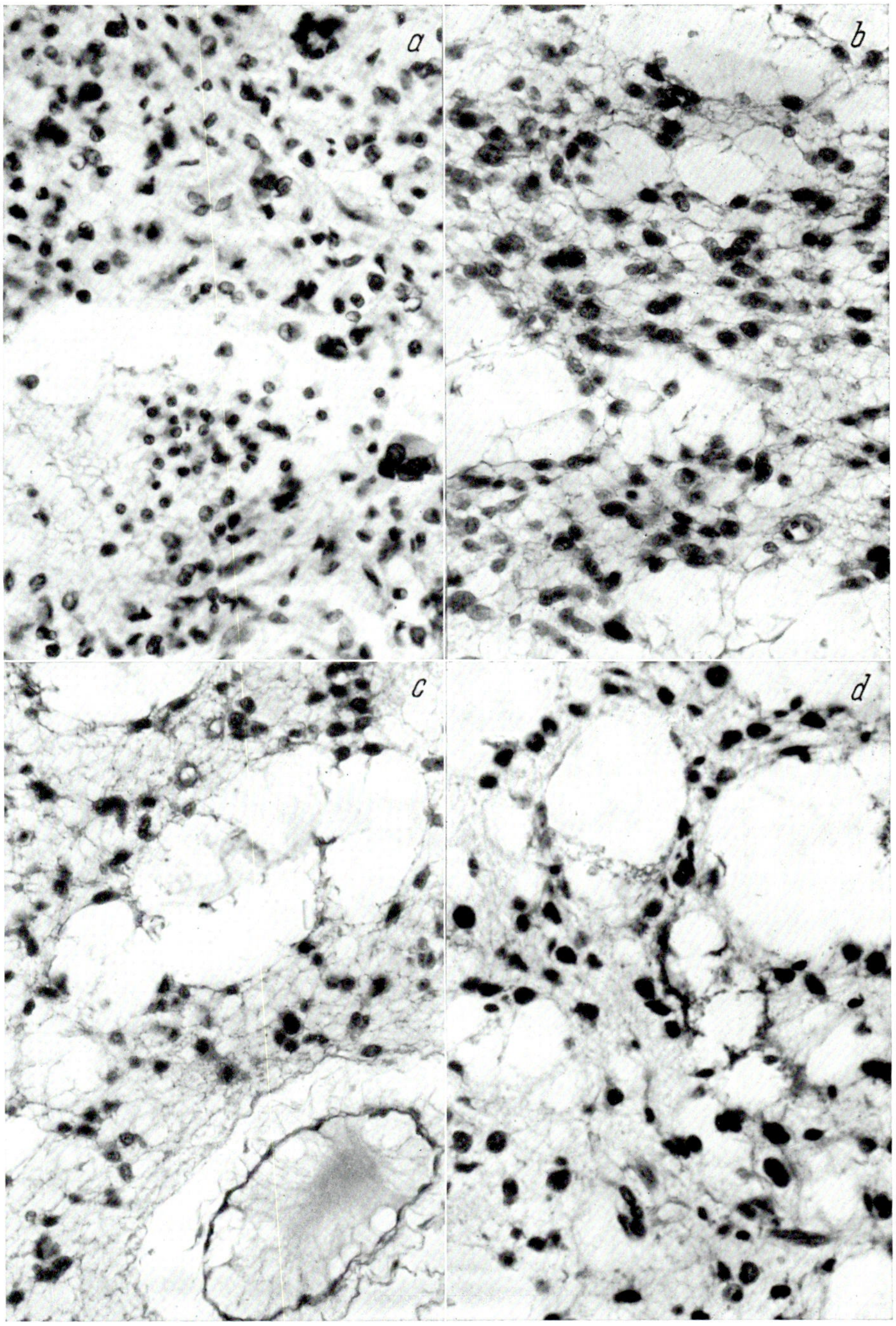

Fig. 25a—d: a, c and d ×272, b ×224
Cresyl violet stain

Fig. 26 — Astrocytomas

a) Typical fibrillary astrocytoma of medium-sized elements. One can still recognize the "sucker feet" of the astrocytes.
b) Very large-bodied, fiber-forming cells of a fibrillary astrocytoma.
c) Partly fibrillary, partly protoplasmic elements, which are very coarse and have few processes.
d) Predominant oblong cells in a fibrillary astrocytoma around the aqueduct.

a) Typisches fibrilläres Astrocytom aus mittelgroßen Elementen. Man erkennt deutlich noch die „Saugfüße“ der Astrocyten.
b) Reichlich großleibige, faserbildende Zellen eines fibrillären Astrocytoms.
c) Teils fibrilläre, teils protoplasmatische Elemente, die sehr plump sind und wenig Fortsätze haben.
d) Überwiegend längliche Zellen in einem fibrillären Astrocytom des Aquädukts.

a) Astrocytome fibrillaire typique, composé d'éléments de taille moyenne. On peut encore reconnaître clairement les «pieds suceurs» des astrocytes.
b) Astrocytome fibrillaire, dont les cellules ont un cytoplasme abondant et produisent les fibres.
c) Astrocytome composé d'éléments fibrillaires et d'éléments protoplasmiques, qui ont un aspect très massif et possèdent peu de prolongements.
d) Astrocytome fibrillaire de l'aqueduc, composé principalement de cellules allongées.

a) Astrocitoma fibrilar típico a base de elementos de mediano tamaño. Se ven claramente los pies chupadores de los astrocitos.
b) Abundantes células grandes, formadoras de fibras, en un astrocitoma fibrilar.
c) Elementos ora fibrilares ora protoplasmáticos, muy groseros y de escasas prolongaciones.
d) Células predominantemente alargadas en un astrocitoma fibrilar del acueducto.

a) Типичная фибриллярная астроцитома с клетками средней величины. Еще четко прослеживаются «сосудистые ножки» астроцитов.
b) Обилие крупных волокнообразующих клеток в фибриллярной астроцитоме.
c) Неправильной формы частично фибриллярные, частично протоплазматические клетки с небольшим количеством отростков.
d) Преимущественно вытянутые клетки фибриллярной астроцитомы области сильвиева водопровода.

a) 中等大細胞からなる定型的線維性星膠細胞腫。星膠細胞の「血管足」が、まだ明瞭である。
b) 線維性星膠細胞腫にみられた、多数の、胞体の大きい、線維形成性細胞。
c) 線維性および形質性細胞混在。後者は腫大し、胞体突起をほとんどもたない。
d) 中脳水道部の線維性星膠細胞腫。多くは細長い細胞によって占められている。

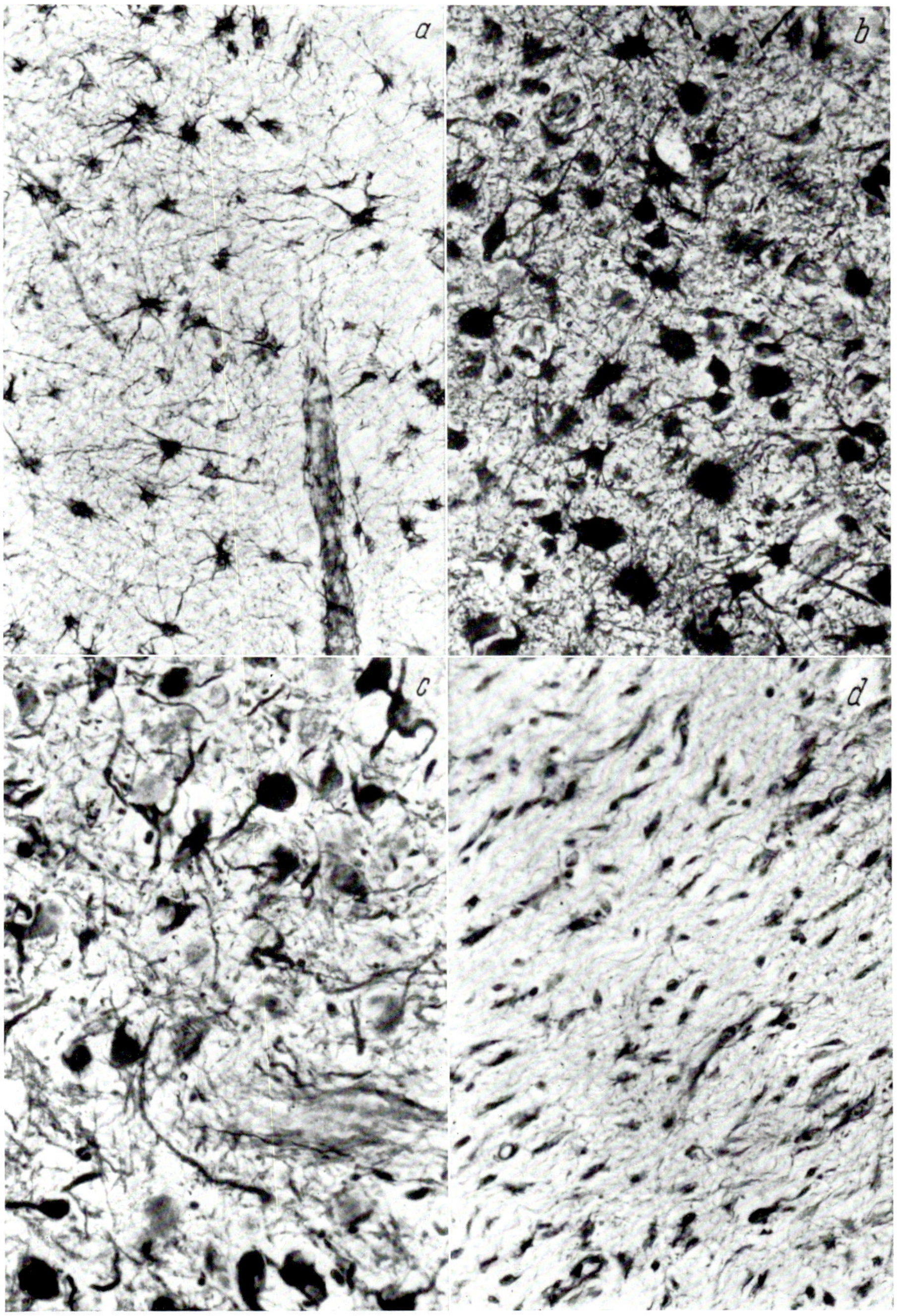

Fig. 26a—d: a ×96. b ×266,
c ×272. Gold sublimate method
d ×272. Cresyl violet stain

Fig. 27 — Astrocytomas

Malignant degeneration of a fibrillary astrocytoma which is still typical in isolated portions.
a) Markedly fibrillary astrocytes in a somewhat unorderly disposition.
b) Nuclear pattern corresponding to a). The beginning of cystic degeneration.
c) and d) In the malignant, degenerated portion, one discerns large-bodied, very polymorphic cells, as well as a cordlike necrosis. The blood vessels are starting to proliferate. Some cells have several, very active ("ganglioid") nuclei.

Maligne Degeneration eines in einzelnen Teilen noch typischen, fibrillären Astrocytoms:
a) Ausgesprochen fibrilläre Astrocyten in einer etwas unruhigen Lagerung.
b) Kernbild zu a). Man sieht den Beginn einer cystischen Entartung.
c) u. d) In dem maligne entarteten Teil erkennt man großleibige, sehr polymorphe Zellen sowie eine strichförmige Nekrose. Die Gefäße beginnen zu wuchern. Einige Zellen haben mehrere, sehr aktive („ganglioide") Zellen.

Dégénérescence maligne d'une tumeur qui présente encore, en plusieurs endroits, l'aspect typique de l'astrocytome fibrillaire.
a) Astrocytes nettement fibrillaires, qui ont peut-être une disposition un peu désordonnée.
b) La coloration cytologique met en évidence le début d'une désintégration kystique.
c) et d) Dans la zone de dégénérescence maligne, on observe des cellules volumineuses et très polymorphes ainsi qu'un foyer allongé de nécrose. Les vaisseaux commencent à proliférer. Quelques cellules possèdent plusieurs noyaux très actifs («ganglioïdes»).

Degeneración maligna de un astrocitoma fibrilar, en algunas zonas aún típico.
a) Astrocitos decididamente fibrilares en una zona quizás algo intranquila.
b) Imagen de los núcleos de a). Se observa el inicio de una degeneración quística.
c) y d) En la zona de transformación maligna se reconocen células grandes muy polimorfas, lo mismo que necrosis en forma de banda. Los vasos empiezan a proliferar. Algunas células tienen núcleos, muy activos (ganglioides).

Малигнизация отдельного участка еще типичной фибриллярной астроцитомы.
a) Участок с наличием выраженных фибриллярных астроцитов, несколько необычно расположенных.
b) К рис. a). Начало кистозного перерождения.
c) и d) В малигнизировавшемся участке крупные очень полиморфные клетки и ограниченные участки некроза. Разрастание сосудов. Наличие очень активных («ганглиоидных») клеток.

ところどころまだ定型的な像を残す線維性星膠細胞腫の悪性化。すべて症例985。
a) 線維性の強い星膠細胞、配列にやゝ乱れがある。
b) 図a)の核染色像。嚢胞形成初期像。
c) および d) 悪性化した部分には、胞体の大きい多形性の細胞と、線維壊死巣をみとめる。血管は増殖しはじめ、若干の細胞は多核性で神経細胞様の明るい核を有する。

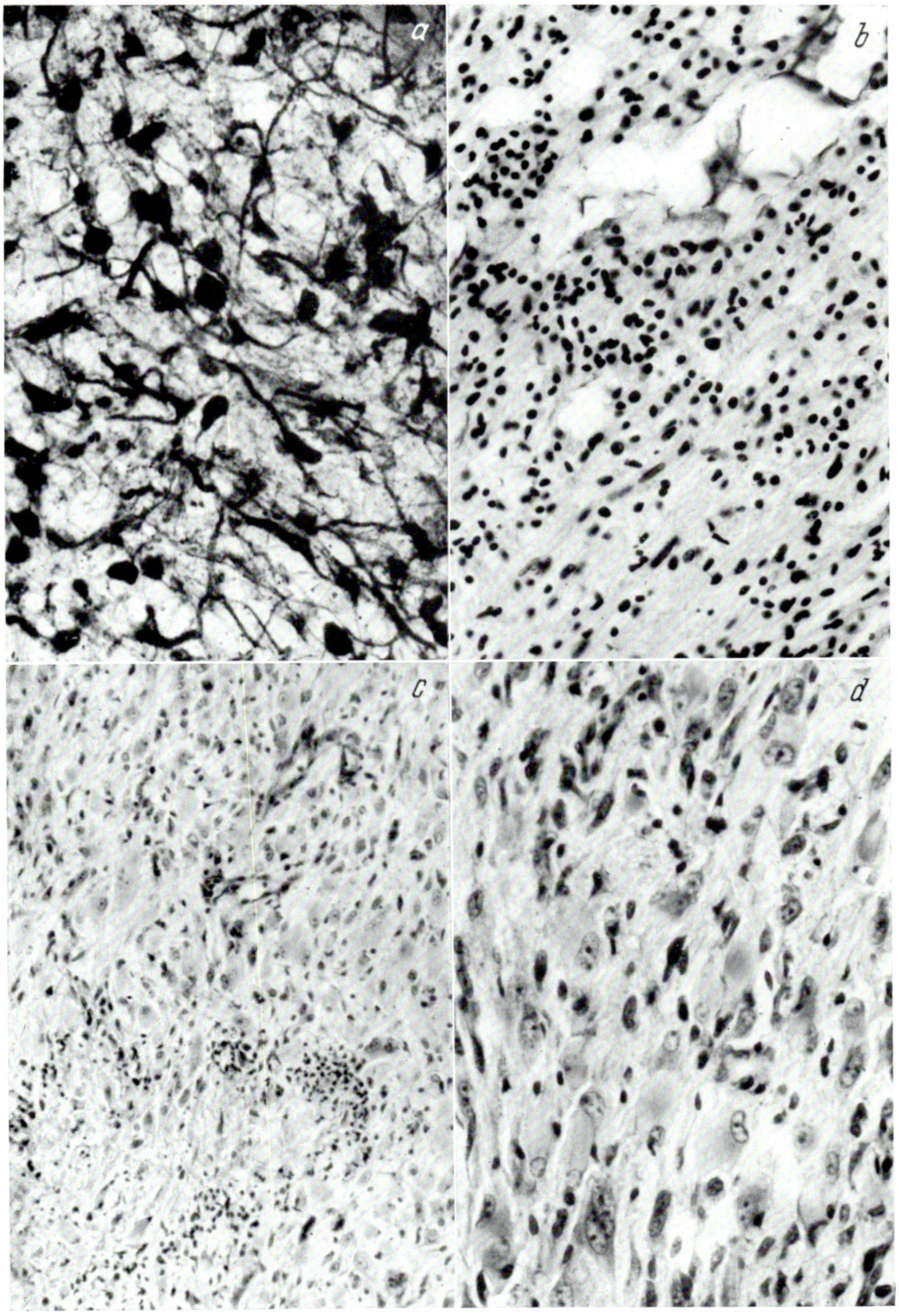

Fig. 27a—d: a ×220. Gold sublimate method
b and d ×112, c ×72. Cresyl violet stain

Oligodendrogliomas

Oligodendroblastoma and oligodendrocytoma, "diffuse glioma", round cell sarcoma, sarcoma angiolithicum, gliome à petites cellules rondes.

Fig. 28 — Oligodendrogliomas

a) and b) Typical honeycomb architecture of an oligodendroglioma embedded in paraffin: "bare" nuclei lie two or more in a vacuole. The pattern is compared to a network of "honeycombs" or "plant cells".
c) The same picture, on impregnation with gold sublimate, reveals the network only vaguely. The cells themselves do not become impregnated.
d) In the oligodendroglioma the axons are usually preserved for a long time.

a) u. b) Typische Honigwabenarchitektur eines Oligodendroglioms bei Paraffineinbettung: „nackte" Kerne liegen zu zwei oder mehreren in einer Vacuole. Das Bild wird mit einem Netz von „Honigwaben" oder „Pflanzenzellen" verglichen.
c) Das gleiche Bild bei Imprägnation mit Goldsublimat läßt das Netzwerk nur verschwommen erscheinen. Die Zellen selbst werden hier nicht imprägniert.
d) Im Oligodendrogliom bleiben die Axone meist lange erhalten.

a) et b) Architecture typique en rayon de miel sur une coupe à la paraffine d'un oligodendrogliome: chaque vacuole contient un et même deux ou plusieurs noyaux «nus». L'image peut être comparée au réseau d'un "rayon de miel" ou de "cellules végétales".
c) La même image n'apparait plus que d'une façon vague par la méthode à l'or sublimé, qui n'imprègne pas les cellules.
d) La plupart des axones persistent longtemps au sein de l'oligodendrogliome.

a) y b) Típica arquitectura en panal de abeja de un oligodendroglioma tras la inclusión en parafina. Núcleos desnudos reunidos en grupos de un a, dos o más, en una vacuola. La imagen se compara a una red en "panal de abeja" o de "células vegetales".
c) La misma imagen con la impregnación con el oro sublimado permite ver la red, hinchada. Las células aquí no se impregnan.
d) En el oligodendroglioma la mayoría de las veces los axones permanecen intactos.

a) и b) Типичное сотовидное строение олигодендроглиомы при заливке в парафин: «голые» ядра по два и больше в одной вакуоле. Картину можно сравнить с сеткой из «сот» или «растительных клеток».
c) При импрегнации той же опухоли золотосулемовым методом сотовидная структура стушовывается, сами клетки не импрегнируются.
d) В олигодендроглиоме в большинстве случаев сохранены длинные аксоны.

a) および b) パラフィン切片にみられる稀突起膠腫特有の蜂窩状構造：「裸」の核が２ないし数個づつ空胞内に存在している。この像は「蜂窩」あるいは「植物細胞」の網状構造と比較出来る。
c) 同様の構造は、金昇汞標本でぼんやり染出されるのみで、胞体は染まらない。
d) 希突起膠腫では、一般に軸索が長期残存する。

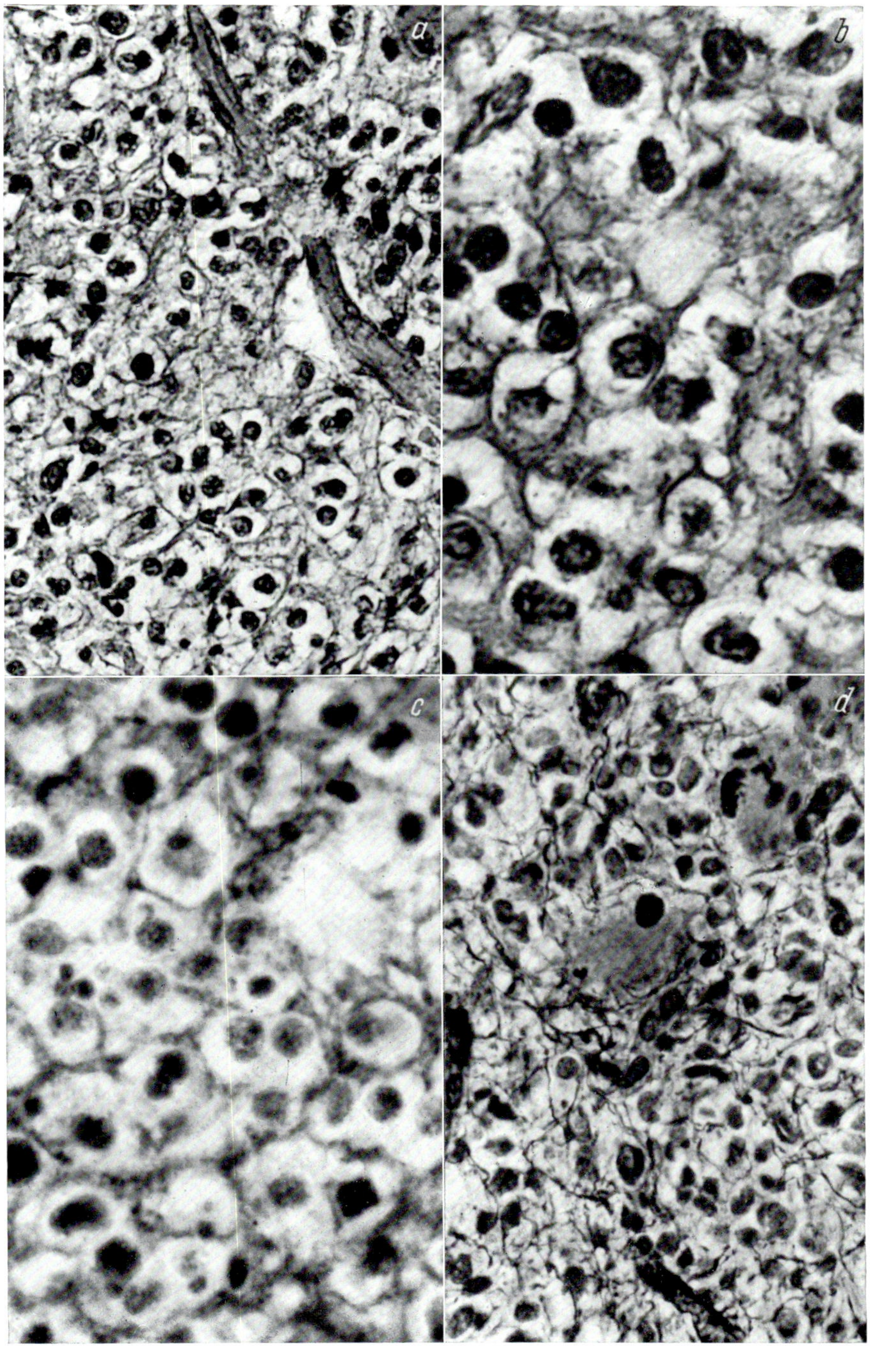

Fig. 28a—d: a ×288, b ×616. H. & E. stain
c × 635. Gold sublimate method
d ×275. Bielschowsky's impregnation

Fig. 29 — Oligodendrogliomas

Various architectures in the same case of an oligodendroglioma:

a) Typical honeycomb architecture.

b) Here, in close apposition to the honeycomb architecture, variations can be seen: Cells rich in cytoplasm with small, round nuclei lie within a vacuolar network; the basic architecture of the "honeycomb formation" is still visible. The cells resemble, however, "ameboid astroglia".

c) and d) In the same case of an oligodendroglioma, peculiar spherical, unipolar or astroblast-like cells are found on impregnation, but the nucleus is not impregnated and appears as a clear space.

Verschiedene Architekturen im gleichen Falle eines Oligodendroglioms:

a) Typische Honigwabenarchitektur.

b) Hier sind dicht neben der erst beschriebenen Architektur Abwandlungen zu sehen: Es liegen cytoplasmareiche Zellen mit kleinen Rundkernen in einem vacuoligen Netz; als Grundarchitektur ist die „Honigwabenbildung" noch sichtbar. Die Zellen gleichen aber „amöboider Astroglia".

c)—d) Im gleichen Fall des Oligodendroglioms finden sich bei Imprägnation eigenartige kugelige unipolare bzw. astroblastenartige Zellen, wobei der Kern nicht imprägniert ist, sondern als helle Lücke erscheint.

Architectures différentes dans le même cas d'oligodendrogliome.

a) Architecture typique en rayon de miel.

b) Image très voisine de l'architecture précédente. Des cellules riches en cytoplasme et contenant un petit noyau arrondi se trouvent dans un réseau vacuolaire; l'architecture fondamentale en «rayon de miel» est encore visible. Toutefois les cellules ressemblent aux «astrocytes amiboïdes».

c) et d) L'imprégnation métallique met en évidence de curieuses cellules globuliformes, unipolaires ou ressemblant à des cellules astroblastiques, dont le noyau n'est pas imprégné, mais apparaît comme une tache vide et claire.

Diferentes arquitecturas en un mismo caso de oligodendroglioma:

a) Típica arquitectura en panal de abeja

b) Aquí, junto a la arquitectura anterior se ven algunas modificaciones: red vacuolar formada por células ricas en protoplasma con pequeños nucleos redondos. Como arquitectura básica, todavía puede apreciarse la estructura en panal de abeja. Las células, sin embargo, parecen «astroglia ameboide».

c) y d) En el mismo caso, por el método del sublimado-oro, se enduentran células singulares, redondas, unipolares, o bien, de tipo astroblástico, en las que el núcleo no se ha impregnado si no que resalta como en una clara laguna.

Различная структура одной и той же олигодендроглиомы:

a) типичное сотовидное строение,

b) некоторые отклонения от предыдущего строения клетки с обильной цитоплазмой и мелкими округлыми ядрами в вакуольной сети; еще видны «соты» как основа структуры, однако клетки похожи на амёбовидную астроглию.

c) и d) В этом же случае олигодендроглиомы при импрегнации видны своеобразные округлые униполярные, астробластоподобные клетки; ядро не импрегнируется и представлено в виде светлого ободка.

稀突起膠腫の同一症例にみられた種々なる構築。

a) 定型的な蜂窩状構造。

b) 上記の定型像に近接して、ここには異型像をみる。空胞状の網状構造の中に、小形の円形核をもった、胞体に富む細胞がある。基本構造としての蜂窩の形成がまだみとめられる。細胞はアメーバ様星膠細胞に似ている。

c) および d) 同上例の稀突起膠腫鍍銀で、特異な球状で単極性、あるいは星膠芽細胞様の細胞をみる。核は染出されないので、その部は淡明な腔としてみられる。

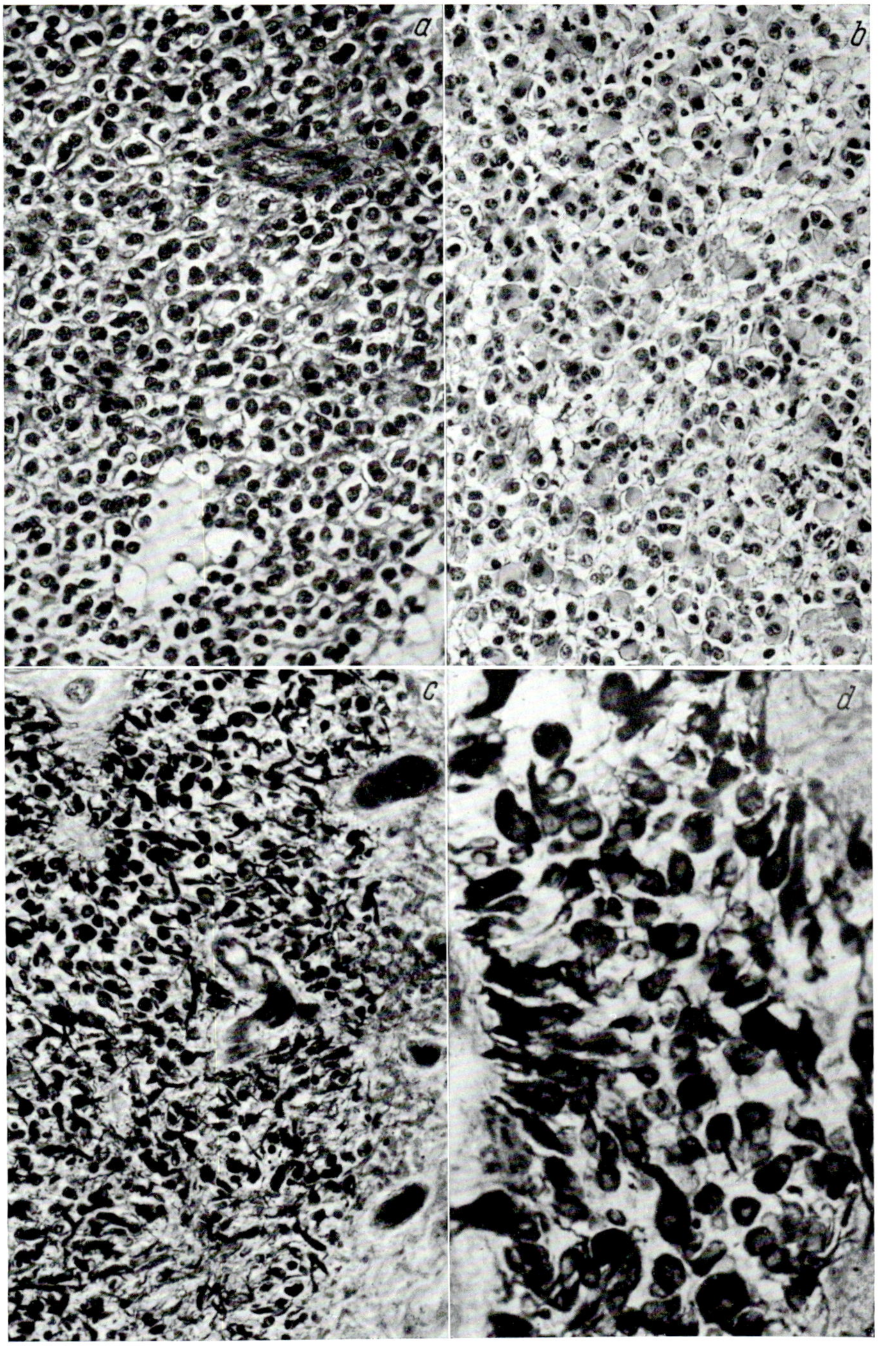

Fig. 29a—d: a and b ×160. H. & E. stain
c ×96, d ×216. Gold sublimate impregnation

Fig. 30 — Oligodendrogliomas

a) Spindle-cell variants of an oligodendroglioma, in which one can still recognize the typical honeycomb architecture.
b) A markedly spindle-celled area in an oligodendroglioma after the spread of the tumor cells into the pia.
c) and d) On impregnation with gold sublimate the majority of the cells can occasionally be demonstrated. There are small, spherical elements, or larger, spindle-or club-shaped elements, whose processes can be impregnated in long sections.

a) Spindelzellige Variante eines Oligodendroglioms, bei dem man noch typisch die Honigwabenarchitektur erkennen kann.
b) Ausgesprochen spindelzelliges Gebiet eines Oligodendroglioms nach Einwachsen der Geschwulstzellen in die weichen Häute.
c) u. d) Bei Imprägnation mit Goldsublimat stellt sich gelegentlich die Mehrzahl der Zellen dar. Es sind kleine kugelige oder größere spindelige oder kolbenförmige Elemente, deren Fortsätze auf lange Strecken imprägniert sein können.

a) Variante à cellules fusiformes dans un cas d'oligodendrogliome, dans lequel on peut encore reconnaître l'architecture typique en rayon de miel.
b) Aspect fusiforme des cellules d'un oligodendrogliome ayant envahi la leptoméninge.
c) et d) Dans certains cas, l'imprégnation à l'or sublimé met en évidence la majorité des cellules. Il s'agit d'éléments soit petits et globuliformes, soit volumineux et fusiformes, soit encore en forme de tête de massue, dont les prolongements peuvent être imprégnés sur une grande longueur.

a) Variante fusiforme de un oligodendroglioma, en el cual se puede reconocer todavía la típica arquitectura en panal de abeja.
b) Zona marcadamente fusiforme en un oligodendroglioma tras el crecimiento de las células tumorales en las leptomeninges.
c) y d) Con el oro sublimado se pueden demostrar la mayoría de las células. Algunas redondas, pequeñas, otras mayores fusiformes o en forma de maza dejan teñir sus prolongaciones en largos trayectos.

a) Веретеноклеточный вариант олигодендроглиомы, еще сохранившей типичное сотовидное строение.
b) Веретеноклеточный участок олигодендроглиомы с прорастанием опухолевыми клетками мягкой мозговой оболочки.
c) и d) Обилие клеток иногда выявляется при импрегнации золото-сулемовым методом. Это мелкие округлые или крупные веретенообразные или колбовидные элементы, отростки которых могут импрегнироваться на больших участках.

a) 紡錘細胞性の稀突起膠腫。しかしまだ定型的な蜂窩状構造をみとめる。
b) 軟膜に浸潤し、高度に紡錘性細胞となった部分。
c) および d) 金昇汞法によって、大多数の細胞が染め出されることもある。小円形またはやゝ大形の紡錘形ないし棍棒状の細胞があり、それらの細胞より長く伸びた突起が染め出されている。

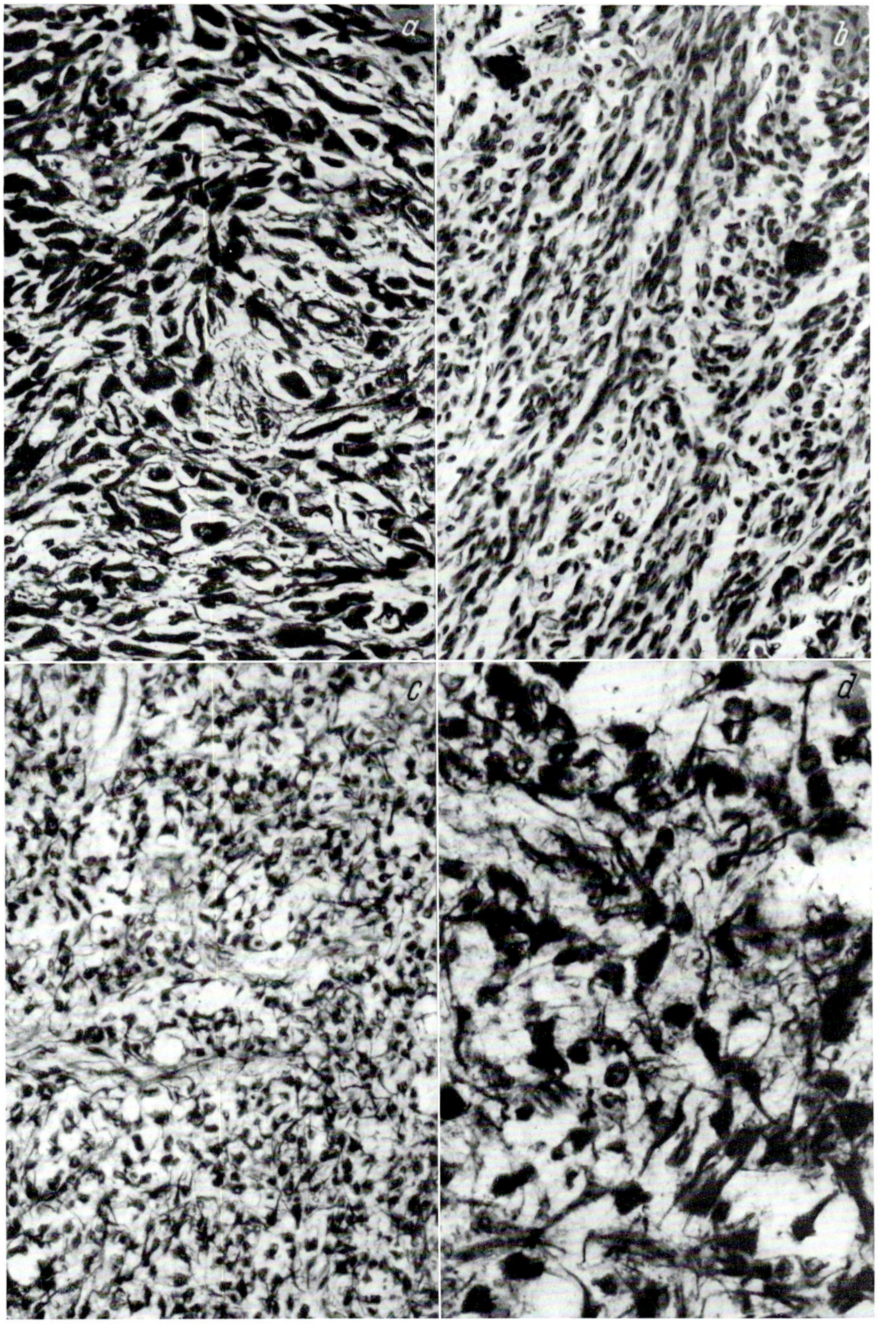

Fig. 30a—d: a ×168, H. & E. stain
b ×224. Cresyl violet stain
c ×96, d ×216. Gold sublimate method

Fig. 31 — Oligodendrogliomas

Variants of an oligodendroglioma:

a) A suggested formation of pseudo-rosettes.

b) Arrangement of the tumor cells in bands along the capillaries.

c) The shape of the nuclei is round, oval, or sometimes oblong. The chromatin is equally distributed; occasionally one nucleolus stands out in particular.

d) The differences in the shapes and sizes of the nuclei are not often seen. The formation of the honeycomb architecture is receding.

Varianten des Oligodendroglioms:

a) Angedeutete Bildung von Pseudorosetten.

b) Anordnung der Geschwulstzellen in Bändern entlang der Capillare.

c) Die Form der Kerne ist rund, oval oder auch nicht zu selten länglich. Das Chromatin ist gleichmäßig verteilt, gelegentlich tritt ein Nucleolus besonders hervor.

d) Den Unterschied der Kerne in Form und Größe sieht man nicht zu selten. Auch tritt die Bildung der Honigwabenarchitektur zurück.

Quelques variantes de l'oligodendrogliome.

a) Disposition cellulaire rappelant les images de pseudorosettes.

b) Rangées de cellules tumorales disposées le long des capillaires.

c) La forme des noyaux est arrondie, ovalaire et parfois allongée. La chromatine est répartie uniformément. Un nucléole est parfois très apparent.

d) Il n'est pas rare d'observer des variations dans la forme et la taille des noyaux. En outre, l'architecture en rayon de miel s'estompe.

Variantes del oligodendroglioma.

a) Formación insinuada de pseudorosetas.

b) Disposición de las células tumoralcs en bandas, a lo largo de los capilares.

c) La forma de los núcleos es oval y frecuentemente alargada. La cromatina está regularmente distribuida; ocasionalmente aparece algún nucleolo.

d) Las diferencias de los núcleos en forma y tamaño es menos frecuente. También la formación de la arquitectura en panal de abejas deja de ser tan evidente.

Варианты олигодендроглиомы:

a) Намечающееся образование псевдорозеток.

b) Расположение опухолевых клеток вдоль капилляров в виде тяжей.

c) Ядра округлые, овальные, но нередко и удлиненные. Хроматин распределен равномерно. Иногда четко выделяется одно ядрышко.

d) Нередко величина и форма ядер различны. Исчезает сотовидное строение.

非定型的な稀突起膠腫の組織像:

a) 偽ロゼッテを思わせる所見。

b) 血管に沿って索状にならんだ腫瘍細胞。

c) 核は円形あるい楕円形、時にはやゝ長めで、クロマチンは均一に分布している。しばしば著明な核小体が1個存在する。

d) 核の形、大きさに差異のあることも稀でない。蜂窩構造も不明となる。

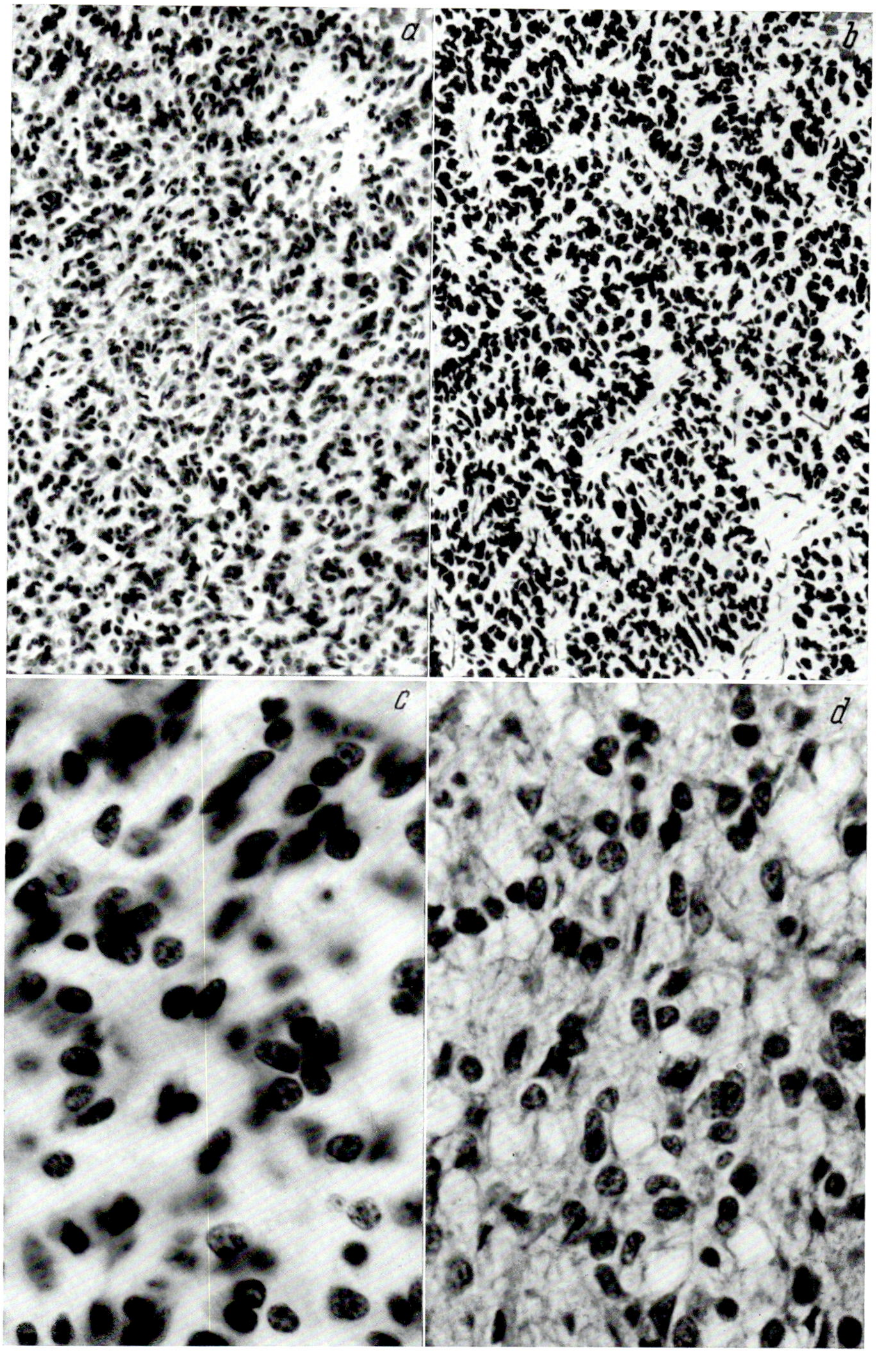

Fig. 31a—d: a ×154, b ×120, c ×420. Cresyl violet stain
d ×342. H. & E. stain

Fig. 32 — Oligodendrogliomas

a) Usually, only single elements are impregnated, while the majority of the tumor cells in an oligodendroglioma show up only as shadows.
b) Here with special stains the majority of the tumor cells can be demonstrated. They correspond predominantly to Types 2 and 3 of Hortega.
c) On impregnation of the smaller tumor cells by special methods, it is apparent that the nucleus does not become impregnated at the same time.
d) The most frequently occurring tumor cells (Type 1 of Hortega) appear usually as bare nuclei. They are the most difficult to impregnate.

a) Meist imprägnieren sich nur einzelne Elemente, während die Mehrzahl der Tumorzellen im Oligodendrogliom nur schattenhaft dargestellt ist.
b) Mit Spezialfärbungen kann man hier die Mehrzahl der Tumorzellen darstellen. Sie entsprechen vorwiegend dem Typus 2 und 3 von Hortega.
c) Auch bei der Imprägnation der kleineren Geschwulstzellen mit Spezialmethoden sieht man, daß der Kern nicht mitimprägniert ist.
d) Die am häufigsten vorkommenden Geschwulstzellen (vom Typus I von Hortega) erscheinen meist nur als nackte Kerne. Sie sind am schwersten zu imprägnieren.

a) En général, la méthode à l'or sublimé imprègne seulement quelques éléments isolés ,tandis que la majorité des cellules tumorales de l'oligodendrogliome sont à peine visibles.
b) Grâçe à des colorations spéciales, on peut mettre en évidence la majorité des cellules tumorales, qui correspondent principalement aux types 2 et 3 de Hortega.
c) On voit également que ces méthodes spéciales n'imprègnent pas le noyau des petites cellules tumorales.
d) Les cellules tumorales, qui sont les plus abondantes (type 1 de Hortega), apparaissent généralement comme des noyaux nus et sont les plus difficiles à imprégner.

a) En los oligodendrogliomas, las más de las veces, sólo se impregnan algunos elementos, mientras la mayoría de las células tumorales se muestran solo vagamente.
b) Con tinciones especiales se puede demostrar aquí la mayoría de las células tumorales. La mayoría corresponden a los tipos dos y tres de Hortega.
c) Incluso con la impregnación de las más pequeñas células tumorales con métodos especiales, se ve que el núcleo no se tiñe.
d) Las células que más comunmente se presentan (tipo 1 de Hortega) aparecen casi siempre como simples núcleos desnudos. Son las más difíciles de impregnar.

a) В основном импрегнируются только единичные элементы, а большинство опухолевых клеток в олигодендроглиоме слабо выражены.
b) Специальными методами окраски выявляется большинство опухолевых клеток, соответствующие преимущественно 2-му и 3-му типам клеток Ортега.
c) Ядро не выявляется даже при импрегнации опухолевых клеток специальными методами.
d) Наиболее распространенные опухолевые клетки (первый тип клеток Ортега) чаще всего представлены лишь в виде голых ядер. Их импрегнация наиболее трудна.

a) 稀突起膠腫では、金昇汞法によって、少数の細胞が染出されるのみで、大部分は陰影状を呈する。
b) 特別の染色法を用いて、大多数の腫瘍細胞を染出することが出来る。細胞の多くはHortegaの第2、3型に一致する
c) 小型の腫瘍細胞は、鍍銀（炭酸銀法）では、核が染まらない。
d) 最も普通にみられる腫瘍細胞（Hortega 第1型）は、単に裸核状に見える。この細胞は、最も鍍銀され難い。

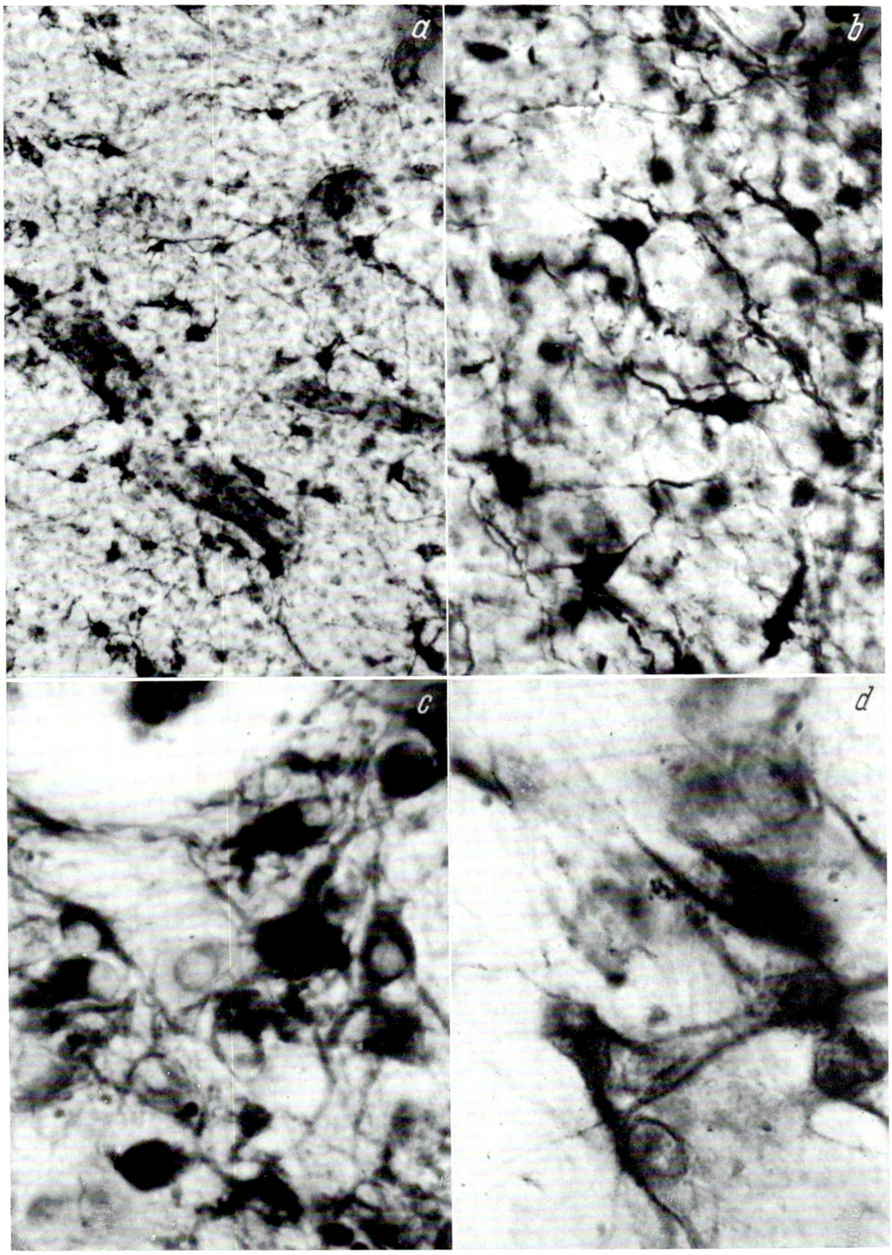

Fig. 32a—d: a ×112, b ×229, c ×600, d ×1,080
a Goldsublimate method
c Silver carbonate
b and d Biondi's impregnation

Fig. 33 — Oligodendrogliomas

a) Heavy calcification (calcium granules) in an oligodendroglioma, which is just infiltrating the cortex from below upward and is already causing subpial accumulation of the cells.
b) Calcification of the cortical capillaries above an infiltration zone of a still very sharply demarcated oligodendroglioma.
c) Higher magnification of the capillary calcification.
d) Rather large calcium granules in the growth zone of an oligodendroglioma, wherein the perivascular infiltration zone can be clearly discerned.

a) Starke Verkalkung (Kalkperlen) in einem Oligodendrogliom, das gerade die Rinde von der Tiefe aus infiltriert und bereits eine subpiale Verdichtung der Zellen herbeiführt.
b) Verkalkung der Rindencapillaren oberhalb einer Infiltrationszone eines noch recht scharf abgesetzten Oligodendroglioms.
c) Höhere Vergrößerung der Capillarverkalkung.
d) Größere Kalkperlen in der Wachstumszone eines Oligodendroglioms, bei dem man die perivasculäre Verdichtungszone deutlich erkennt.

a) Nombreuses précipitations calcaires (calcophérites) dans un oligodendrogliome, qui infiltre le cortex à partir de la profondeur et provoque déjà une accumulation cellulaire sous la pie-mère.
b) Calcification des capillaires corticaux au-dessus d'une zone d'infiltration d'un oligodendrogliome, qui est encore bien délimité.
c) Calcification des capillaires, à un grossissement plus élevé.
d) Calcophérites plus volumineux dans la zone de croissance d'un oligodendrogliome, où l'on reconnaît bien la condensation périvasculaire des cellules tumorales.

a) Intensa calcificación (perlas calcáreas) en un oligodendroglioma que acaba de infiltrar la corteza y que ha dado lugar a un engrosamiento subpial de las células.
b) Calcificación de los capilares corticales por encima de una zona de infiltración, todavía bastante bien limitada.
c) Mayor aumento de las calcificaciones capilares.
d) Perlas calcáreas mayores en la zona de crecimiento de un oligodendroglioma en el que se ve claramente la zona de engrosamiento perivascular.

a) Обильное обызвествление (глыбки кальция) в олигодендроглиоме, инфильтрирующей кору из глубины. Субпиальное скопление клеток.
b) Обызвествление корковых капилляров над зоной инфильтрации четко ограниченной олигодендроглиомы.
c) Обызвествление капилляров под бо́льшим увеличением.
d) Крупные глыбки из кальция в зоне роста олигодендроглиомы. Четкие периваскулярные скопления.

a) 稀突起膠腫内の高度石灰化（真珠様石灰化）。腫瘍は深部より皮質内に浸潤し、すでに軟膜下に細胞の緻密化をみとめる。
b) 皮質内毛細血管の石灰沈着。稀突起膠腫の浸潤はまだ限局性で、石灰化巣とは境界をもっている。
c) 毛細血管石灰沈着の強拡大。
d) 稀突起膠腫の発育部にみとめた、やゝ大きな真珠様石灰化巣。血管周囲の濃縮をみとめる。

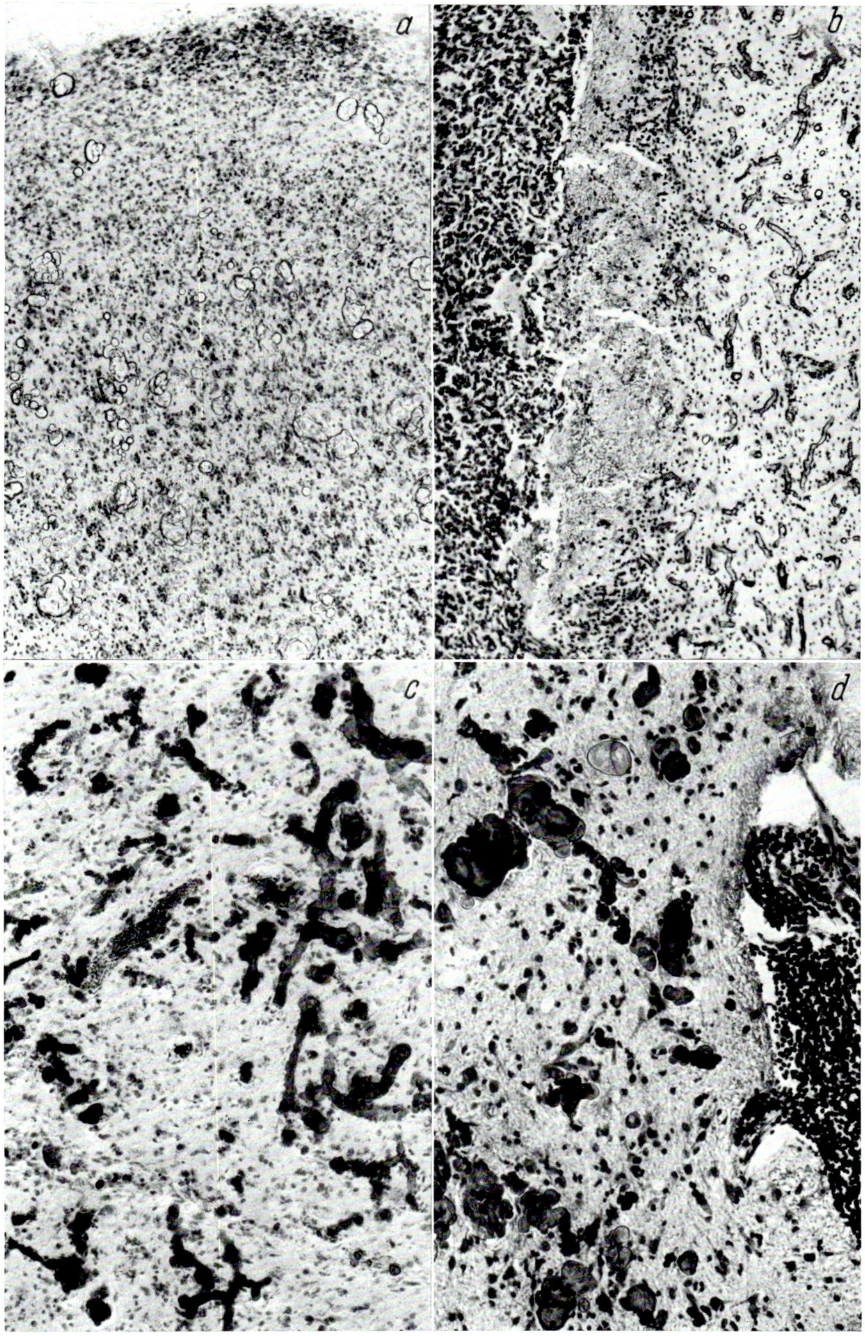

Fig. 33a—d: a ×78. Cresyl violet stain
b ×72, c ×92, d ×172. H. & E. stain

Fig. 34 — Oligodendrogliomas

a) Subpial thickening by the cells with formation of "warts" in an oligodendroglioma. Here a glial fiber stain shows the heavy fiber content. The "wart" feels hard to the palpating finger of the operating surgeon.
b) The wart formation in cell staining.
c) and d) Cortical "warts" in an oligodendroglioma at different magnifications.

a) Subpiale Verdichtung der Zellen mit Bildung von „Warzen“ in einem Oligodendrogliom. Hier zeigt eine Gliafaserfärbung den starken Gehalt an Fasern. Die „Warze“ scheint dem tastenden Finger des Operateurs hart.
b) Die Warzenbildung in Zellfärbung.
c) u. d) Rinden„warzen“ in einem Oligodendrogliom bei verschiedener Vergrößerung.

a) Dans l'oligodendrogliome, l'accumulation sous-piale de cellules provoque la formation de «verrues», qui contiennent de nombreuses fibres gliales. A la palpation, le chirurgien constate que la «verrue» a une consistance indurée.
b) La formation de «verrues» mise en évidence par une coloration cytologique.
c) et d) «Verrues» corticales dans un oligodendrogliome à des grossissements différents.

a) Engrosamiento subpial de las células con la formación de «verrugas», en un oligodendroglioma. Con una tinción para la glía puede verse el gran contenido en fibras. La «verruga» aparece como dura al tacto del cirujano.
b) La formación verrucosa coloreada por células.
c) y d) Verrugas marginales en un oligodendroglioma, bajo distintos aumentos.

a) Субпиальное уплотнение клеток олигодендроглиомы с образованием «сосочков». Обилие глиальных волокон при специальной окраске. Пальцами хирурга в этих случаях прощупывается твердый «сосочек».
b) Образование сосочков при избирательной окраске.
c) и d) Врастание «сосочковидных» участков олигодендроглиомы в кору при различном увеличении.

a) 稀突起膠腫における皮質表層の細胞緻密化と「乳頭」の形成。グリア線維染色で、高度な線維増殖をみる。この「乳頭」は手術時、固くふれる。
b) 細胞染色でみた乳頭。
c) および d) 種々の拡大でみた稀突起膠腫の皮質乳頭。

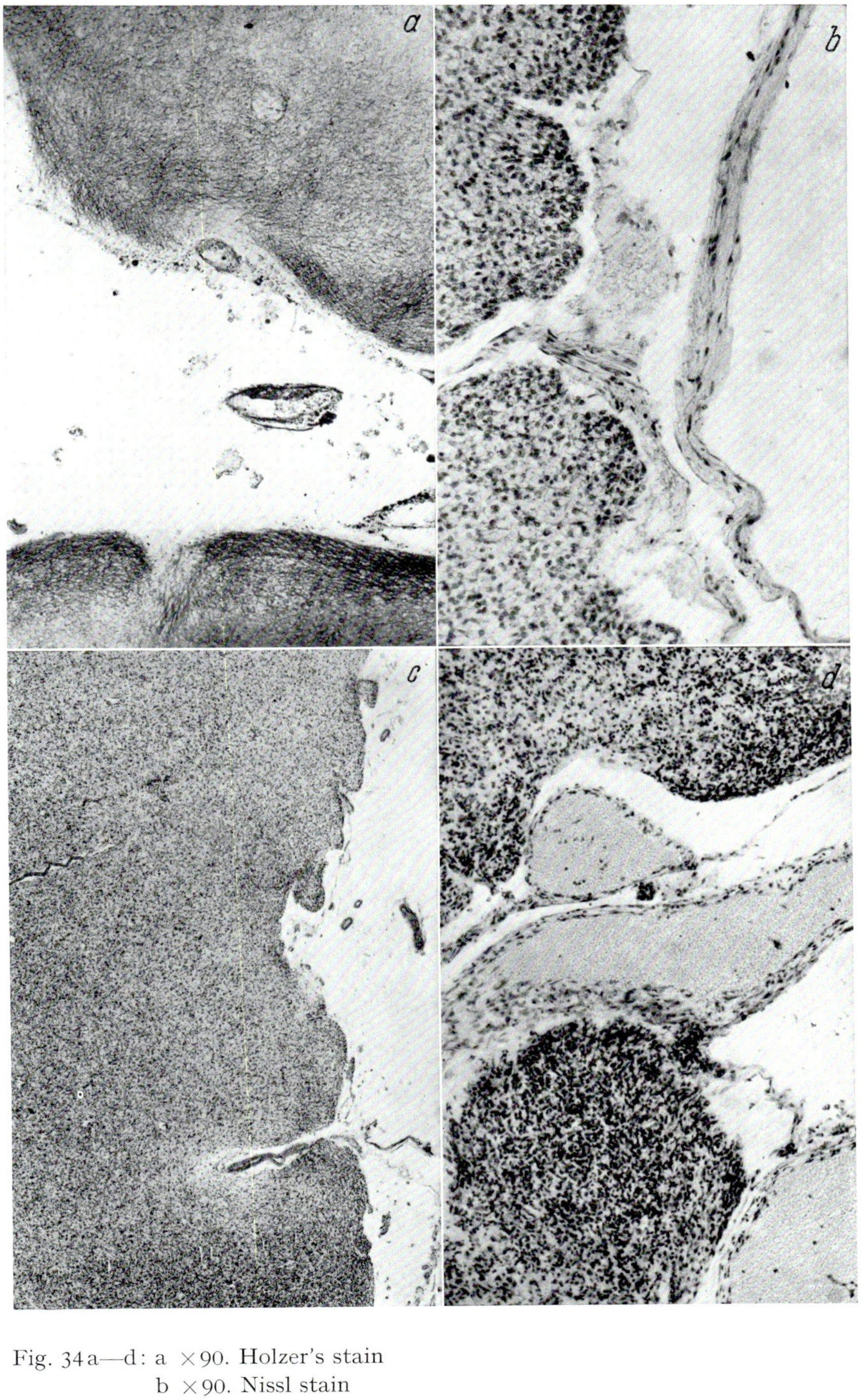

Fig. 34a—d: a ×90. Holzer's stain
b ×90. Nissl stain
c ×20, d ×90. Cresyl violet stain

Fig. 35 — Oligodendrogliomas

a), c) and d) In the marginal zone of an oligodendroglioma the tumor cells tend to accumulate around the ganglion cells (satellitosis).
b) Proliferation of the macroglia at the border of an oligodendroglioma.

a), c) u. d) In der Randzone eines Oligodendroglioms neigen die Geschwulstzellen zur Ansammlung um die Ganglienzellen (Satellitose).
b) Proliferation der Makroglia am Rande eines Oligodendroglioms.

a), c) et d) A la périphérie d'un oligodendrogliome, les cellules tumorales ont tendance à se rassembler autour des cellules nerveuses (satellitose).
b) Prolifération de la macroglie à la périphérie d'un oligodendrogliome

a), c) y d) En la periferia de un oligodendroglioma las células tumorales tienden a acumularse alrededor de las células ganglionares (satelitosis).
b) Proliferación de la macroglia al borde de un oligodendroglioma.

a), c) и d) В краевой зоне олигодендроглиомы опухолевые клетки склонны скапливаться вокруг ганглиозных (сателлитоз).
b) Пролиферация макроглии в окружности олигодендроглиомы.

a), c) および d) 稀突起膠腫の辺縁部で、腫瘍細胞は神経細胞周囲にあつまる傾向を示す（随伴細胞症）。
b) 稀突起膠腫周辺のマクログリア増殖。

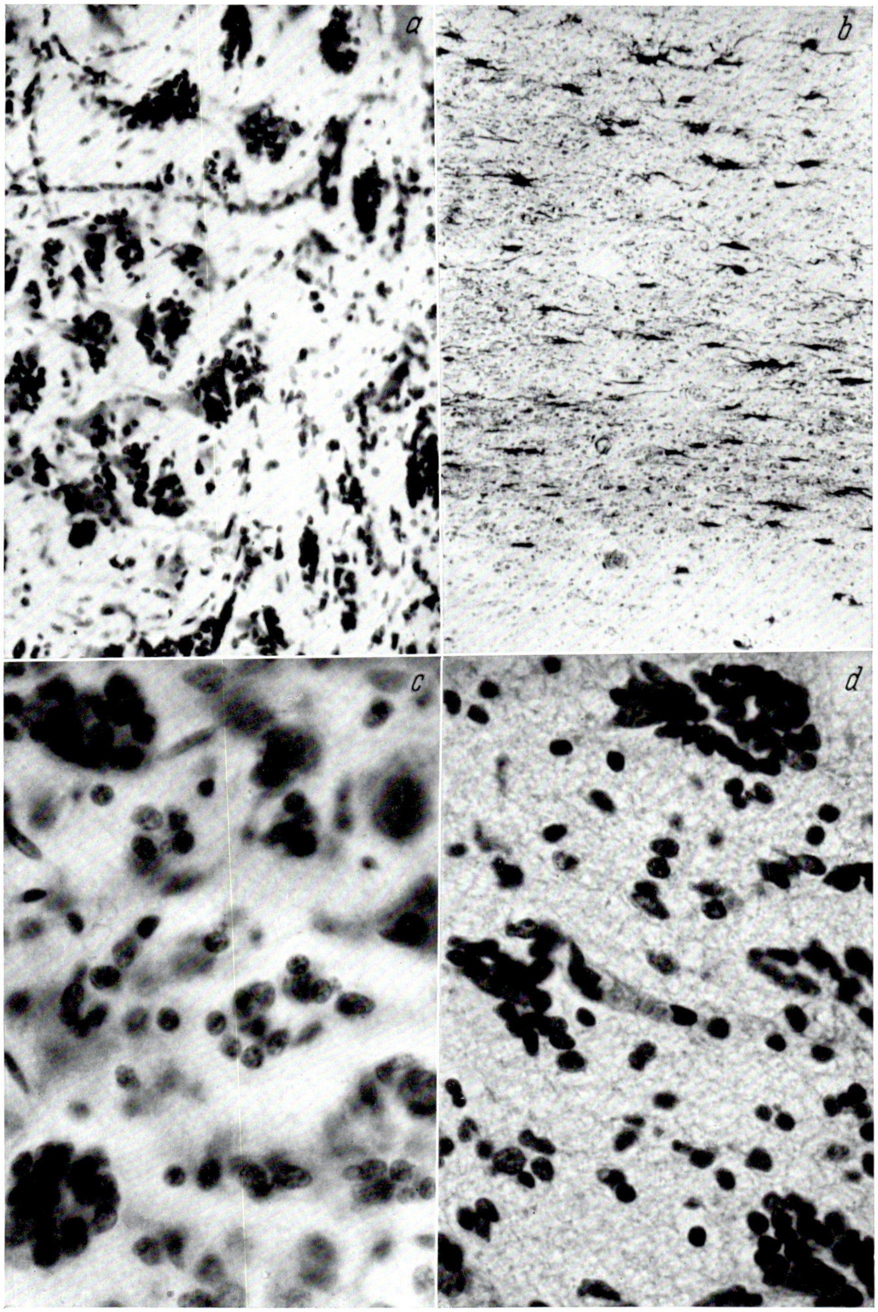

Fig. 35a—d: a ×72. Cresyl violet stain
b ×78. Gold sublimate method
c ×212. Nissl stain
d ×180. H. & E. stain

Fig. 36 — Oligodendrogliomas

a) Calcification and complete occlusion of a large vessel in an oligodendroglioma.
b) Calcification of a large vessel and calcium plaques in a large vein(?)
c) Obstruction of a calcified vessel by loose tissue which fills the lumen. Only two small remnants of lumen remain patent.
d) Delicate proliferations of tissue within a calcified vessel leaving only part of the lumen patent.

a) Verkalkung und völliger Verschluß eines großen Gefäßes in einem Oligodendrogliom.
b) Verkalkung eines großen Gefäßes und Kalkplatteneinlagerung in eine große Vene (?).
c) Verschluß eines verkalkten Gefäßes mit einem lockeren Füllgewebe. Nur zwei kleine Restlumina blieben bestehen.
d) Zart gewuchertes Füllgewebe mit kleinem Restlumen in verkalkten Gefäßen.

a) Calcification et occlusion complète d'un gros vaisseau dans un oligodendrogliome.
b) Calcification d'un grand vaisseau et plaques calcifiées dans une grosse veine(?).
c) Obturation d'un vaisseau calcifié par du tissu lâche. A la place de la lumière, il persiste seulement deux petits pertuis.
d) Obstruction de vaisseaux calcifiés par la prolifération de tissu conjonctif lâche dans la lumière, dont il persiste encore quelques petits pertuis.

a) Calcificación y completa oclusión de un grueso vaso en un oligodendroglioma.
b) Calcificación de un grueso vaso y placas de calcificación en una vena(?) grande.
c) Oclusión de un vaso calcificado con tejido laseo. Sólo permenecen dos restos de luz.
d) Crecimiento delicado de tejido con resto de luz en vasos calcificados.

a) Обызвествление и полная закупорка крупного сосуда в олигодендроглиоме.
b) Обызвествление крупного сосуда и отложение извести в крупной вене.
c) Закупорка обызвествленного сосуда рыхлой заполняющей тканью. Видны только два мелких остаточных просвета сосудов.
d) Незначительное разрастание заполняющей ткани с мелкими остаточными просветами в обызвествленных сосудах.

a) 稀突起膠腫内の太い血管の石灰化と完全な閉塞。
b) 太い血管の石灰化と太い静脈内への石灰板の流入（？）。
c) 粗大な充填組織をともなった石灰化血管の閉塞、わずかに２個の小腔が残存している。
d) 石灰化した血管内に増生した充填組織、小さな残腔をみとめる。

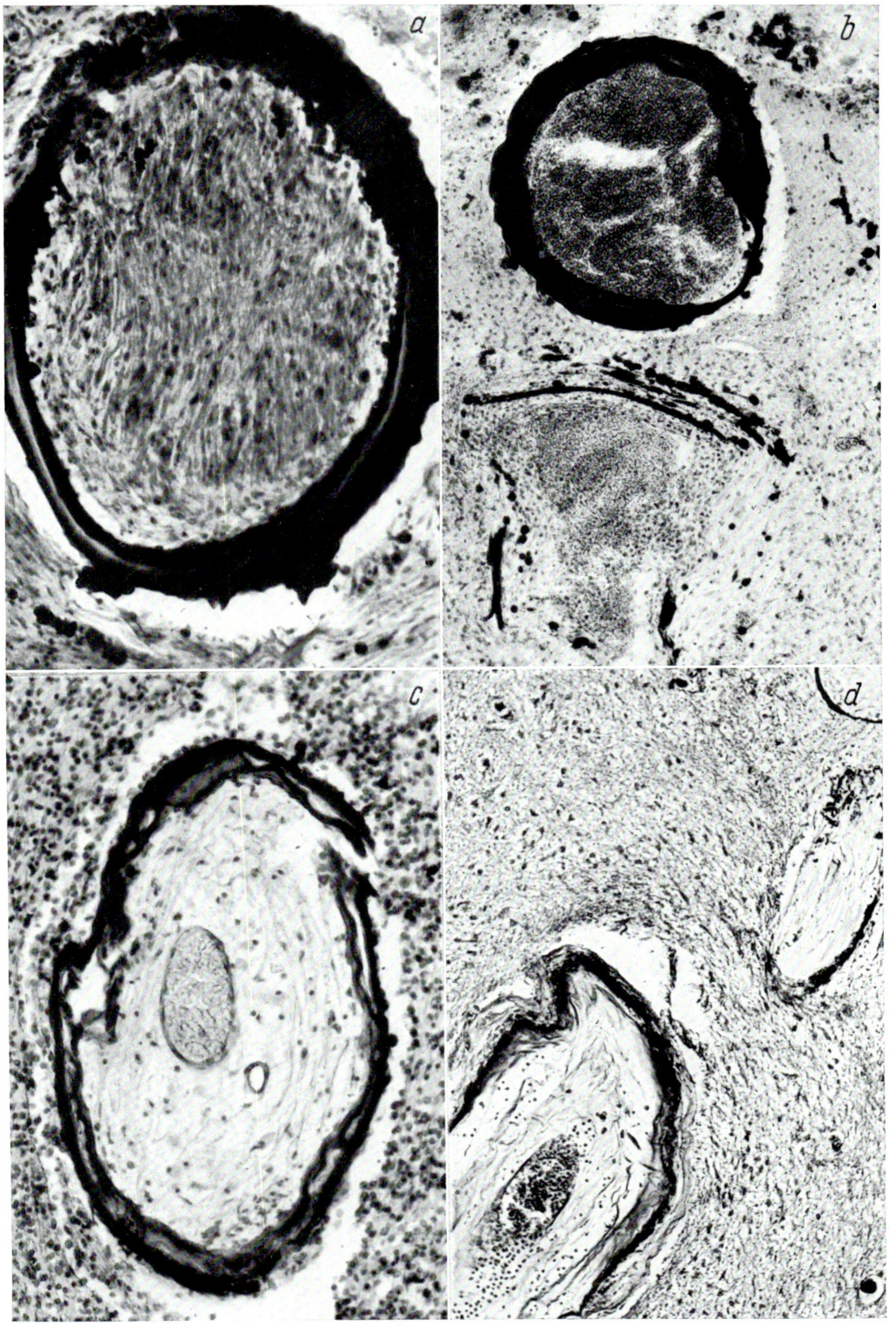

Fig. 36a—d: a ×128, b ×75, c ×121, d ×92
H. & E. stain

Fig. 37 — Oligodendrogliomas

a) and b) Peculiar giant cells rich in cytoplasm grow in a manner similar to "glial rasen". The majority of the cells have a ganglioid nucleus.

c) Formation of large tumor cells with a peculiar "epithelial" growth pattern in an otherwise still typical oligodendroglioma.

d) Nest- and cone-shaped advancing tumor in the marginal zone of a recurring originally typical oligodendroglioma.

a) u. b) Eigenartige cytoplasmareiche Riesenzellen, die ähnlich ,,Gliarasen" wachsen. Die Mehrzahl der Zellen hat einen ganglioiden Kern.

c) Bildung eigenartig ,,epithelial" wachsender großer Geschwulstzellen in einem sonst noch typischen Oligodendrogliom.

d) Nest- und zapfenartig vordringende Geschwulstteile in der Randzone eines Rezidives eines früher typischen Oligodendroglioms.

a) et b) Curieuses cellules géantes, riches en cytoplasme et ressemblant à des «Gliarasen». La plupart des noyaux ont un aspect ganglioïde.

c) Dans ce cas par ailleurs typique d'oligodendrogliome, on note la prolifération de grandes cellules tumorales d'aspect curieusement «épithélial».

d) Dans ce cas de récidive d'un oligodendrogliome précédemment typique, des îlots et des languettes de tissu tumoral pénètrent dans le parenchyme environnant.

a) y b) Células gigantes especiales, ricas en citoplasma, que crecen como un résped de glia. La mayoría de las células tienen un núcleo ganglioide.

c) Formación de células tumorales especiales «epiteliales», grandes, en un oligodendroglioma, por lo demás típico.

d) Zona invasora con formación de nidos y espigas de células tumorales en la zona marginal de la recidiva de un oligodendroglioma, inicialmente típico.

a) и b) Своеобразные, богатые на цитоплазму гигантские клетки, растущие в виде «глиальных газонов». Наличие ганглиоидного ядра в большинстве клеток.

c) Образование своеобразных «эпителиальных» крупных опухолевых клеток в еще типичной олигодендроглиоме.

d) Гнездное и клиноподобные проникновение опухоли в краевую зону ранее типичной олигодендроглиомы.

a) および b) 小群集をなして増殖する、胞体の多い独特な巨細胞。大多数の細胞は神経細胞様の核を有する。

c)「上皮様」に増殖する、大型の腫瘍細胞。他の部分は、まだ定型的な稀突起膠腫の像を呈している。

d) 初発時は定型的であった稀突起膠腫。その再発辺縁部における、胞巣状ないし栓状浸潤部分。

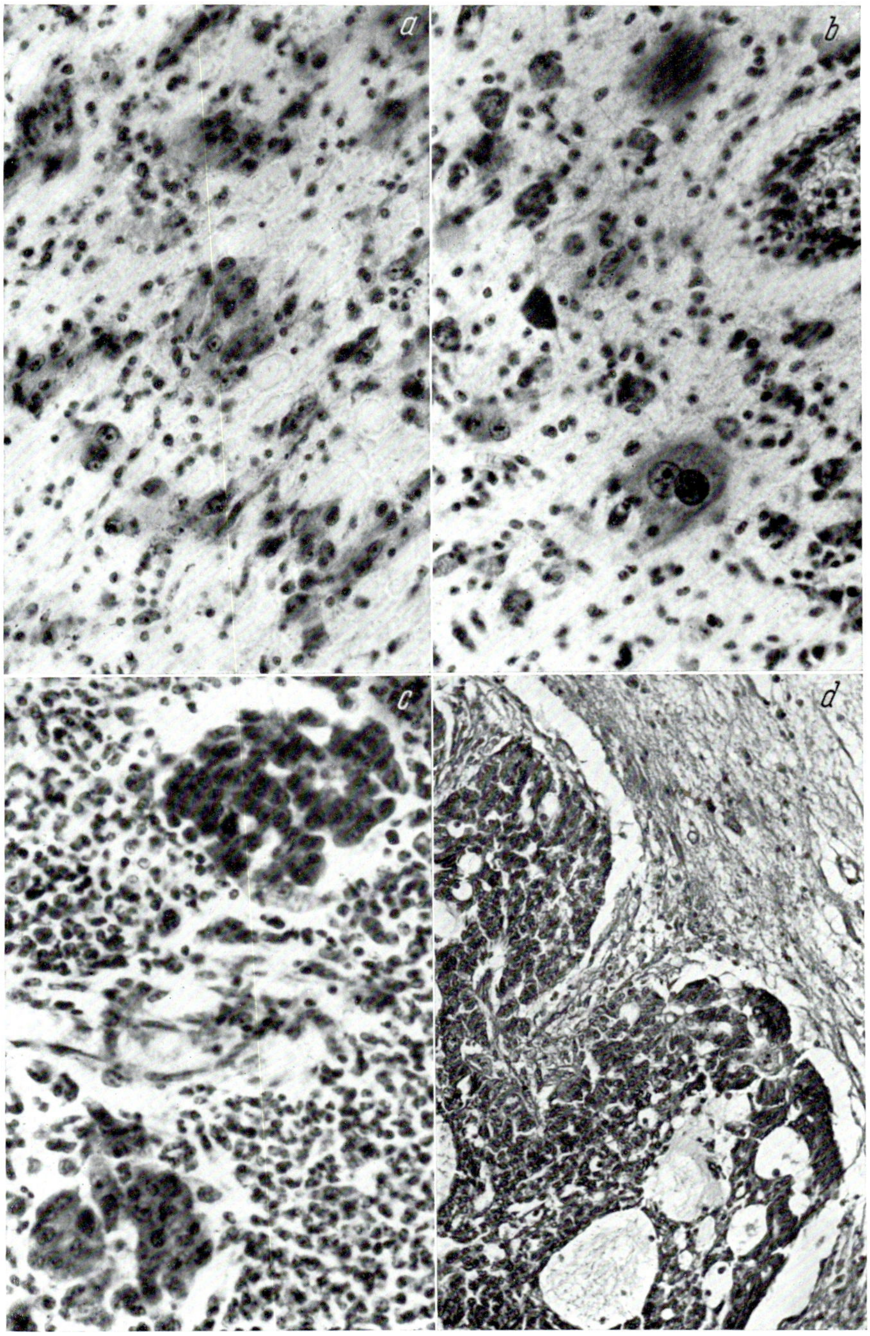

Fig. 37a—d: a and b ×205, c ×210. Nissl stain
d ×85. H. & E. stain

Fig. 38 — Oligodendrogliomas

Numerous, very heterogeneous elements in a polymorphous oligodendroglioma.

a) From the marginal zone of a circumscribed nodule: a cell rich section with small round-cells and very large-bodied polymorphic cells, in which a honeycomb architecture is still suggested.
b) An area of predominantly small nuclei from the marginal zone. Sharp demarcation.
c) Elongated spindle shaped and very large-bodied cells, which are located along the capillaries.
d) A predominantly spindle celled area in the same tumor.

Zahlreiche, sehr verschiedenartige Elemente in einem polymorphen Oligodendrogliom.

a) Aus der Randzone eines umschriebenen Knotens: zellreicher Teil mit kleinen Rundzellen und sehr großleibigen polymorphen Zellen, bei denen eine Honigwabenarchitektur noch angedeutet ist.
b) Vorwiegend kleinkerniger Bezirk aus der Randzone. Scharfe Abgrenzung.
c) Langgezogene spindelige und sehr großleibige Zellen, die entlang den Capillaren gelagert sind.
d) Vorwiegend spindelzelliger Teil des gleichen Tumors.

Nombreux éléments de formes variées dans un oligodendrogliome polymorphe.

a) A la périphérie d'un nodule circonscrit, on note une zone très cellulaire, composée de petits éléments arrondis et de cellules polymorphes très volumineuses. L'architecture en rayon de miel est encore visible.
b) Dans cette zone bien délimitée de la périphérie, la plupart des cellules ont un petit noyau.
c) Cellules alongées, fusiformes, riches en cytoplasme et disposées le long des capillaires.
d) Zone constituée principalement de cellules fusiformes dans la même tumeur.

Gran variación y ríqueza en células en un oligodendroglioma polimorfo.

a) En la perifería de un nódulo circunscrito se ve: zona multicelular con células redondas pequeñas y otras grandes muy polimorfas, en las que aun se puede reconocer una arquitectura en panal de abeja.
b) Zona predominantemente micronuclear en los bordes. Demarcación acusada.
c) Células fusiformes de gran protoplasma, situadas a lo largo de los vasos.
d) Zona predominantemente fusiforme del mismo tumor.

Многочисленные очень разнообразные элементы в полиморфной олигодендроглиоме

a) Краевая зона ограниченного узла. Участок, изобилующий мелкими округлыми и очень крупными полиморфными клетками, еще сохранившими сотовидное строение.
b) Краевая зона. Резко ограниченный участок с преимущественно мелкоядерным строением.
c) Вытянутые веретенообразные и очень крупные клетки, расположенные по ходу капилляров.
d) Участок с преимущественно веретенообразными клетками в той же опухоли.

1例の多形性稀突起膠腫にみられた、多様な組織像。

a) 限局性腫瘍結節の辺縁部。小円形細胞と大きな多形細胞からなる多細胞部分。蜂窩構造も伺われる。
b) 辺縁における、主として小核性細胞巣。境界は鮮明である。
c) 血管沿いに位置する、大きな紡錘状の細胞。
d) 紡錘細胞の多い部分。

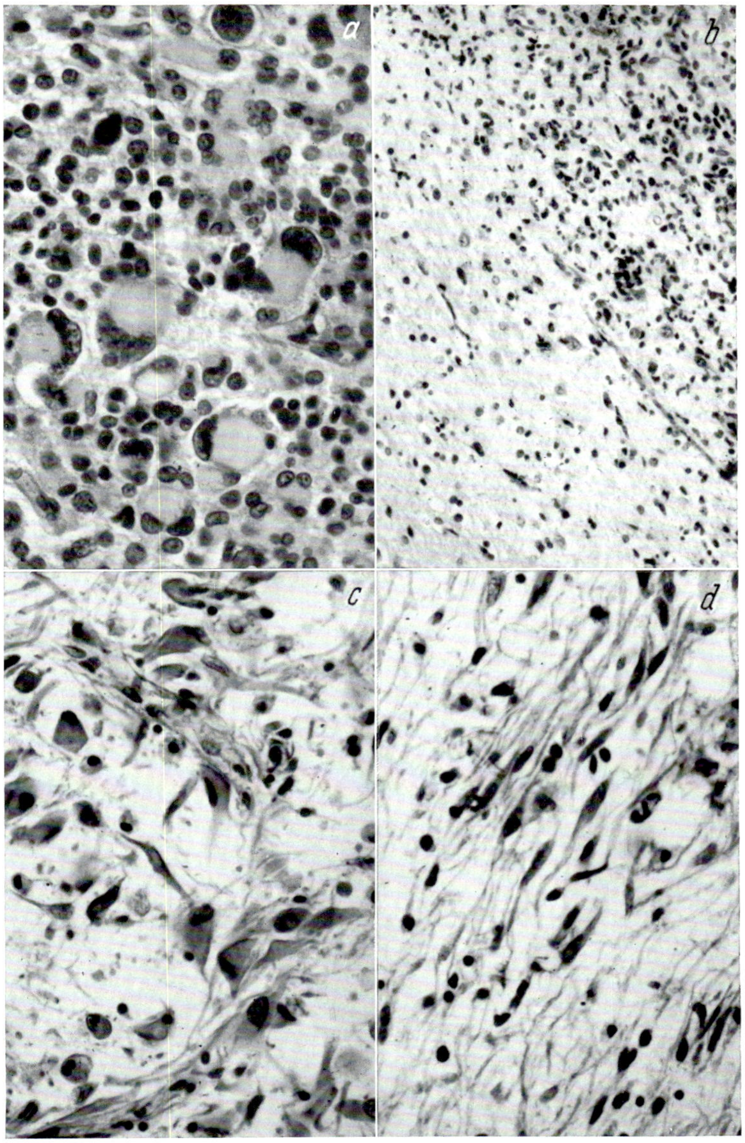

Fig. 38a—d: a, c and d ×220, b ×110. H & E. stain

Fig. 39 — Oligodendrogliomas

In the polymorphous form of oligodendroglioma, one is able to distinguish the "classical" basic architecture amidst a marked degree of polymorphism.

a) Distinct "honeycomb" appearance with individual hyperchromatic giant cells.

b) In this area, there is an increased number of giant cells in addition to the basic "honeycomb" architecture. The giant cells are generally multinucleated and have hyperchromatic nuclei.

c) and d) In this region the polymorphism is even more marked, however, rests of the honeycomb architecture are still present.

Die polymorphe Form des Oligodendroglioms erkennt man an der noch ,,klassischen" Grundarchitektur, in der aber Zeichen hochgradiger Polymorphie auftreten.

a) Deutliches Honigwabennetz, einzelne hyperchromatische Riesenzellen.

b) In diesem Gebiet sieht man zwar auch noch die Grundstruktur des ,,Honigwabennetzes", doch nimmt die Zahl der polymorphen Riesenzellen zu, sie sind z.T. mehrkernig und haben hyperchromatische Kerne.

c) u. d) In diesen Gebieten wird die Polymorphie immer größer, wenn man auch Reste der Honigwabenarchitektur noch erkennen kann.

La forme polymorphe de l'oligodendrogliome se reconnaît à l'architecture de fond encore «classique», dans laquelle cependant des signes nets de polymorphisme apparaissent.

a) Architecture évidente en «nids d'abeilles», quelques cellules géantes hyperchromatiques.

b) A cet endroit, on voit encore bien la structure fondamentale en «nids d'abeilles», mais les cellules géantes polymorphes sont plus nombreuses: certaines d'entre elles contiennent plusieurs noyaux et d'autres ont des noyaux hyperchromatiques.

c) et d) Dans ces régions, le polymorphisme s'accentue, bien qu'on puisse encore reconnaître des traces de l'architecture en «nids d'abeilles».

Las formas polimorfas de los oligodendrogliomas muestran siempre la «clásica» arquitectura aunque estén en camino de alto grado de polimorfismo.

a) Claro aspecto en «panal de abeja» con células grandes hipercromáticas.

b) En esta zona se ve todavía la estructura en «panal de abeja» apesar del polimorfismo celular, con varios nucleos, muchos hipercromáticos.

c) y d) En este campo el polimorfismo es mayor y con todo aún son visibles los restos de la arquitectura «en panal de abeja».

Полиморфную форму олигодендроглиомы еще можно узнать по «классической» структуре, в которой, однако, уже есть признаки выраженного полиморфизма.

a) Четкое сотовидное строение опухоли. Единичные гиперхромные гигантские клетки.

b) В этом участке еще прослеживается »сотовидное» строение опухоли, но количество полиморфных гигантских клеток уже увеличено. Эти клетки частично многоядерны, а ядра гиперхромны.

c) и d) В этих участках отмечается все увеличивающийся полиморфизм, хотя видны еще следы сотовидной структуры.

稀突起膠腫の多形型は、古くから知られている基本構造のほかに高度の多形性を示す。

a) 著明な蜂窩状構造と、2～3の濃染性巨細胞。

b) この領域には、基本構造である蜂窩網をみとめるが、さらに多形性巨細胞の数が増している。この細胞は多核で濃染核を有する。

c) およびd) この領域では多形性がさらに著明であるが、蜂窩構造の残存部をまだみとめる。

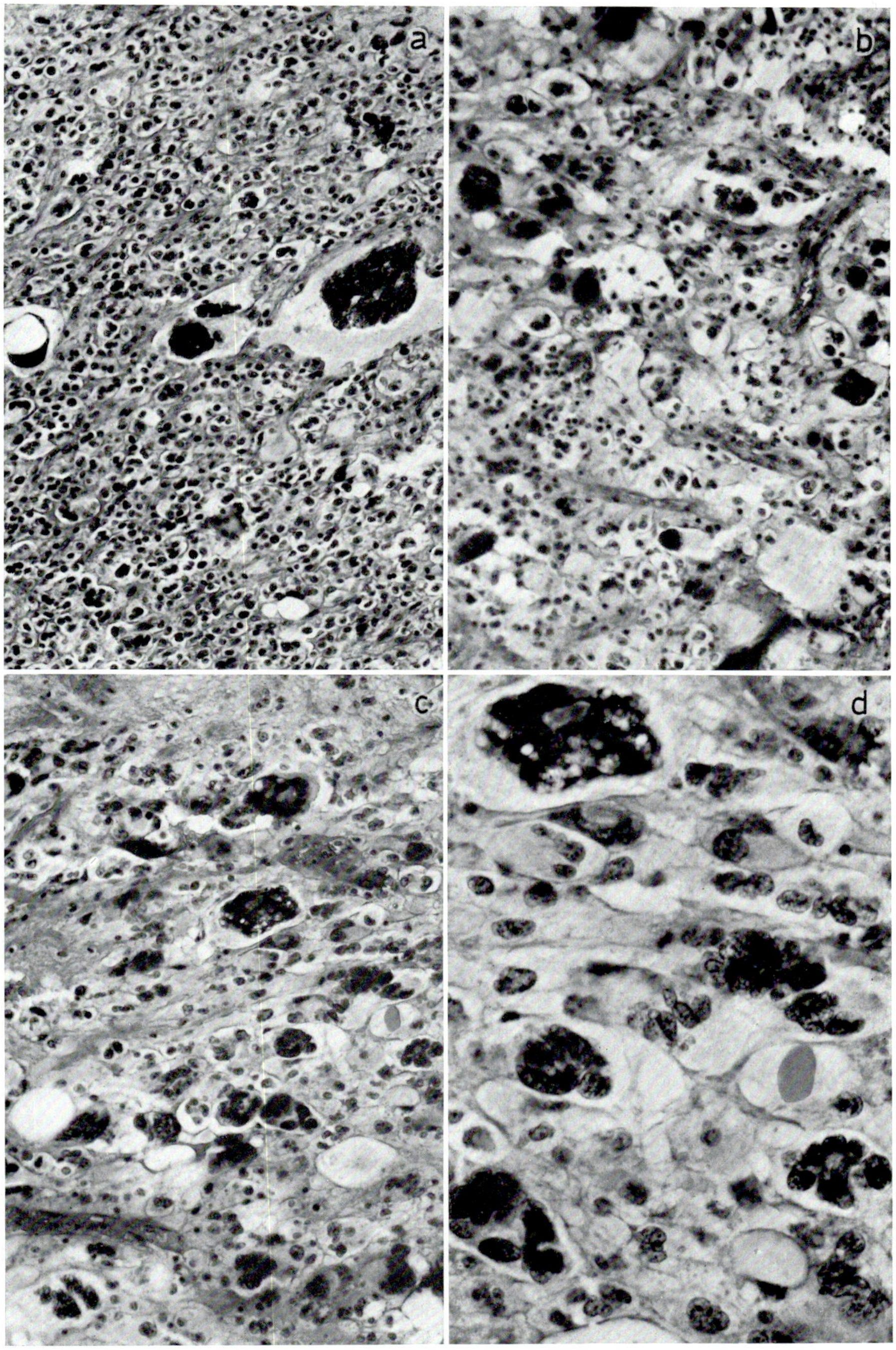

Fig. 39a—d: a—c × 125, d × 500. H. & E. stain

Fig. 40 — Oligodendrogliomas

a) and b) The final proof of an oligodendroglioma is dependent upon the typical basic architecture and silver staining (MELLER's method). One can see also multinucleated cells (b) which possess the distinct features of oligodendroglia cells.

c) In addition to the type of oligodendroglioma which is polymorphous as a result of the dysmorphism of the cells, there is another type in which the tissue architecture is polymorphic. In this latter type, necrotic areas appear and evoke a stromal proliferation, thus, characteristics of the glioblastoma become noticeable.

d) Langhans' type of giant cells with marginal, hyperchromatic nuclei occur quite frequently in polymorphous oligodendrogliomas.

a) u. b) Den endgültigen Beweis für die Zugehörigkeit zum Oligodendrogliom liefert neben der typischen Grundarchitektur auch noch die Versilberung (Verfahren nach MELLER). Hier sieht man auch die mehrkernigen Zellen (b) deutlich nach dem typischen Bild der Oligodendrogliazellen dargestellt.

c) Neben dem Typus, der durch die Dysmorphie der *Zelle* polymorph wird, gibt es auch noch den Typus des Oligodendroglioms, dessen Gewebs*architektur* polymorph wird. Hier treten strichförmige Nekrosen auf und das Stroma antwortet mit erheblicher Proliferation, so daß die Merkmale des Glioblastoms sichtbar werden.

d) Sehr häufig findet sich in den polymorphen Oligodendrogliomen der Typus der Langhans'schen Riesenzellen mit randständigen hyperchromatischen Kernen.

a) et b) Outre l'architecture fondamentale typique, l'imprégnation argentique (selon la méthode de MELLER) fournit la preuve décisive que ces tumeurs appartiennent au groupe des oligodendrogliomes. On voit clairement que les cellules multinucléées (b) sont mises en évidence de la même façon que les cellules oligodendrogliales.

c) Outre la variété d'oligodendrogliomes appelés polymorphes par suite du «dysmorphisme cellulaire», il existe un type d'oligodendrogliomes devenant polymorphes à cause de la disposition architecturale. Dans ce cas, on note des nécroses de forme linéaire et une prolifération accrue du stroma, ce qui confère à ces tumeurs les caractères du glioblastome.

d) Dans les oligodendrogliomes polymorphes, on voit très souvent des cellules géantes du type Langhans, contenant des noyaux hyperchromatiques disposés à la périphérie.

a) y b) La impregnación argéntica (MELLER) comprueba la arquitectura del oligodendroglioma. Aquí se ven también células polinucleadas (b) con aspecto general típico de la oligodendroglia.

c) Al lado de células dismórficas existen las células del oligodendroglioma típico a pesar tejido polimorfo. Aqui existe tejido en necrobiosis y el estroma reacciona proliferando dando la impresión de un glioblastoma.

d) Con frecuencia en los oligodendrogliomas polimorfos se encuentran las células de tipo Langhans, con núcleos periféricos hipercromáticos.

a) и b) Окончательное доказательство принадлежности к олигодендроглиоме, наряду с типичной гистроструктурой, дает также и импрегнация серебром (по МЕЛЛЕРУ). Здесь видны также многоядерные клетки (b), четко соответствующие типичной схеме олигодендроглиальных клеток.

c) Наряду с типом олигодендроглиомы, ставшей полиморфной вследствие «дисморфии клеток», имеется также олигодендроглиома с полиморфной структурой. Здесь появляются полоски некроза, отмечается значительная пролиферация стромы и начинают прослеживаться черты глиобластомы.

d) Довольно часто в полиморфной олигодендроглиоме обнаруживают гигантские клетки типа клеток Лангханса с гиперхромными, расположенными по краям, ядрами.

a) および b) 稀突起膠腫の最終的な証明には、特徴的な組織構造のほかに、鍍銀法が必要である（Meller 鍍銀法）。ここでは稀突起膠細胞の定型的特質をもった多核細胞（図b）をみとめる。

c) 希突起膠腫には、腫瘍細胞が非定形となって多形性を示す型と、腫瘍構造が多形性をとる型とがある。ここには索状に壊死が現われ、間質が増殖をおこし、その結果膠芽腫の特徴がでている。

d) 多形性稀突起膠腫には、Langhans 型巨細胞をしばしばみとめる。この細胞は濃染核をもち、核は細胞体の辺縁部に位置する。

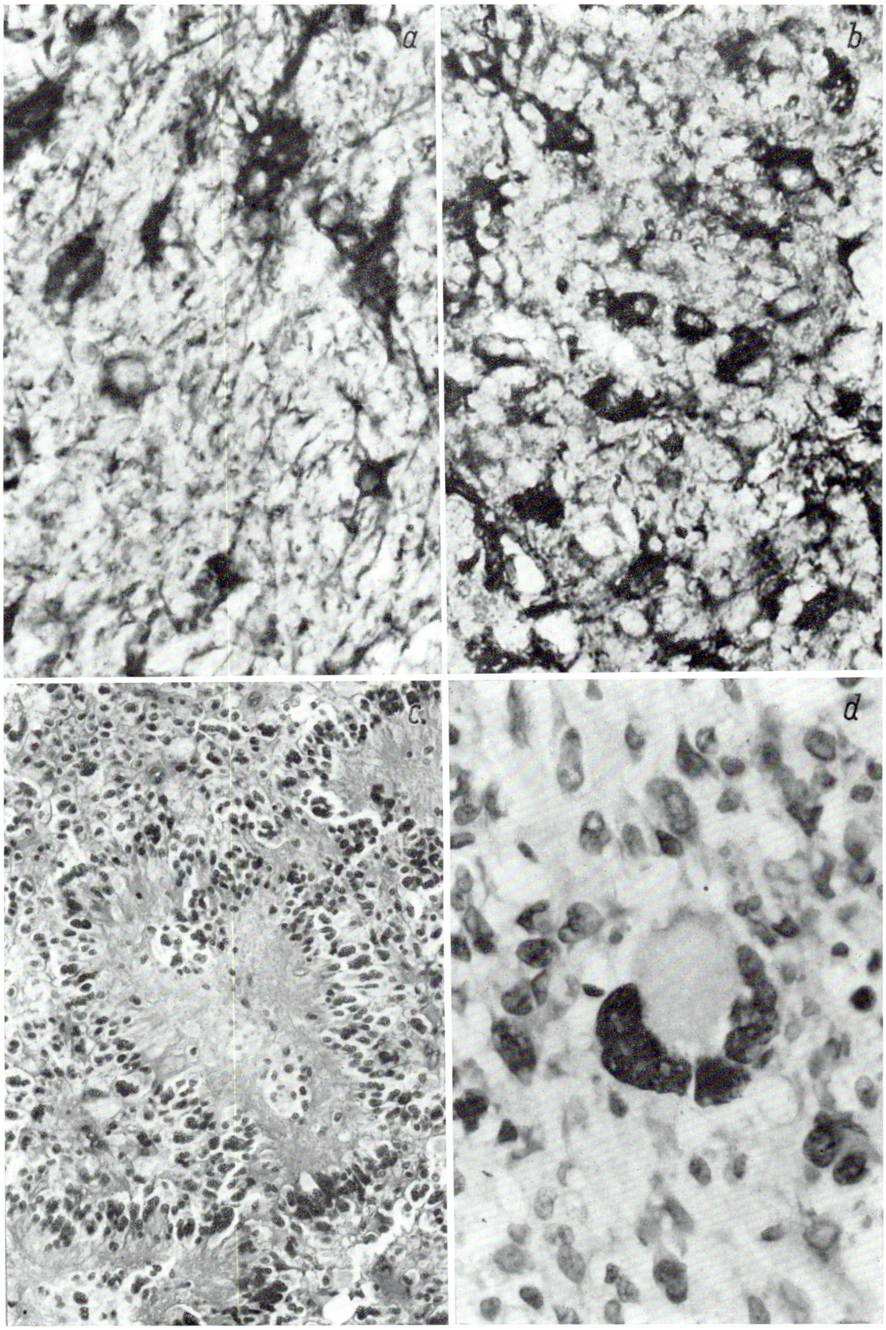

Fig. 40a—d: a and b × 500. Meller's impregnation.
c × 125, d × 500. H. & E. stain

Fig. 41 — Oligodendrogliomas

a) Increased amount of lactate dehydrogenase in large, dysmorphic cells in a polymorphic oligodendroglioma.
b)—d) Impregnation of the various tumor cells in the polymorphic oligodendroglioma. In addition to the typical forms of the small cells containing single nuclei, multinucleated giant cells are also impregnated. As is true of oligodendroglia, the nucleus always remains visible as a small, clear "vesicle".

a) Starker Gehalt großer dysmorph gebauter Zellen an Lactatdehydrogenase in einem polymorphen Oligodendrogliom.
b)—d) Imprägnation verschiedener Tumorzellen im polymorphen Oligodendrogliom. Man sieht kleinere einkernige, sehr typische Formen, aber auch mehrkernige Riesenzellen ausreichend imprägniert. Immer bleibt — wie bei der Oligodendroglia — der Kern hell als kleine „Blase" sichtbar.

a) Taux élevé de lactate-déshydrogénase des grandes cellules dysmorphiques dans un oligodendrogliome polymorphe.
b)—d) Imprégnation de différentes cellules tumorales dans un oligodendrogliome polymorphe. Non seulement de petites cellules mononucléées, très typiques, mais aussi des cellules géantes multinucléées sont suffisamment imprégnées. Le noyau reste toujours clair, semblable à une petite «vésicule», comme c'est le cas pour l'oligodendroglie.

a) Marcado contenido en lactatodehidrogenasa en un oligodendroglioma polimorfo.
b)—d) Impregnación de varias células tumorales en un oligodendroglioma polimorfo. Pueden verse pequeños núcleos de forma típica pero también células multinucleadas. Siempre aparece, como en la oligodendroglia, el núcleo claro como una pequeña burbuja.

a) Большое содержание лактат-дегидрогеназы в крупных дисморфных клетках полиморфной олигодендроглиомы.
b)—d) Импрегнация различных опухолевых клеток в полиморфной олигодендроглие. Видны мелкие одноядерные весьма типичные структуры, однако импрегнировано немало многоядерных гигантских клеток. Как и в олигодендроглиоме светлое ядро имеет вид маленького «пузырка»

a) 多形性稀突起膠腫内の大形で異型を示す細胞は、乳酸脱水素酵素をより多量に含む。
b) —d) 多形性稀突起膠腫内の各種腫瘍細胞の鍍銀。小形で一核の定型的な像をみとめるが、さらに多核の巨細胞が鍍銀されている。核は常に稀突起膠細胞の場合と同じく小胞のように明るい。

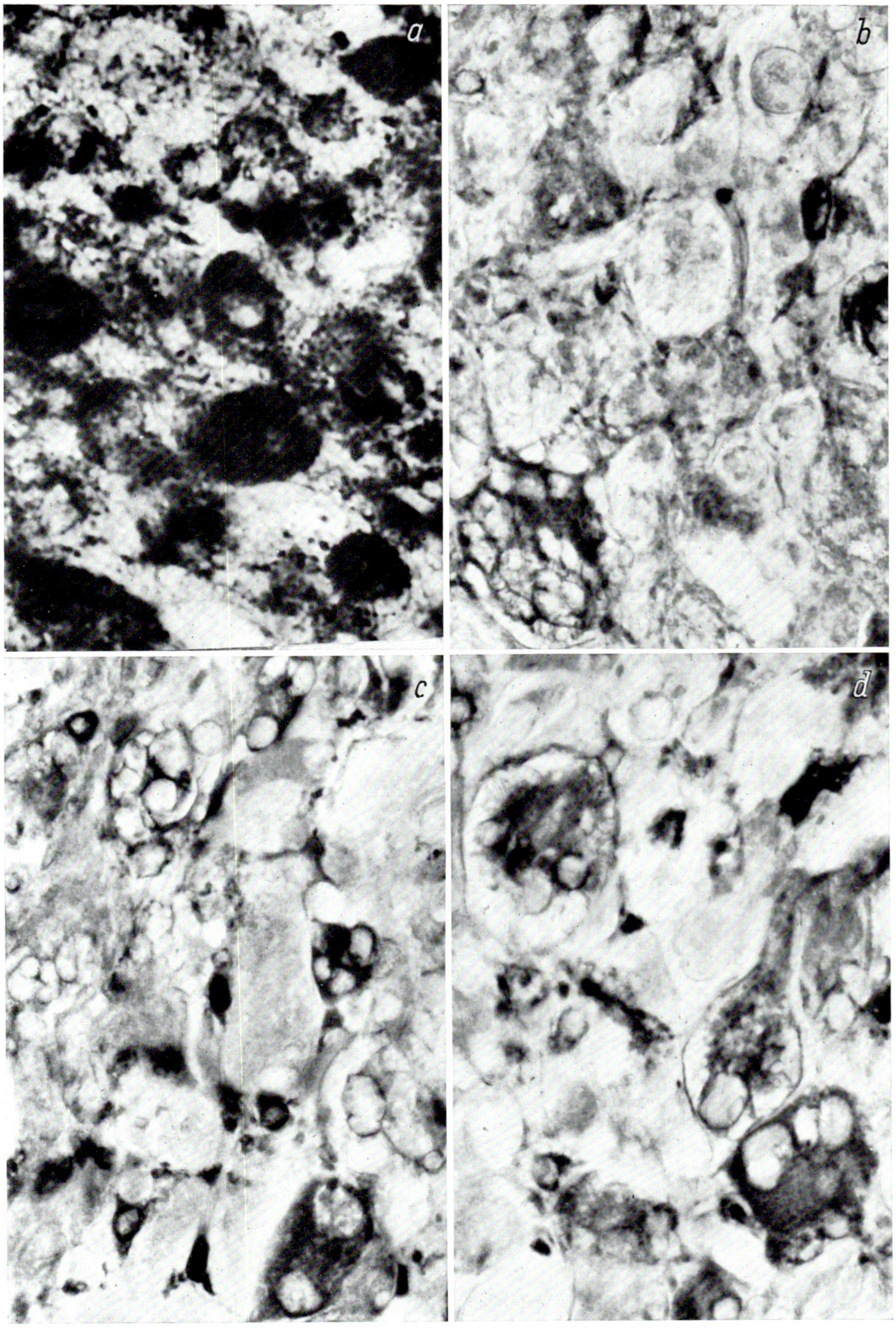

Fig. 41 a—d: a × 600. lactate dehydrogenese
b—d × 750. Meller's impregnation

Glioblastomas, Malignant

Glioblastoma/spongioblastoma multiforme, giant-cell glioblastoma, astrocytoma grade IV, polymorphic glioma, gliosarcoma, "Buntes Gliom". — A large part of the „glioma telangiectaticum" and the glioma "apoplecticum" group belongs to the glioblastoma, a smaller part to the oligodendroglioma

Fig. 42 — Glioblastomas, Malignant

Markedly polymorphic glioblastoma with extensive proliferation of the adventitial and endothelial cells. One sees partly uninucleated, partly multinucleated, hyperchromatic giant cells, or nuclear conglomerates, as well as the numerous, partly atypical mitoses. The tissue is polymorphic to a high degree because of the mixture of neuroepithelial and mesodermal elements.

Ausgesprochen polymorphes Glioblastom mit reichlicher Wucherung der Adventitial- und Endothelzellen. Man sieht teils ein-, teils mehrkernige hyperchromatische Riesenzellen bzw. Kernkonglomerate sowie die zahlreichen, zum Teil atypischen Mitosen. Das Gewebe ist hochgradig polymorph durch die Mischung neuroepithelialer und mesodermaler Elemente.

Dans un glioblastome très polymorphe, présentant une importante prolifération des cellules adventitielles et endothéliales, on observe des cellules géantes hyperchromatiques, uninucléées ou multinucléées ainsi que des amas de noyaux agglomérés et de nombreuses mitoses parfois atypiques. Le mélange d'éléments épithéliaux et mésodermiques donne au tissu un aspect très polymorphe.

Glioblastoma marcadamente polimorfo con abundante crecimiento de células adventiciales y endoteliales. Se ven células gigantes uni y multinucleadas, o bien formando conglomerados nucleares, igualmente que abundantes mitosis, parte de ellas atípicas. El tejido es altamente polimorfo por la mezcla de elementos neuroepiteliales y mesodermales.

Выраженная полиморфноклеточная глиобластома с сильным разрастанием адвентициальных и эндотелиальных клеток. Видны одно- и многоядерные гигантские клетки с гиперхромными ядрами, а также многочисленные частично атипичные митозы. Вследствие смешения нейроэпителиальных мезодермальных элементов — ткань очень полиморфна.

血管外膜および内皮細胞の著しい増殖を伴った高度多形性膠芽腫。1個あるいは数個の濃染核をもつ巨細胞、核集塊、ならびに多数の核分裂をみとめる。核分裂は一部異型的。外胚葉性および間葉性要素の混合により、著しい多形像を示している。

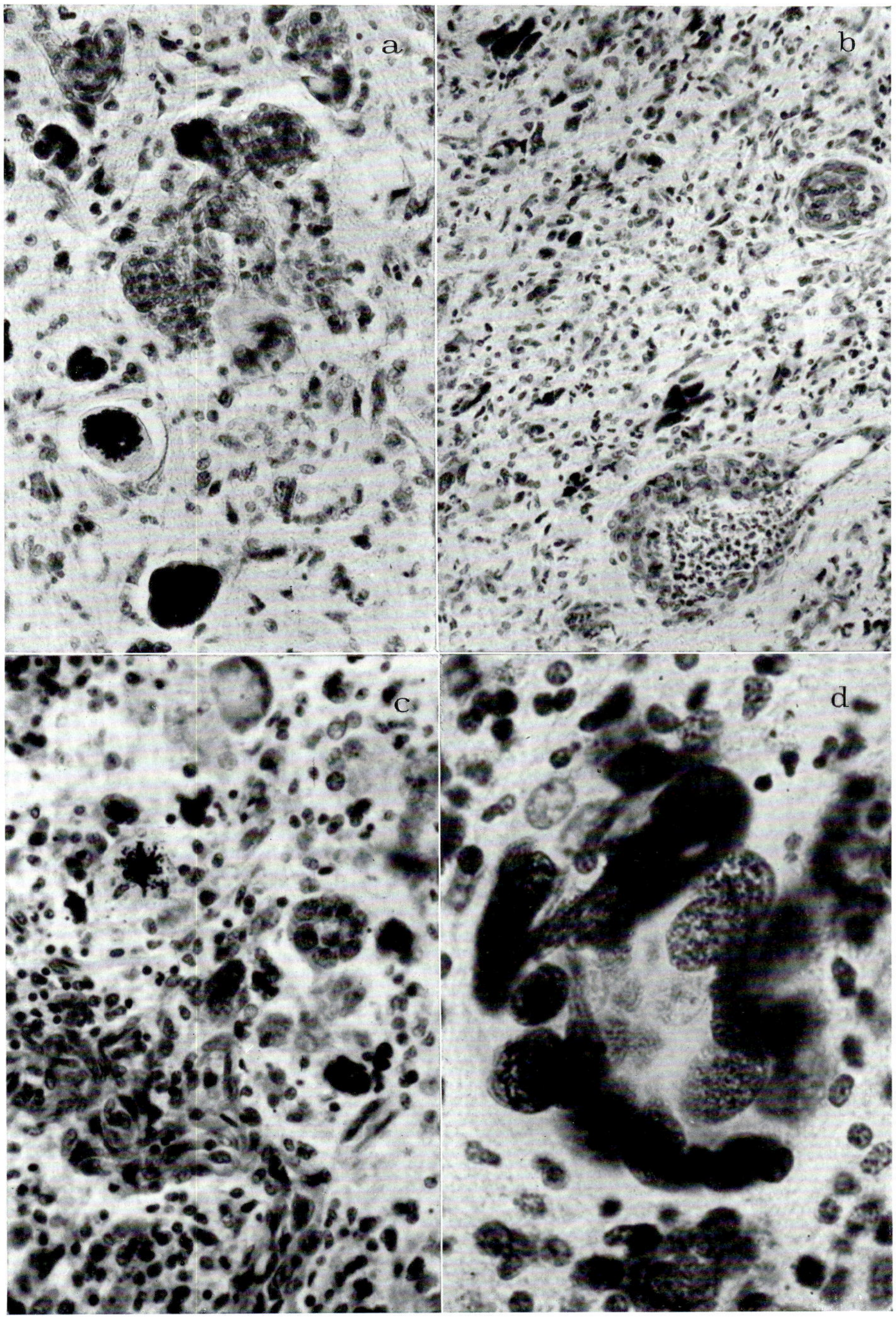

Fig. 42a—d: a and b ×84, c ×168, d ×640
Cresyl violet stain

Fig. 43 — Glioblastomas, Malignant

a) Round-cell glioblastoma consisting of very isomorphic elements.
b) Spindle-celled, very polymorphic glioblastoma with numerous mitoses.
c) and d) Pronounced multiform glioblastomas with hyperchromatic giant cells and multinucleated cell complexes.

a) Rundzelliges Glioblastom aus recht isomorphen Elementen.
b) Fusiformes, sehr polymorphes Glioblastom mit zahlreichen Mitosen.
c) u. d) Ausgesprochen multiforme Glioblastome mit hyperchromatischen Riesenzellen und mehrkernigen Zellkomplexen.

a) Glioblastome globuliforme composé d'éléments très isomorphes.
b) Glioblastome fusiforme très polymorphe et riche en mitoses.
c) et d) Glioblastome très multiforme contenant des noyaux géants hyperchromatiques et des cellules multinucléées.

a) Glioblastoma de células redondos con células bastante isomorfas.
b) Glioblastoma de células fusiformes muy polimorfo, con numerosas mitosis.
c) y d) Glioblastoma declaradamente multiforme, con células gigantes hipercromáticas y complejos celulares multinucleares.

a) Круглоклеточная глиобластома с выраженными изоморфными элементами.
b) Круглоклеточная, очень полиморфная глиобластома с многочисленными митозами.
c) и d) Выраженная мультиформная глиобластома с гиперхромными гигантскими клетками и многоядерными клеточными комплексами.

a) 全く同形の細胞からなる、円形細胞性膠芽腫。
b) 多形性のつよい、紡錘細胞性膠芽腫。核分裂像が多数。
c) および d) 濃染核をもつ巨細胞や多核合胞体を混じた、高度多形性膠芽腫。

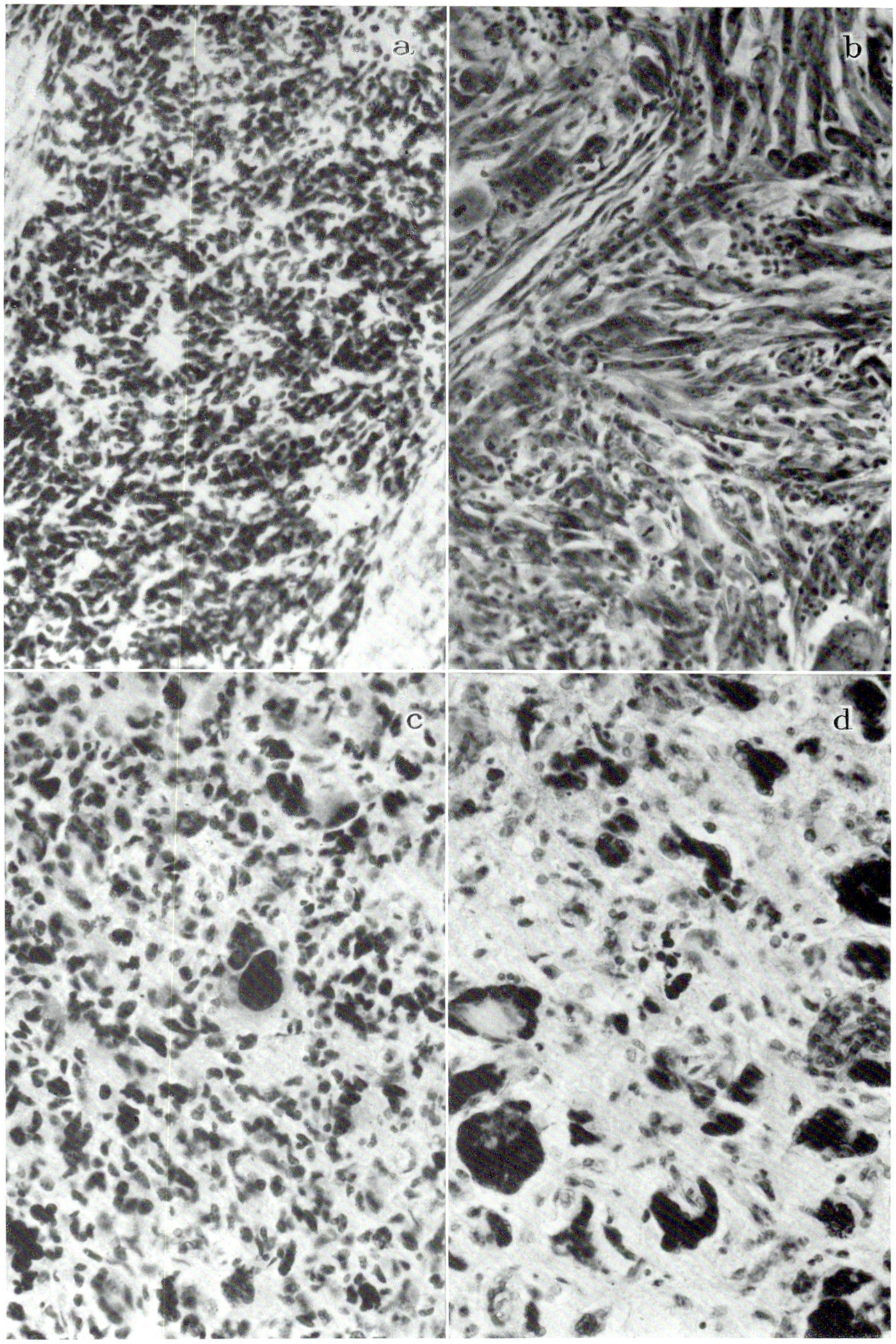

Fig. 43 a—d: a ×120. Nissl stain
b ×120, c and d ×148, Cresylviolet stain

Fig. 44 — Glioblastomas, Malignant

Fusiform glioblastoma:

a) Arrangement of the cells in columns and streams.

b) and c) Among the spindle-shaped nuclei are found extensive mitotic configurations.

d) At high magnification one can discern the delicate chromatin reticulum of the nuclei and the protoplasmic processes of the spindle cells.

Fusiformes Glioblastom.

a) Anordnung der Zellen in Zügen und Strömen.

b) u. c) Unter den spindeligen Kernen finden sich reichlich mitotische Figuren.

d) Bei hoher Vergrößerung erkennt man das zarte Chromatingerüst der Kerne und die protoplasmatischen Fortsätze der spindeligen Zellen.

Glioblastome fusiforme.

a) Les cellules sont disposées en faisceaux et en courants.

b) et c) Parmi les noyaux fusiformes, on observe de nombreuses figures de mitoses.

d) A un plus fort grossissement, on voit le réseau délicat de la chromatine nucléaire ainsi que les prolongements protoplasmiques des cellules fusiformes.

Glioblastoma multiforme.

a) Disposición de las células en corrientes y bandas.

b) y c) Bajo los núcleos fusiformes se encuentran abundantes figuras mitóticas.

d) A mayor aumento se reconoce el delicado armazón cromatínico de los núcleos y las prolongaciones protoplasmáticas de las células fusiformes.

Веретеноклеточная глиобластома:

a) Клетки расположены тяжами и пучками.

b) и c) Обилие митотических фигур в веретенообразных ядрах.

d) Под бóльшим увеличением видна нежная хроматиновая сеть в ядрах и протоплазматические отростки веретенообразных клеток.

紡錘細胞性膠芽腫。

a) 細胞の列状ないし流線状の配列。

b) および c) 紡錘状の細胞核に混じて、多数の核分裂がみられる。

d) 強拡大で、紡錘形の細胞は胞体突起をもち、核にせん細なクロマチン網をみとめる。

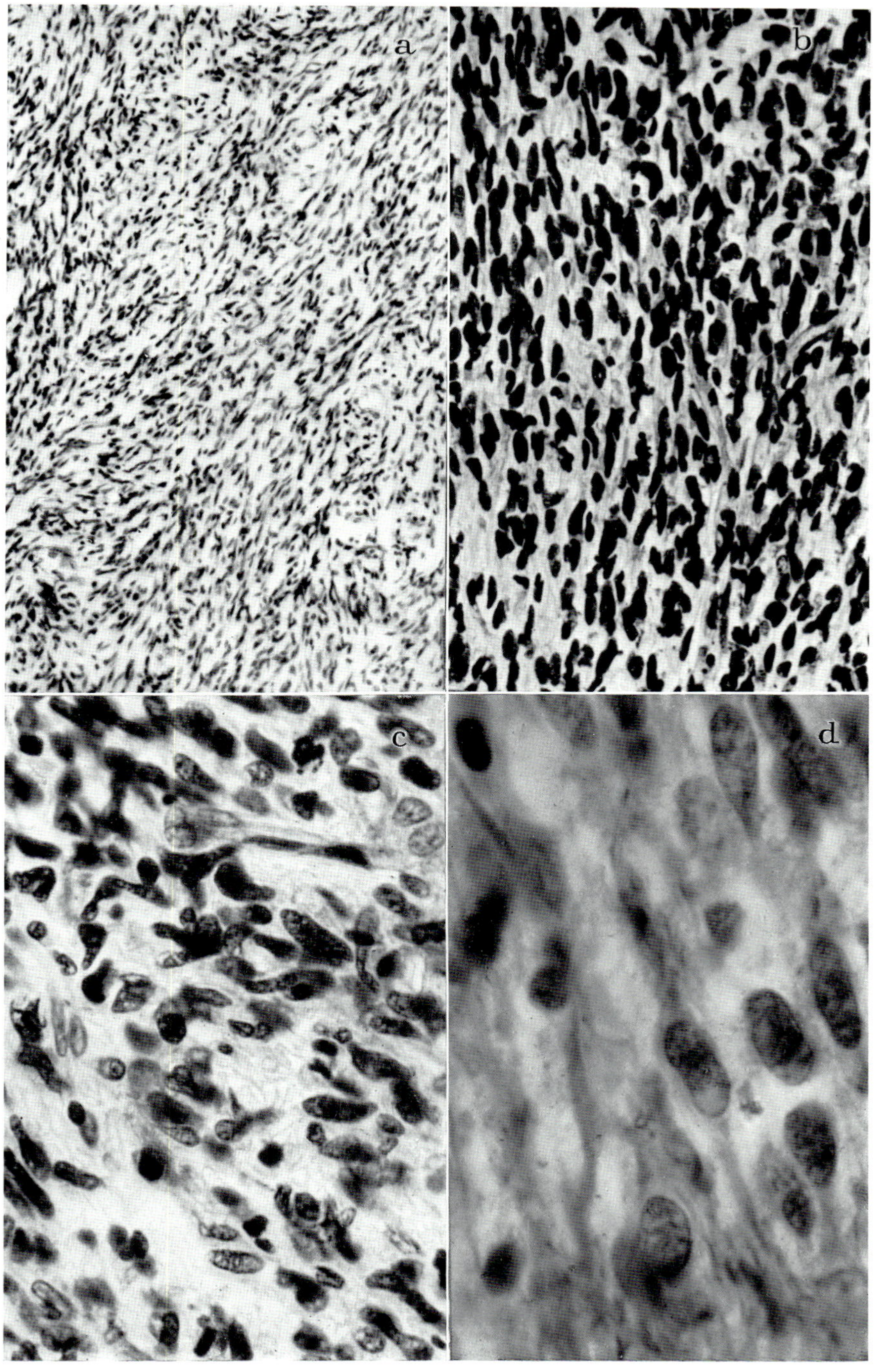

Fig. 44a—d: a ×120. Nissl stain
b ×240, c ×480. Cresyl violet stain
d ×840. Impregnation with silver carbonate

Fig. 45 — Glioblastomas, Malignant

Typical glomerulus formation in a glioblastoma. One usually sees the efferent and afferent vessel as well as the proliferation of edematous connective tissue cells, occasionally with numerous mitoses.

Typische Glomerulusbildung in einem Glioblastom. Man sieht meist das ab- und zuführende Gefäß sowie die Wucherung saftiger Bindegewebszellen, gelegentlich mit zahlreichen Mitosen.

Formations glomérulaires typiques dans le glioblastome. On reconnaît souvent les vaisseaux afférents et efférents. Les cellules conjonctives sont gonflées et prolifèrent. Elle présentent parfois beaucoup de mitoses.

Típica formación de glomérulos en un glioblastoma. La mayoría de las veces se ven los vasos aferente y eferente, lo mismo que la proliferación de celulas conectivas en ocasiones con abundantes mitosis.

Типичные гломеролуподобные образования в глиобластоме. Виден отводящий и приводящий сосуды и разрастание интенсивно-окрашенных соединительно-тканных клеток, многочисленные митозы.

膠芽腫における、定型的な糸球体様内皮増殖。しばしば輸出入血管、増殖した浮腫状結合組織細胞、ときに多数の核分裂をみとめる。

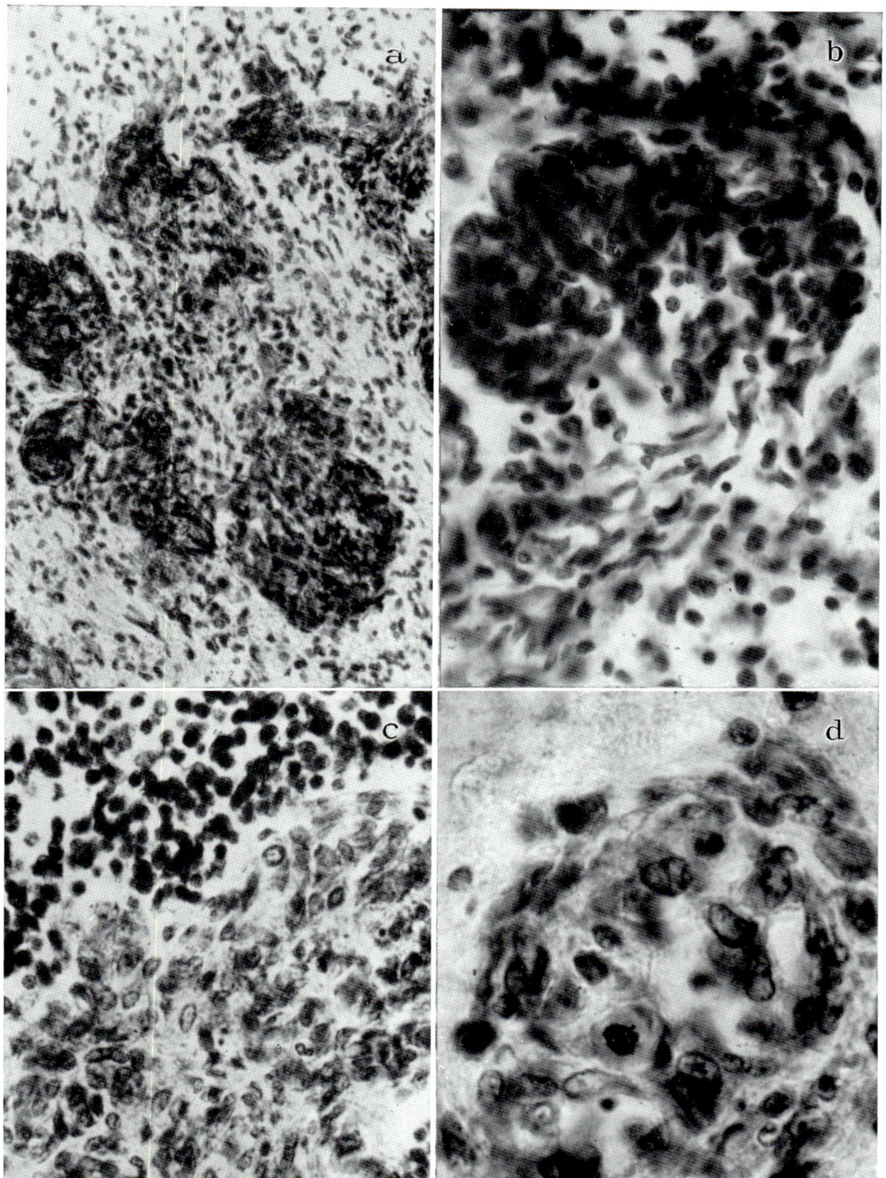

Fig. 45a—d: a ×96. Cresyl violet stain
b ×180, c ×240, d ×680. Nissl stain

Fig. 46 — Glioblastomas, Malignant

Various forms of mesodermal proliferation in a glioblastoma.
a) Irregularly constructed capillary systems with thickening of the walls.
b) Small sinusoid vessels with only slight proliferation of the walls.
c) Coil- and loop formation of blood vessels in a typical glioblastoma.
d) Cavernoma-like vascular systems at the border of necrosis.

Verschiedene Formen mesodermaler Wucherung in einem Glioblastom.
a) Unruhig gebaute Capillarsysteme mit Wandverdickung.
b) Kleine sinusoide Gefäße mit nur geringer Wandwucherung.
c) Knäuel- und Schlingenbildung an Gefäßen in einem typischen Glioblastom.
d) Cavernomartige Gefäßsysteme am Rande einer Nekrose.

Différents aspects de la prolifération mésodermique dans le glioblastome.
a) Système capillaire à paroi épaisse et à disposition désordonnée.
b) Petits vaisseaux sinusoïdes dont la paroi prolifère très peu.
c) Vaisseaux pelotonnés et enlacés dans un cas typique de glioblastome.
d) Aspect caverneux du système vasculaire au voisinage d'une nécrose.

Distintas formas de crecimiento mesodermal en un glioblastoma.
a) Sistema capilar de características inquietas, con engrosamiento de sus paredes.
b) Vasos pequeños sinusoidales, con escasa proliferación de sus paredes.
c) Formación de ovillos y lazos vasculares en un típico glioblastoma.
d) Sistema vascular de tipo cavernoso al borde de una necrosis.

Различные формы разрастания мезодермы в глиобластоме.
a) Активные системы капилляров с утолщенной стенкой.
b) Мелкие синусоидные сосуды с маловыраженным разрастанием стенки.
c) Образование сосудистых клубков и петель в типичной глиобластоме.
d) Кавернономоподобные сосудистые системы в окружности некроза.

膠芽腫における、間葉系組織増殖の種々の形態。
a) 無秩序に増殖した毛細血管。壁が肥厚している。
b) 小さな、類洞状血管。内皮細胞増殖は僅少。
c) 定型的な膠芽腫にみられた、血管球と係蹄の形成。
d) 壊死周辺部の海綿腫様血管。

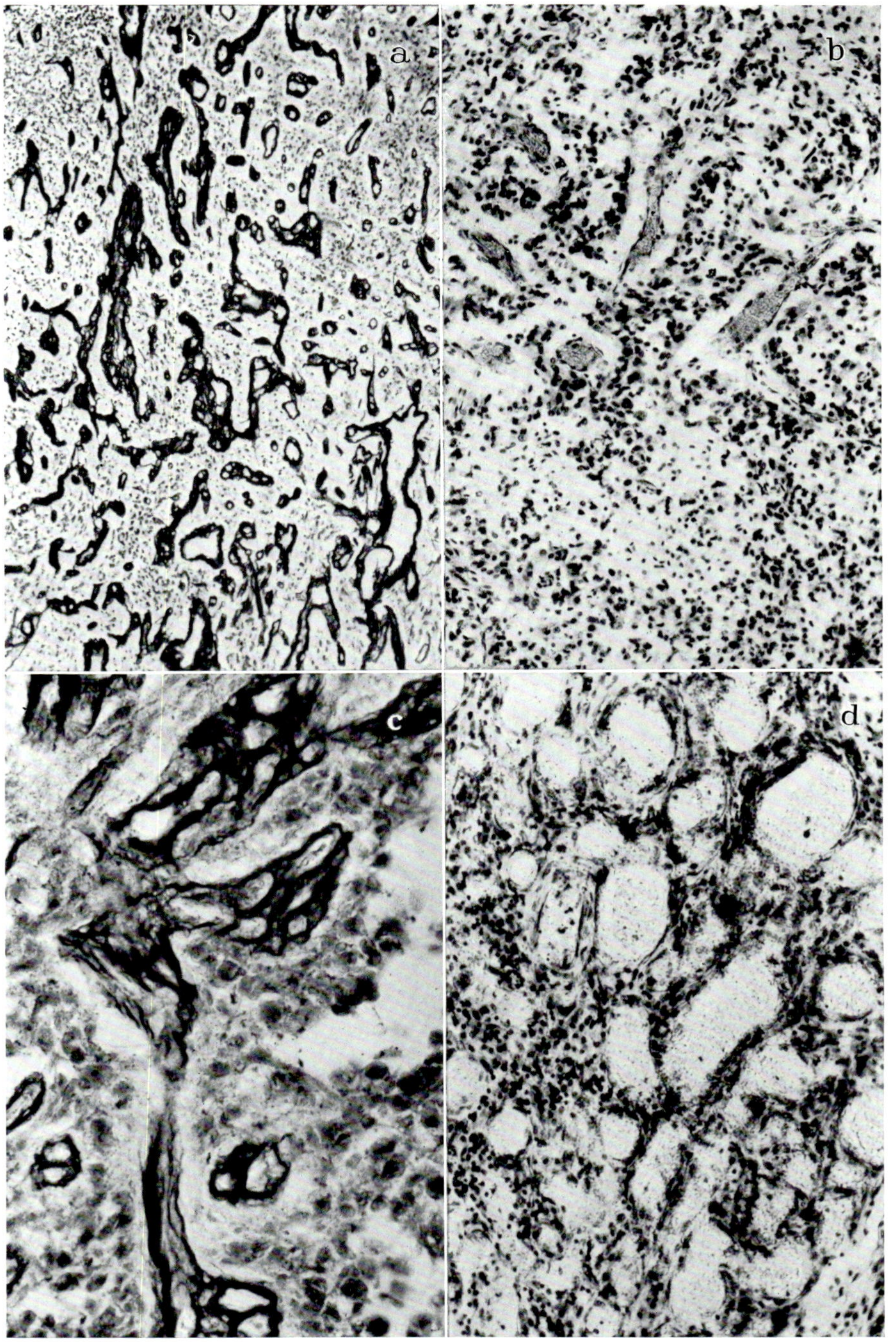

Fig. 46a—d: a ×72, c ×156. Perdrau's impregnation
b × 156, d ×96. Cresyl violet stain

Fig. 47 — Glioblastomas, Malignant

a) Large, lacunar vessels with recent thrombus formation.
b) The vessel, of about the thickness of a knitting needle, has a thin wall, consisting of only a few cell layers.
c) In a vessel of similar size, numerous small lumina have been formed, probably by the rechanneling of a former thrombosis.
d) A somewhat older thrombosis in a lacunar blood vessel. These vessels are visible particularly clearly in angiography as so-called "fistulae".

a) Große lacunäre Gefäße mit frischer Thrombenbildung.
b) Das etwa stricknadeldicke Gefäß hat eine dünne Gefäßwand, nur aus wenigen Zellagen.
c) In einem ähnlich großen Gefäß haben sich zahlreiche kleinere Lumina gebildet, wahrscheinlich durch Rekanalisation einer früheren Thrombose.
d) Etwas ältere Thrombose in einem lacunären Gefäß. Diese Größe der Gefäße ist besonders deutlich als sog. „Fisteln" bei der Angiographie sichtbar.

a) Thrombose récente dans un gros vaisseau lacunaire.
b) La paroi de ce vaisseau, gros comme une aiguille à tricoter, est mince et n'est constituée que par quelques couches de cellules.
c) Dans un vaisseau de taille similaire, on note de nombreuses petites lumières, qui correspondent probablement à la recanalisation d'une thrombose préalable.
d) Thrombose un peu plus ancienne dans un vaisseau lacunaire. Ce genre de vaisseaux donne des images de «fistules», particulièrement bien visibles à l'angiographie.

a) Vasos grandes lacunares, con reciente formación de trombos.
b) El vaso, del grosor aproximado de una aguja de hacer media, tiene una pared delgada, formada sólo por algunas células.
c) En un vaso de tamaño parecido se han formado numerosos lúmenes pequeños probablemente por recanalización de una trombosis anterior.
d) Trombosis algo antigua en un vaso lacunar. Estos vasos se ven especialmente claros como «fístulas», en la angiografía.

a) Крупные лакуноподобные сосуды со свежими тромбами.
b) Сосуд толщиной в вязальную спицу с тонкой сосудистой стенкой, состоящей из немногих клеточных слоев.
c) Такой же сосуд, в котором, по-видимому, вследствие реканализации тромба возникли многочисленные мелкие просветы.
d) Старый тромбоз в лакуноподобном сосуде. На ангиограмме эти сосуды четко прослеживаются в виде так называемых «анастомозов».

a) 新鮮血栓をいれた大きな洞状血管。
b) 編物針大の血管。壁は薄く、数層の細胞からなるのみである。
c) 同様な血管内にできた多数の小血管腔。おそらく、血栓の再疎通によると思われる。
d) 洞状血管内の、やゝ古い血栓。このような血管は、いわゆる「瘻管」として、血管撮影の場合特にはっきり見出される。

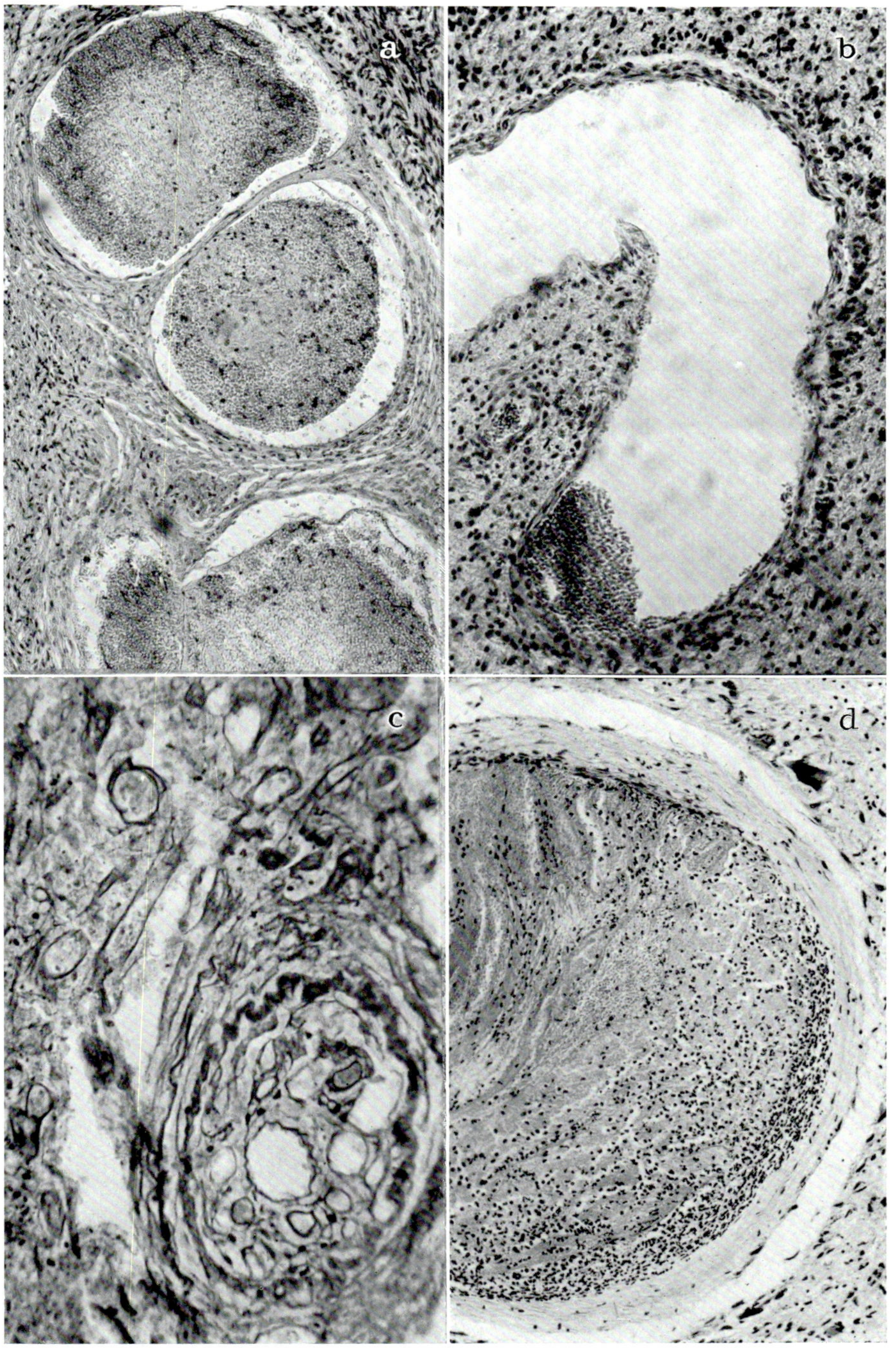

Fig. 47a—d: a, b and d ×84. Cresyl violet stain
c ×78. Gold sublimate impregnation

Fig. 48 — Glioblastomas, Malignant

Various types of proliferation of the adventitia in a glioblastoma:

a) Umbillicated proliferations of the outermost marginal zone of a medium-sized blood vessel.
b) Numerous newly-formed capillaries, often with glomerulus formation.
c) Systematic network of capillary proliferations arranged in clusters around a fairly small blood vessel.
d) Extreme proliferation of the intima and enlargement and swelling of the media.

Verschiedene Typen der Adventitiaproliferation im Glioblastom:

a) Doldenförmige Wucherungen der äußersten Randzone an einem mittelgroßen Gefäß.
b) Zahlreiche neugebildete Capillaren, oft mit Glomerulusbildung.
c) Systematisches Netz von traubenartig angeordneten Capillarwucherungen um ein kleineres Gefäß.
d) Hochgradige Intimawucherung und Mediaverbreiterung mit Verquellung.

Différents types de la prolifération adventitielle dans le glioblastome.

a) Prolifération ombelliforme au niveau de la couche externe d'un vaisseau de calibre moyen.
b) Nombreux capillaires néoformés, qui constituent très souvent des images glomérulaires.
c) Réseau systématisé de capillaires proliférant en forme de grappes autour d'un petit vaisseau.
d) Prolifération importante de l'intima, épaississement et gonflement de la média.

Distintos tipos de proliferación adventicial en un glioblastoma.

a) Proliferaciones eflorescentes en la zona más periférica, en un vaso de mediano tamaño.
b) Abundantes capilares neoformados, con frecuente formación de glomérulos.
c) Red sistematizada constituida a base de proliferaciones capilares en forma de racimo, alrededor de un pequeño vaso.
d) Crecimiento extremo de la íntima y engrosamiento e hinchazón de la media.

Различные типы пролиферации адвентиции в глиобластоме:

a) Грибовидные разрастания наружной краевой зоны сосуда средней величины.
b) Многочисленные новообразованные капилляры с нередкими гломерулоподобными образованиями.
c) Типичная сеть гроздевидно-расположенных разросшихся капилляров вокруг мелкого сосуда.
d) Выраженное разрастание интимы. Расширение и набухание медии.

膠芽腫における、血管外膜細胞増殖の諸型。

a) 中等大血管最外層をとりまく、繖形花状の増殖。
b) 新生した多数の毛細血管。しばしば糸球体様構造を示す。
c) 小血管周囲に増殖した、ぶどう状毛細血管網。
d) 著明な血管内膜細胞増殖と、中膜の拡大、膨化。

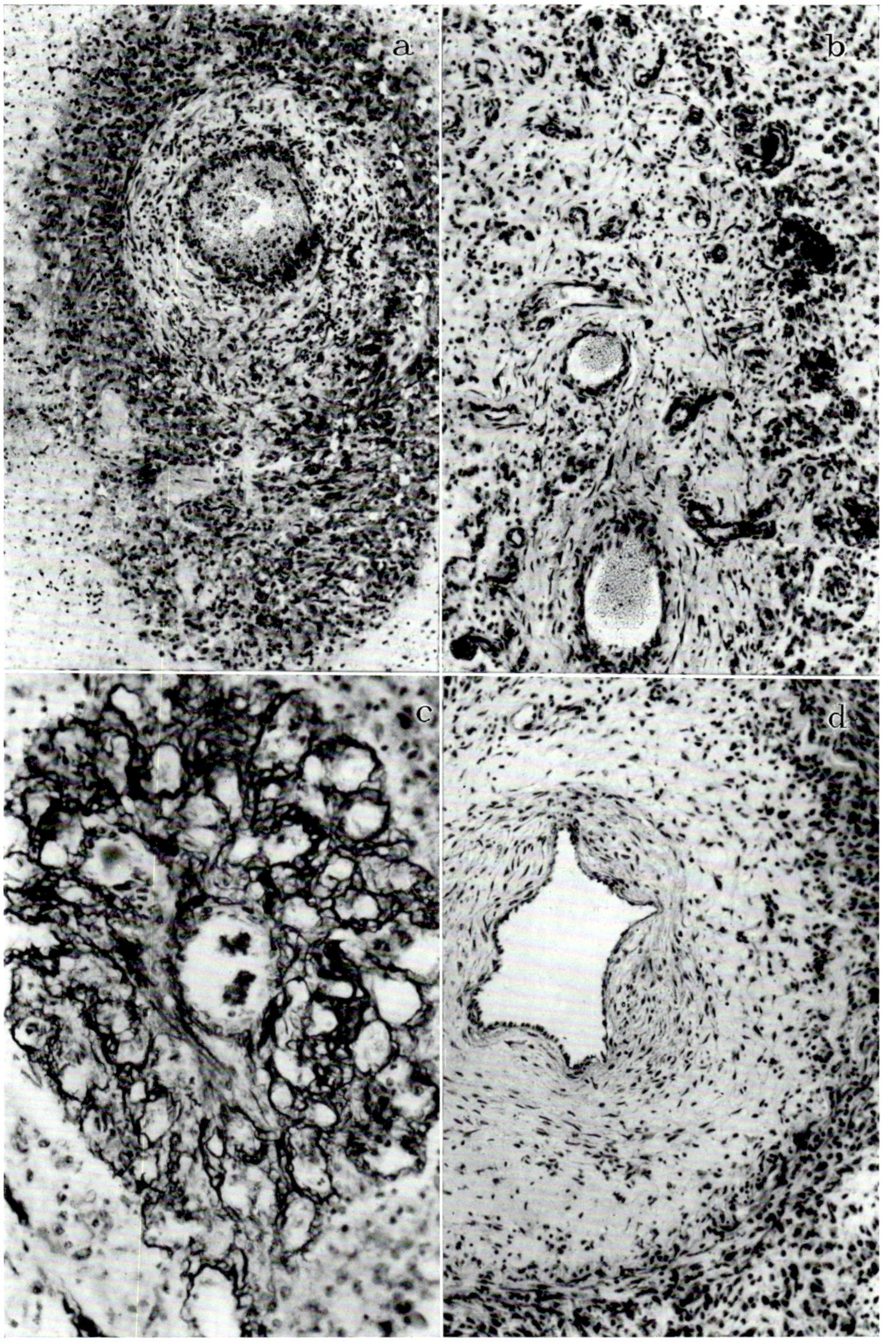

Fig. 48a—d: a, b and d ×78. Cresyl violet stain
c ×78. Perdrau's impregnation

Fig. 49 — Glioblastomas, Malignant

a)—c) Vascular architecture in a frontobasal glioblastoma. Clearing method according to Spalteholz. One can clearly discern in the marginal zone the garland of lacunar and sinusoid vessels, which end in an increased growth in the zone.
b) and c) are turned 90 degrees to the right. Note the large sinusoid vessel, which makes an orientation in the vascular systems possible.
d) Lacunar, sinusoid and capillary vessels in a glioblastoma.

a)—c) Gefäßarchitektur in einem frontobasalen Glioblastom. Aufhellung nach Spalteholz. Man erkennt deutlich in der Randzone den Kranz von lacunären und sinusoiden Gefäßen, die in der Zone in einem vermehrten Wachstum enden.
b) und c) sind um 90° nach rechts gedreht. Man beachte das große sinusoide Gefäß, das in den Gefäßsystemen eine Orientierung ermöglicht.
d) Lacunäre, sinusoide und capilläre Gefäße in einem Glioblastom.

a)—c) Architecture vasculaire dans un glioblastome fronto-basal (préparation selon Spalteholz). A la périphérie, on reconnaît nettement la couronne de lacunes et sinus vasculaires.
b) et c) Images tournées de 90° vers la droite. Le gros vaisseau sinusoïde permet de s'orienter dans le système vasculaire.
d) Réseaux lacunaires, sinusoïdes et capillaires.

a)—c) Arquitectura vascular en un glioblastoma frontobasal. Transparencia según Spalteholz. En los bordes se ve claramente la corona de vasos lacunares y sinusoides, que terminan en la zona de un crecimiento intenso.
b) y c) Tienen un giro de 90° hacia la derecha. Los grandes vasos sinusoidales permiten orientarse en el sistema vascular.
d) Vasos lacunares, sinusoidales y capilares

a)—c) Сосудистая сеть лобно-базальной глиобластомы (Просветление по ШПАЛЬТЕГОЛЬЦУ). В краевой зоне четко виден венок из лакуноподобных и синусоидных сосудов, оканчивающихся в зоне усиленного роста b) и c) повернуты на 90°. Виден крупный синусоидный сосуд, служащий ориентиром в сосудистой системе.
d) Лакуноподобные, синусоидные и капиллярные сосуды глиобластомы.

a)—c) 前頭葉下部膠芽腫の血管構築。Spalteholz による透徹法。腫瘍周辺には、空洞あるいは類洞状血管が明瞭にみとめられる。これらは、腫瘍増殖帯に終っている。
b) と c) は 90° 右に回してある。大きな類洞状血管を目標にすれば、位置は容易にきめられる。
d) 別な膠芽腫例の空洞状、類洞状血管および毛細血管。

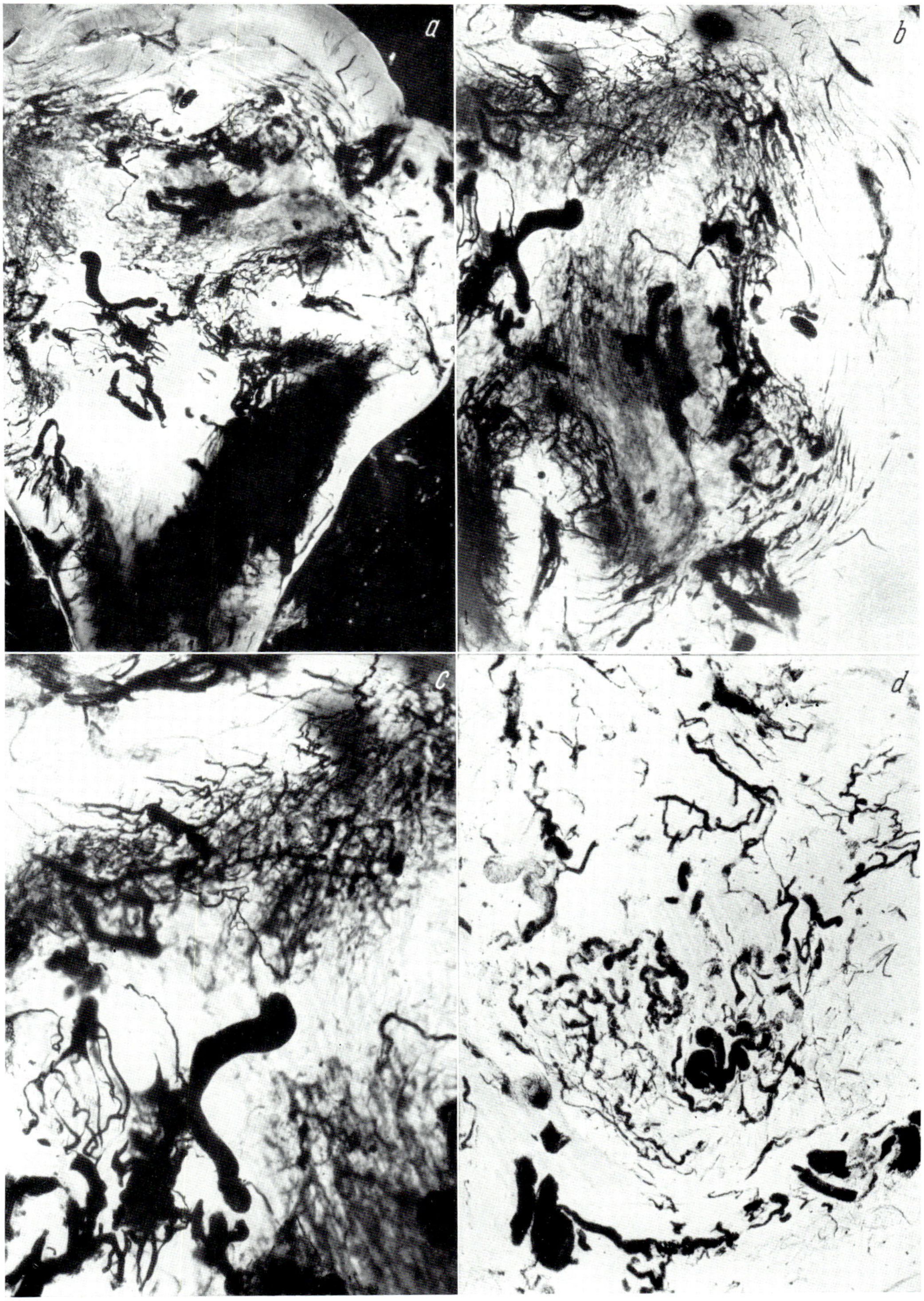

Fig. 49a—d: a ×2, b ×6, c ×10, Clearing method of Spalteholz, d ×12, Pickworth stain.

Fig. 50 — Glioblastomas, Malignant

Regressive tissue change of the necrotic type:

a) The necroses lie between the vessels. Thus a perivascular, occasionally ring-shaped, well-nourished marginal zone around the vessel is preserved ("perivascular cell-wreath", "perivascular cuffing").
b) Pseudo-palisading of nuclei at the border of a band-like necrosis
c) Band-like, proliferated blood vessels at the border of the necrosis.
d) Strikingly large-celled proliferation of the vascular adventitia in a necrosis.

Regressive Gewebsveränderungen vom Typus der Nekrose:

a) Die Nekrosen liegen zwischen den Gefäßen. Dadurch bleibt eine perivasculäre, gelegentlich ringförmige, gut ernährte Ringzone um das Gefäß erhalten („perivasculärer Zellkranz").
b) Pseudo-Palisadenstellung der Kerne am Rande einer strichförmigen Nekrose.
c) Bandartig gewucherte Gefäße am Nekroserand.
d) Auffällig großzellige Wucherung der Gefäßadventitia in einer Nekrose.

Altérations tissulaires régressives du type nécrosant.

a) Vu que les nécroses s'étendent entre les vaisseaux, il persiste une zone périvasculaire mieux nourrie, qui a parfois une forme annulaire («couronne cellulaire périvasculaire»).
b) Disposition pseudo-palissadique des noyaux au bord d'une nécrose allongée.
c) Guirlande de vaisseaux proliférés le long d'une nécrose.
d) Dans une nécrose, la prolifération adventitielle aboutit à la formation de cellules extrêmement volumineuses.

Procesos regresivos de tipo necrótico.

a) Les necrosis están entre los vasos. Por ello alrededor de éstos se mantiene una zona anular, bien nutrida (coronas celulares perivasculares).
b) Proliferación vascular en banda en los bordes de la necrosis.
c) Guirlanda de vasos proliferados a lo largo de una necrosis.
d) En una necrosis, la proliferación adventicial mena a la formación de celulas voluminosas.

Регрессивные изменения ткани по типу некроза:

a) Некрозы между сосудами, вокруг которых располагаются в виде кольца опухолевые клетки («периваскуляризация клеточной короны»).
b) Ядра расположены по краям некроза в виде псевдопалисадов.
c) Разрастание сосудов в виде тяжей по краям некроза.
d) Выраженное разрастание клеток адвентиции сосудов в некрозе.

腫瘍組織の壊死と退行性変化。

a) 壊死は血管からはなれた部位におこっている。血液供給のよい血管周囲に、腫瘍組織が輪状にのこる（血管周囲細胞冠)。
b) 線状壊死をふちどる核の偽柵状配列。
c) 壊死辺縁に、帯状に増殖した血管。
d) 壊死部の血管外膜にみられた、きわめて大きな細胞の増殖。2個の脂肪変性に陥った細胞がみとめられる。

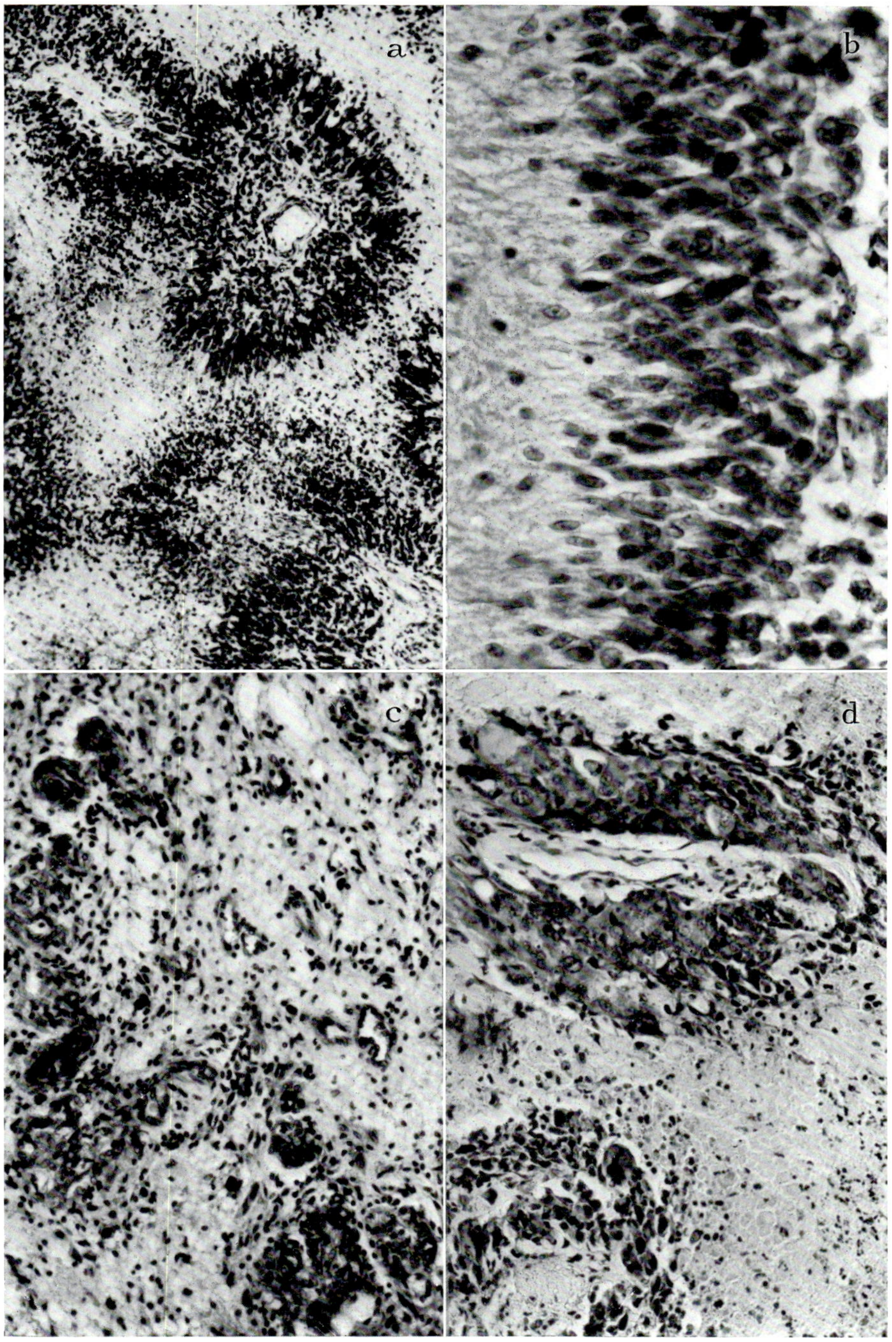

Fig. 50a—d: a ×78, b ×240, c and d ×120.
Cresyl violet stain

Fig. 51 — Glioblastomas, Malignant

Sudan fat stain in a glioblastoma.

a) Single fat-granule cells at the border of a necrosis.
b) Diffuse accumulation of fat-granule cells in a tumor that has undergone cystic disintegration.
c) Massive foci of fat-granule cells.
d) Fat-bearing rod cells.

Sudanfettfärbungen in einem Glioblastom.

a) Einzelne Fettkörnchenzellen am Rande einer Nekrose.
b) Diffuse Ansammlung von Fettkörnchenzellen in einem cystisch zerfallenen Tumor.
c) Massive Fettkörnchenzellherde.
d) Fettführende Stäbchenzellen.

Coloration des graisses par le soudan dans un glioblastome.

a) Présence de quelques corps granulo-graisseux au bord d'une nécrose.
b) Corps granulo-graisseux dispersés dans une tumeur en état de dégénérescence kystique.
c) Accumulation massive de corps granulo-graisseux.
d) Cellules en bâtonnet, bourrées de graisses.

Coloracíon con Sudán en un glioblastoma.

a) Algunos corpúsculos gránuloadiposos al borde de una necrosis.
b) Acúmulo difuso de corpúsculos gránuloadiposos en un tumor con procesos de degeneración quística.
c) Focos masivos de corpúsculos gránuloadiposos.
d) Células en bastoncito portadoras de grasa.

Окраска суданом водном глиобластомы.

a) Единичные клетки с липоидными включениями по периферии некроза.
b) Диффузное скопление клеток с липоидными включениями в кистозно-перерожденной опухоли.
c) Массивные скопления клеток с липидными включениями.
d) Палочковидные клетки, содержащие липидные включения.

スダン染色した膠芽腫

a) 壊死辺縁に散在する脂肪顆粒細胞。
b) 嚢胞状に崩壊した腫瘍組織のなかの、多数の脂肪顆粒細胞。
c) 脂肪顆粒細胞の密集塊。
d) 脂質を有する桿状細胞。

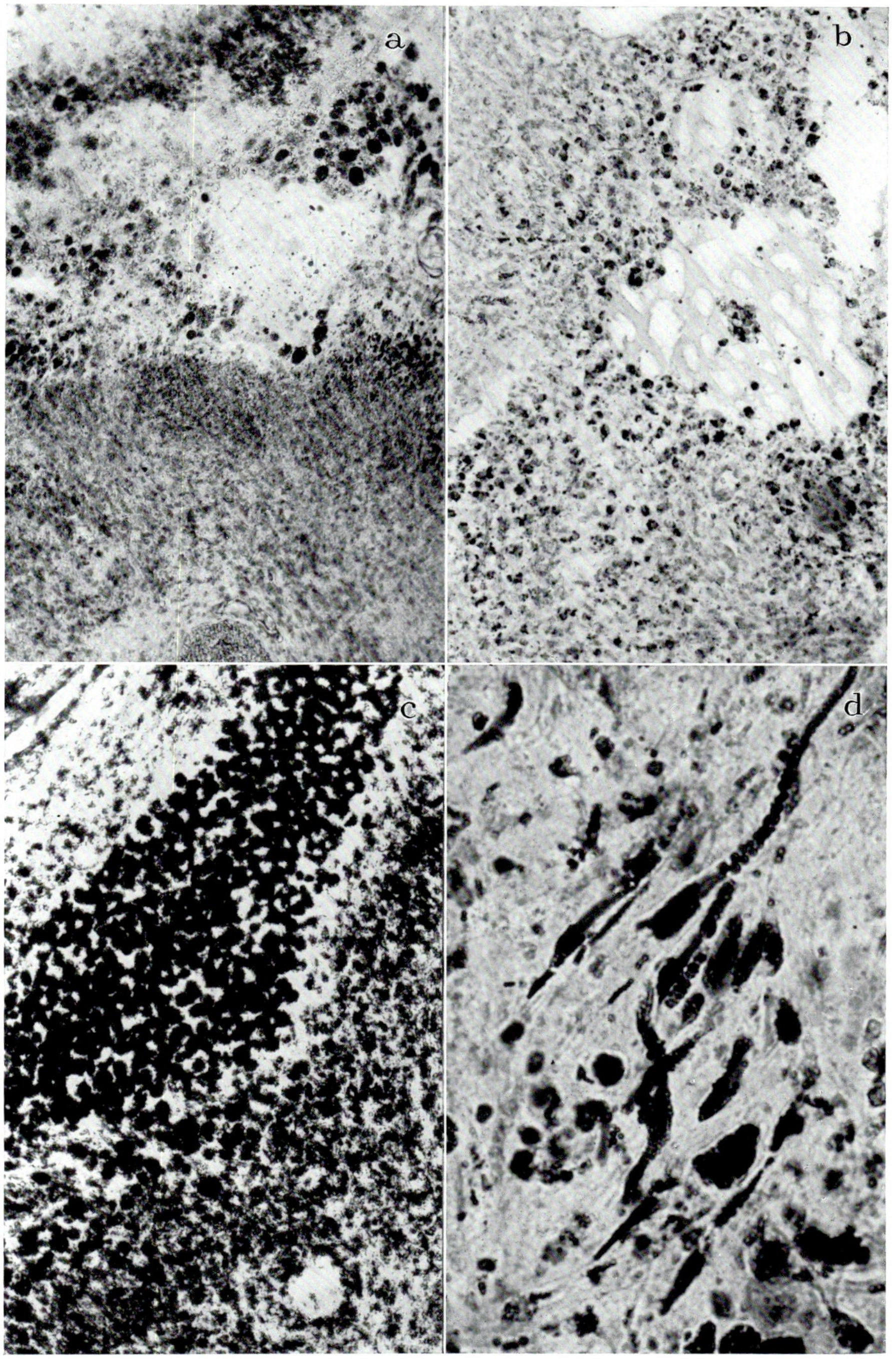

Fig. 51a—d: a and b ×78, c ×84, d ×880
Sudan fat stain

Spongioblastomas, Polar

Pilocytic or piloid astrocytoma, astrocytoma of juvenile type, optic nerve glioma, gliomyxoma, myxosarcoma, fusicellular oligodendrocytoma, "central neurinoma", gliome muqueux, polar glioma.

Fig. 52 — Spongioblastomas, Polar

a) The typical architecture of a spongioblastoma shows the oblong cells arranged in long streams. Individual blood vessels are dilated. Free calcium granules are seen in the tissue.
b) In a spongioblastoma of the optic nerve one finds the tumor cells especially elongated and arranged in parallel between the myelin sheaths.
c) Spongioblastoma of the retina shows, besides the typical spindle-shaped tumor cells (*bottom*), separations of the retinal epithelium (*top*), which are often described as "rosettes".
d) By impregnation the elongated tumor cells are revealed in their parallel position.

a) Die typische Architektur eines Spongioblastoms zeigt die länglichen Zellen in langen Strömen geordnet. Einzelne Gefäße sind verbreitert. Man sieht aber auch im Gewebe freie Kalkperlen.
b) In einem Spongioblastom des Fasc. opticus findet man die Geschwulstzellen besonders lang ausgezogen und zwischen den Markscheiden parallel ausgerichtet.
c) Das Spongioblastom der Retina zeigt neben den typischen spindeligen Geschwulstzellen (unten) auch noch Abschnürungen des Retinaepithels (oben), die oft als ,,Rosette" bezeichnet werden.
d) Durch Imprägnation lassen sich die langausgezogenen Geschwulstzellen in ihrer parallelen Lagerung darstellen.

a) L'architecture typique d'un spongioblastome est caractérisée par des faisceaux de cellules allongées, parmis lesquels on observe quelques vaisseaux dilatés et des dépôts de calcophérites.
b) Dans un spongioblastome du nerf optique, on note l'aspect particulièrement étiré des cellules tumorales, qui se disposent parallèlement aux gaines de myéline.
c) Dans un spongioblastome de la rétine, outre l'aspect typiquement fusiforme des cellules tumorales (au bas de l'image), on observe également des cordons d'épithélium rétinien (à la partie supérieure de l'image), auxquels on donne souvent le nom de «rosettes».
d) La forme étirée et la disposition parallèle des cellules tumorales sont bien mises en évidence par une imprégnation métallique.

a) La arquitectura típica de un espongioblastoma muestra las células alargadas, ordenadas en largas corrientes. Algunos vasos están ensanchados. En el tejido se ven también perlas calcáreas libres.
b) En un espongioblastoma del fascículo óptico las células tumorales son especialmente alargadas y están dispuestas paralelamente a lo largo de las vainas medulares.
c) Un espongioblastoma de la retina mostrando además de las típicas células fusiformes (abajo), restos de epitelio retiniano (arriba) que frecuentemente son catalogados de «rosetas».
d) A través de la impregnación, las alargadas células tumorales, se muestran dispuestas en situación paralela.

a) Типичное строение спонгиобластомы с вытянутыми в длину крупными клетками. Отдельные сосуды расширены. В тканях видны свободные глыбки из солей кальция.
b) В спонгиобластоме fasc. opticus обнаруживаются резко вытянутые в длину и параллельно расположенные между миелиновыми оболочками опухолевые клетки.
c) В спонгиобластоме сетчатки наряду с типичными веретенообразными опухолевыми клетками (внизу) видны перетяжки эпителия сетчатки (вверху), так называемые «розетки».
d) Импрегнация дает возможность проследить параллельное расположение вытянутых в длину опухолевых клеток.

a) 海綿芽細胞腫の定型的組織像。細長い細胞が流線状にならんでいる。いくつかの血管は拡大している。組織内には真珠様石灰沈着がみとめられる。
b) 視束の海綿芽細胞腫。腫瘍細胞は非常に細長く、髄鞘間に平行にならんでいる。
c) 網膜の海綿芽細胞腫。定型的な紡錘状腫瘍細胞（図下）のほかに、とり残された網膜上皮（図上）がみられる。これはときに「ロゼッテ」の形をとる。
d) 鍍金によって、平行に並んだ長い腫瘍細胞が染出される。

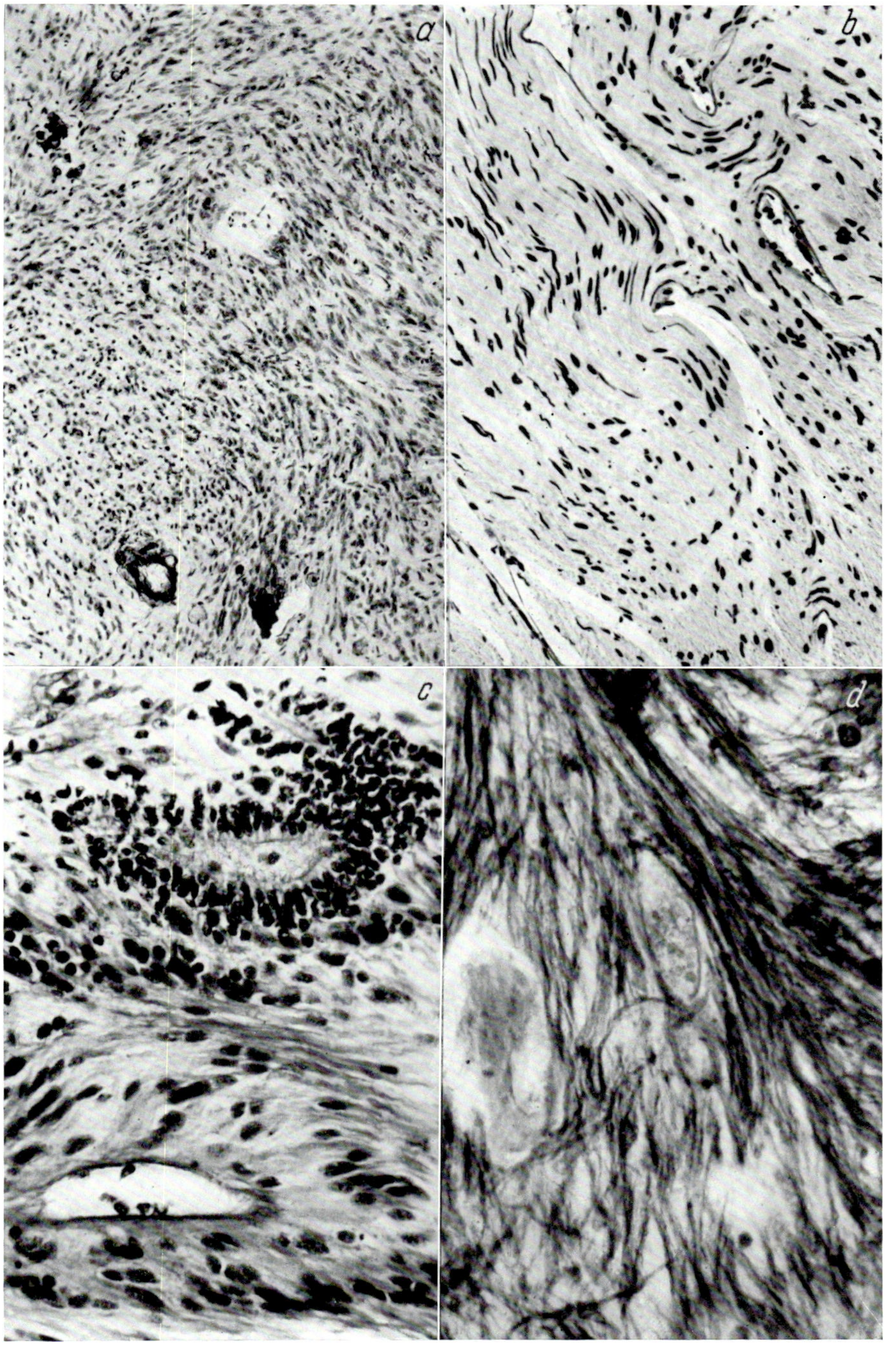

Fig. 52a—d: a ×90, b ×136. Cresyl violet stain
c ×262. H. E. stain
d ×288. Gold sublimate method

Fig. 53 — Spongioblastomas, Polar

a), b) and c) By impregnation, more astrocyte-like cells with long fibrils are revealed in some parts, in other parts more bipolar cells, which have arranged their processes in narrow, wavy bands. These patterns are clearly different from those of the cerebral astrocytoma.
d) Wire-thin glial fibers can be demonstrated in the spongioblastoma in paraffin embedded material and Heidenhain's hematoxylin.

a), b) u. c) Durch Imprägnation lassen sich teils mehr astrocytenartige Zellen mit langen Ausläufern, teils mehr bipolare Zellen darstellen, die ihre Fortsätze in schmalen Bändern angeordnet haben und wellig verlaufen. Diese Bilder sind von denen des Großhirnastrocytoms deutlich verschieden.
d) Dünne, drahtige Gliafasern lassen sich im Spongioblastom bei Paraffineinbettung mit dem Heidenhainschen Hämatoxylin darstellen.

a), b) et c) Par une imprégnation métallique, on voit certaines cellules de type astrocytaire, munies de longs prolongements, ainsi que des cellules bipolaires, dont les prolongements ondulants se groupent en petits faisceaux. Cet aspect est nettement différent de celui d'un astrocytome cérébral.
d) Dans le spongioblastome, des fibres gliales minces et filiformes sont bien mises en évidence par l'hématoxyline de Heidenhain sur des coupes à la paraffine.

a), b) y c) Gracias a la técnica del sublimado-oro pueden verse unas células en parte más astrocíticas con largas prolongaciones y otras más bipolares, que ordenan sus prolongaciones en estrechas bandas que transcurren onduladamente. Estas imágenes son totalmente diferentes de las correspondientes al astrocitoma de los hemisferios cerebrales.
d) En los espongioblastomas, con la hematoxilina de Heidenhain y inclusión en parafina, pueden demostrarse finas fibras gliales, que semejan alambre.

a), b) и c) Импрегнация дает возможность увидеть то астроцитоподобные клетки с длинными отростками, то биполярные клетки, отростки которых образуют узкие волнообразные тяжи. Эта картина существенно отличается от той, которую мы наблюдаем при астроцитомах больших полушарий.
d) Тонкие проволокообразные глиальные волокна в спонгиобластоме, залитой в парафин и окрашенной гематоксилином Гейденгайна.

a), b) および c) 鍍金によって、いくつかの、長い胞体突起をもった星膠細胞様の細胞と、より二極性の細胞が染出される。後者は、細い束状の突起を有し、波状の走向を示す。これは大脳の星膠細胞腫と明らかに異なる点である。
d) 海綿芽細胞腫では、パラフィン切片のHeidenhain ヘマトキシリン染色によって、細い針金状のグリヤ線維が見出される。

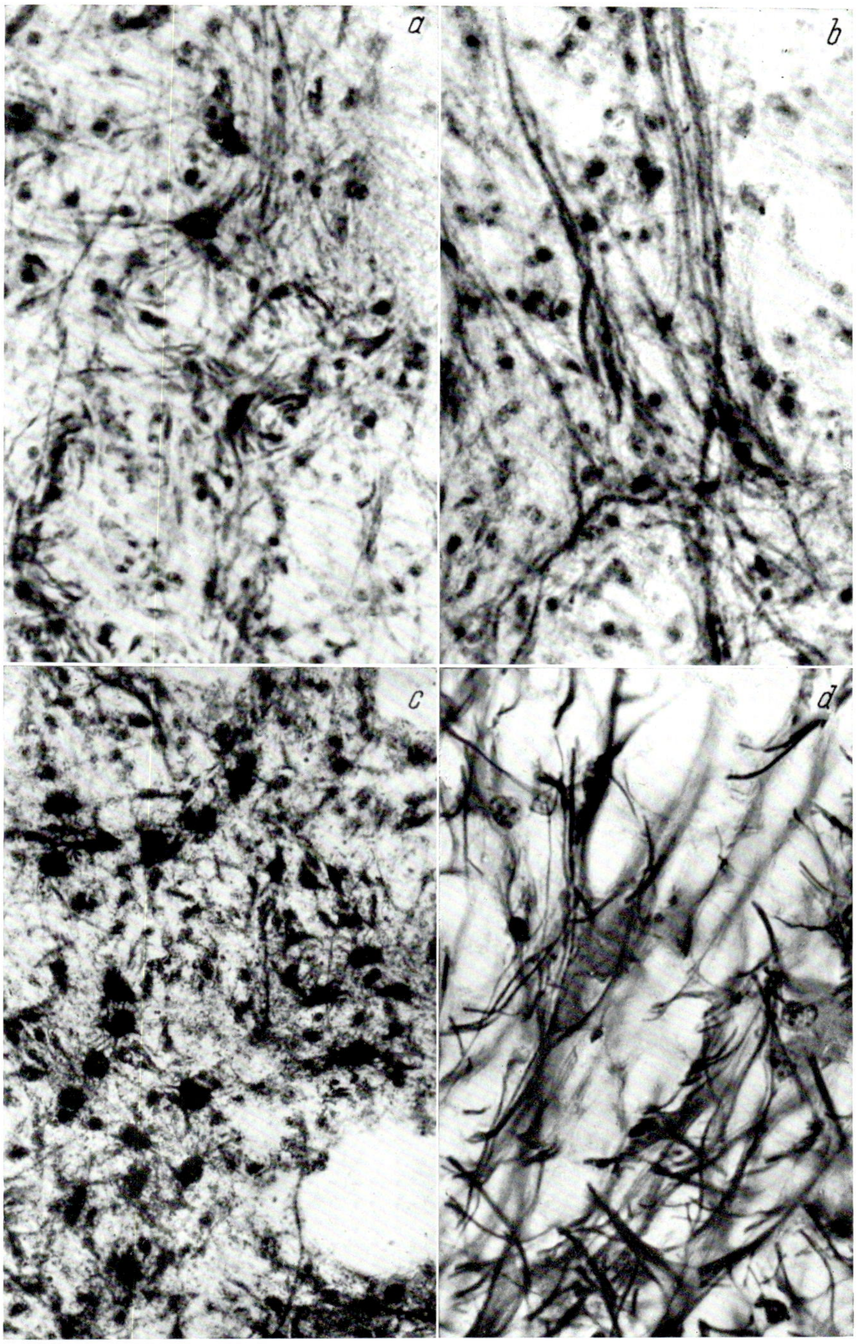

Fig. 53 a—d: a—c ×288. Gold sublimate impregnation
d ×576. Heidenhain's hematoxylin

Fig. 54 — Spongioblastomas, Polar

a) When the regressive processes set in, complete mucoid degeneration of the spongioblastoma may ensue. Then the nuclei are round and extremely pyknotic, the tissue is in a state of loose decomposition, and lakes of mucin appear.
b) In a spongioblastoma the formation of giant cells and multinucleated cell complexes may result. Here one sees also Rosenthal fibers beginning to form.
c) A variant of the spindle-cell spongioblastoma leads to marked palisading of the nuclei.
d) In the cerebellar spongioblastoma apparently "multinucleated" formations may result by the fusing of chromatin-rich nuclei.

a) Wenn die regressiven Vorgänge einsetzen, kann es zur völligen Verschleimung des Spongioblastoms kommen. Dann sind die Kerne rund und hochgradig pyknotisch, das Gewebe ist in einem lockeren Zerfall und es treten ganze Mucinseen auf.
b) Es kann im Spongioblastom zur Bildung von Riesenzellen und mehrkernigen Zellkomplexen kommen. Hier sieht man auch den Beginn der Bildung Rosenthalscher Fasern.
c) Eine Variante des spindelzelligen Spongioblastoms führt zur Bildung von ausgesprochenen Palisadenstellungen der Kerne.
d) Im Kleinhirnspongioblastom kann es auch durch Zusammensintern chromatinreicher Kerne zu anscheinend „mehrkernigen“ Bildungen kommen.

a) Lorsque des phénomènes régressifs s'installent, on assiste à un empâtement complet (une lyse) du spongioblastome: les noyaux deviennent arrondis et fortement pycnotiques, le tissu subit une dégradation lâche et on voit apparaître des flaques de substance mucoïde.
b) Dans le spongioblastome, on peut observer des cellules géantes et des complexes cellulaires multinucléés. Dans cette image, on observe également le début de la formation des fibres de Rosenthal.
c) Une variante du spongioblastome à cellules fusiformes est caractérisée par la disposition nettement palissadique des noyaux.
d) Dans un spongioblastome du cervelet, l'agglutination de noyaux riches en chromatine donne des images ressemblant à des cellules «multinucléées».

a) Cuando se instauran los procesos regresivos se puede llegar a una total degeneración mucosa del espongioblastoma. Los núcleos entonces se redondean y se hacen altamente picnóticos, el tejido se encuentra laxamente desintegrado y se forman extensas lagunas de mucina.
b) En el espongioblastoma se pueden formar células gigantes y complejos celulares multinucleares. Aquí se observa además el inicio de la formación de las fibrillas de ROSENTHAL.
c) Una variante del espongiblastoma fusicelular lleva a una exagerada disposición de los nucleos en empalizada.
d) En el espongioblastoma del cerebelo puede llegarse también por la agrupación de núcleos ricos en cromatina a la formación aparente de complejos multinucleados.

a) Развитие регрессивных процессов приводит к полному мукоидному перерождению спонгиобластомы. Ядра округлые и резко гиперхромны; ткань в состоянии рыхлого распада; появление слизистого расплавления.
b) Гигантские клетки и многоядерные клеточные комплексы в ткани спонгиобластомы. Начальная стадия образования волокон Розенталя.
c) Вариант веретеноклеточной спонгиобластомы, ядра которой образуют четкие палисады.
d) Наличие в спонгиобластоме мозжечка гиперхромных ядер создает картину «многоядерных» структур.

a) 海綿芽細胞腫に退行変性がおこると、完全な粘液様変化が現われる。その場合、核は円形となり、高度に濃縮し、腫瘍組織は崩壊して、粘液様、疎鬆となる。
b) 海綿芽細胞腫には、巨細胞、多核合胞細胞もみられることがある。ここではRosenthal線維形成の初期像も又みられる。
c) 紡錘細胞性海綿芽細胞の異型のひとつとして、核の著明は柵状配列もみられる。
d) 小脳海綿芽細胞腫で、濃染核の癒合によって、見かけ上、「多核細胞」を思わせる像のできることがある。

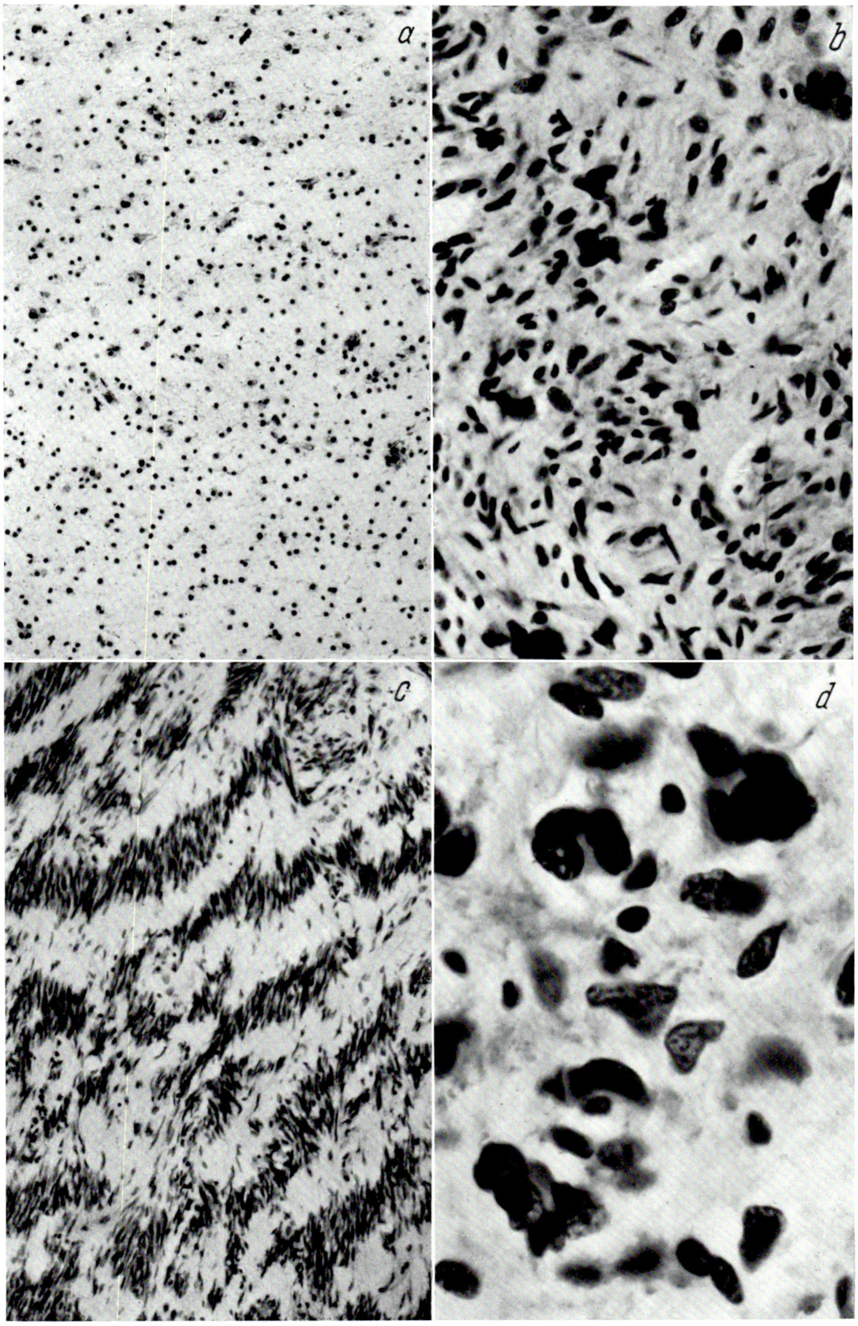

Fig. 54a—d: a ×72, b and c ×112, d ×604
Cresyl violet stain

Fig. 55 — Spongioblastomas, Polar

a) and b) The mucoid transformation of a spongioblastoma of the cerebellum leads to the formation of a network with single pyknotic nuclei between the tissue bridges. Frequently cystic formation is found in the spongioblastoma, with coil-like, proliferated blood vessels lying at the border of the cyst.
c) Because of the deposit of racemose calcium granules, the calcification may also be demonstrated radiologically.
d) Within the framework of the mucoid transformation of the otherwise typical spongioblastoma of the cerebellum, the honeycomb architecture of an oligodendroglioma can be simulated.

a) u. b) Die schleimige Umbildung des Spongioblastoms des Kleinhirns führt zu einem Netz mit einzelnen pyknotischen Kernen zwischen den Gewebsbrücken. Häufig findet sich im Spongioblastom eine Cystenbildung, dabei liegen am Cystenrand knäuelartig gewucherte Gefäße.
c) Durch Einlagerung von traubenartigen Kalkperlen kommt es auch röntgenologisch zur Verkalkung.
d) Im Rahmen der schleimigen Umwandlung sonst typischer Spongioblastome des Kleinhirns kann die Honigwabenarchitektur des Oligodendroglioms vorgetäuscht werden.

a) et b) La transformation muqueuse du spongioblastome du cervelet aboutit à la formation d'un réseau dont les mailles tissulaires contiennent des noyaux pycnotiques isolés. Le spongioblastome contient souvent un kyste, autour duquel on observe des pelotons de vaisseaux proliférés.
c) Des grappes de calcophérites se déposent dans la tumeur, qui présente ainsi des calcifications visibles à la radiographie.
d) Dans un cas par ailleurs typique de spongioblastome du cervelet, la transformation muqueuse peut être facilement confondue avec l'image en rayon de miel de l'oligodendrogliome.

a) y b) La transformación mucosa del espongioblastoma del cerebelo se traduce en una red con algunos núcleos picnóticos entre los puentes tisulares. En el espongioblastoma se observa con frecuencia la formación de quistes; en sus paredes se ven proliferaciones vasculares en ovillo.
c) Debido al depósito de perlas calcáreas arracimadas se llega también a la visión radiográfica de la calcificación.
d) En el cuadro de la transformación mucosa de un espongioblastoma de cerebelo, por lo demás típico, puede quedar confundida la arquitectura en panal de abeja de un oligodendroglioma.

a) и b) Мукоидное перерождение спонгиобластомы мозжечка ведет к появлению сетки с отдельными гиперхромными ядрами между тканевыми мостиками. Часто в спонгиобластоме видны кисты, по краям которых расположены разросшиеся в виде клубка сосуды.
c) Отложение гроздеподобных глыбок из кальция обусловливает рентгенологическое распознавание обызвествления.
d) Вследствие мукоидного перерождения типичная спонгиобластома мозжечка может быть принята за олигодендроглиому сотовидной структуры.

a) 小脳海綿芽細胞腫の粘液様変性の結果、空隙をともなった網状構造ができ、その隔壁に濃縮核がみとめられる。
b) 海綿芽細胞腫には、しばしば嚢胞が形成され、嚢胞壁には糸球体状に増殖した血管がみられる。
c) ぶどう状の石灰沈着。これはレ線によっても証明される。
d) 定型的な小脳海綿芽細胞腫でも、粘液様変性部では、稀突起膠腫にみる蜂窩状構造に似た像が生じうる。

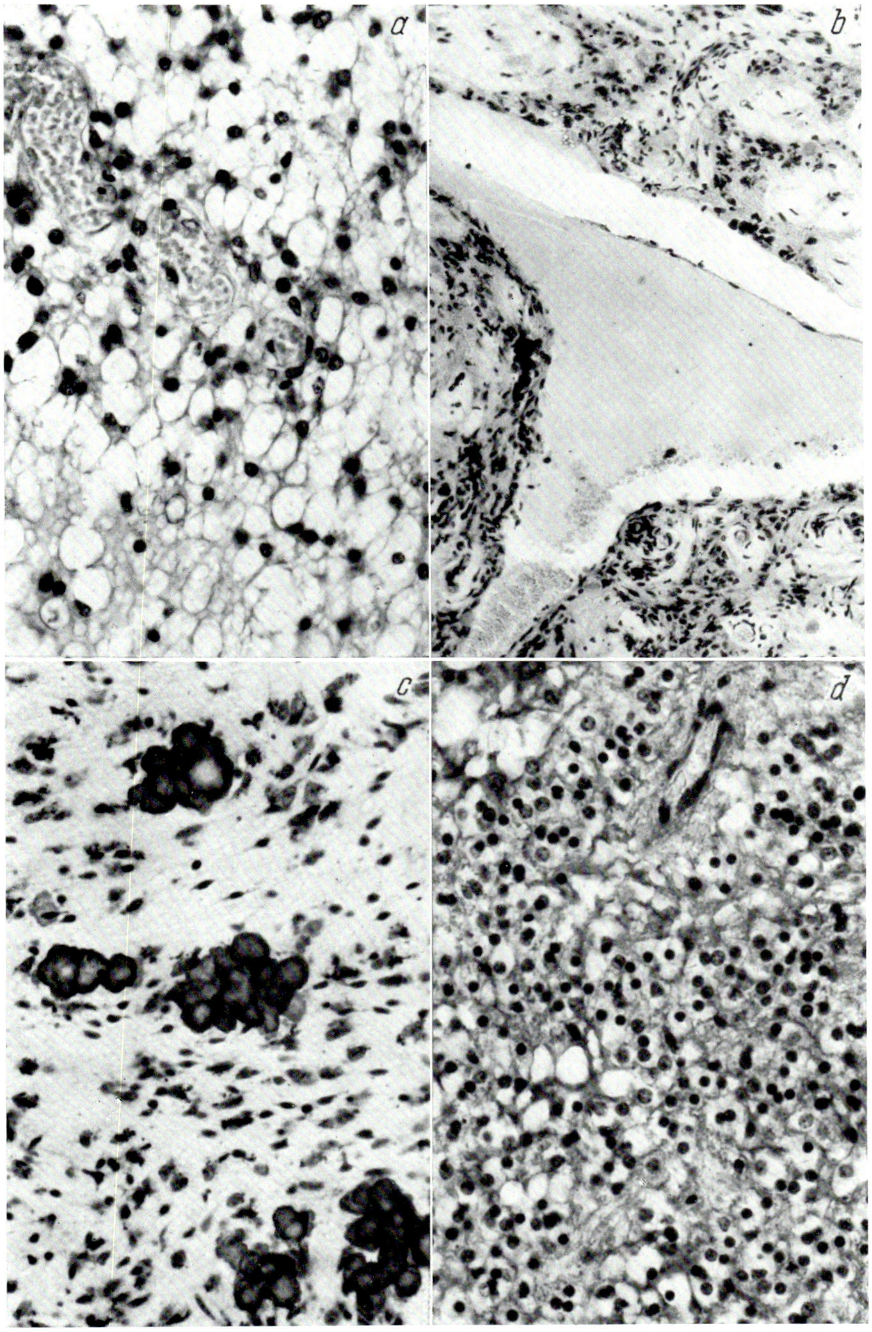

Fig. 55a—d: a ×262, b ×96, c ×240, d ×272
Cresyl violet stain

Fig. 56 — Spongioblastomas, Polar

The blood vessels of a spongioblastoma may exhibit noteworthy formations:

a) Large cavernoma-like convolutions.
b) The spread of the mucoid swelling of the blood vessel leads to enlargement and mucoid transformation of the vessel wall.
c) As a consequence of complete mucoid degeneration of the tumor tissue, only "cell wreaths" (cuffings) remain around the vessels. Thus the architecture of "pseudo-rosettes" is formed, just as in an ependymoma.
d) Many spongioblastomas are characterized by great vascularity. In this case there are sinusoid and capillary vessels.

Die Gefäße des Spongioblastoms können besonders merkwürdige Bildungen aufweisen:

a) Große kavernomartige Konvolute.
b) Die schleimige Verquellung des Gewebes führt auch zur Verbreiterung und mukösen Umwandlung der Gefäßwand.
c) Infolge völliger Verschleimung des Geschwulstgewebes bleiben nur um die Gefäße „Zellkränze" stehen. So bildet sich die Architektur von „Pseudopapillen" ähnlich wie in einem Ependymom.
d) Manche Spongioblastome sind durch großen Gefäßreichtum gekennzeichnet. Dabei sieht man sinusoide und capilläre Gefäße.

Les vaisseaux du spongioblastome peuvent présenter des aspects très particuliers.

a) Volumineux amas vasculaires de type caverneux.
b) Le gonflement œdémateux provoque l'épaississement et la métamorphose muqueuse de la paroi des vaisseaux.
c) A la suite de l'œdème important du tissu tumoral, il ne persiste plus que des «couronnes cellulaires» autour des vaisseaux. Ces «pseudopapilles» ressemblent à l'architecture de l'épendymome.
d) Beaucoup de spongioblastomes sont caractérisés par une vascularisation abondante, dans laquelle on trouve des vaisseaux sinusoïdes et capillaires.

Los vasos del espongioblastoma pueden constituir imágenes especialmente notables:

a) Grandes convoluciones de tipo cavernoso.
b) La degeneración mucosa del tejido contribuye a la difusión del proceso en las pared del vaso.
c) A consecuencia de la total degeneración mucosa del tejido tumoral sólo quedan alrededor de los vasos «coronas vasculares». Asi se forman las pseudopapilas, parecidas a las de un ependimoma.
d) Algunos espongioblastomas se caracterizan por su gran vascularización. Aquí se ven al mismo tiempo vasos capilares y sinusoidales.

Своеобразное строение сосудов спонгиобластомы:

a) Большие кавернподобные конволюты.
b) Слизистое набухание сосудов ведет к увеличению мукоидного перерождения стенки сосудов.
c) Вследствие полного мукоидного перерождения опухолевой ткани «венки клеток» остаются только вокруг сосудов. Так возникает «псевдопапиллярное» строение, аналогичное эпендимоме.
d) Обилие сосудов в спонгиобластоме. Видны синусоиды и капилляры.

海綿芽細胞腫内の血管は、ときに注目すべき変化を示す。

a) 大きな、海綿腫様の血管結節。
b) 腫瘍組織の粘液様膨化の結果、血管壁の粘液変性がおこる。
c) 腫瘍組織の完全な粘液様変性によって、血管周囲にのみ「細胞冠」が残存する。その結果、上衣細胞腫に似た「偽乳頭」がつくられる。
d) 多くの海綿芽細胞腫は非常に血管にとんでいる。これは類洞様血管及び毛細血管が主である。

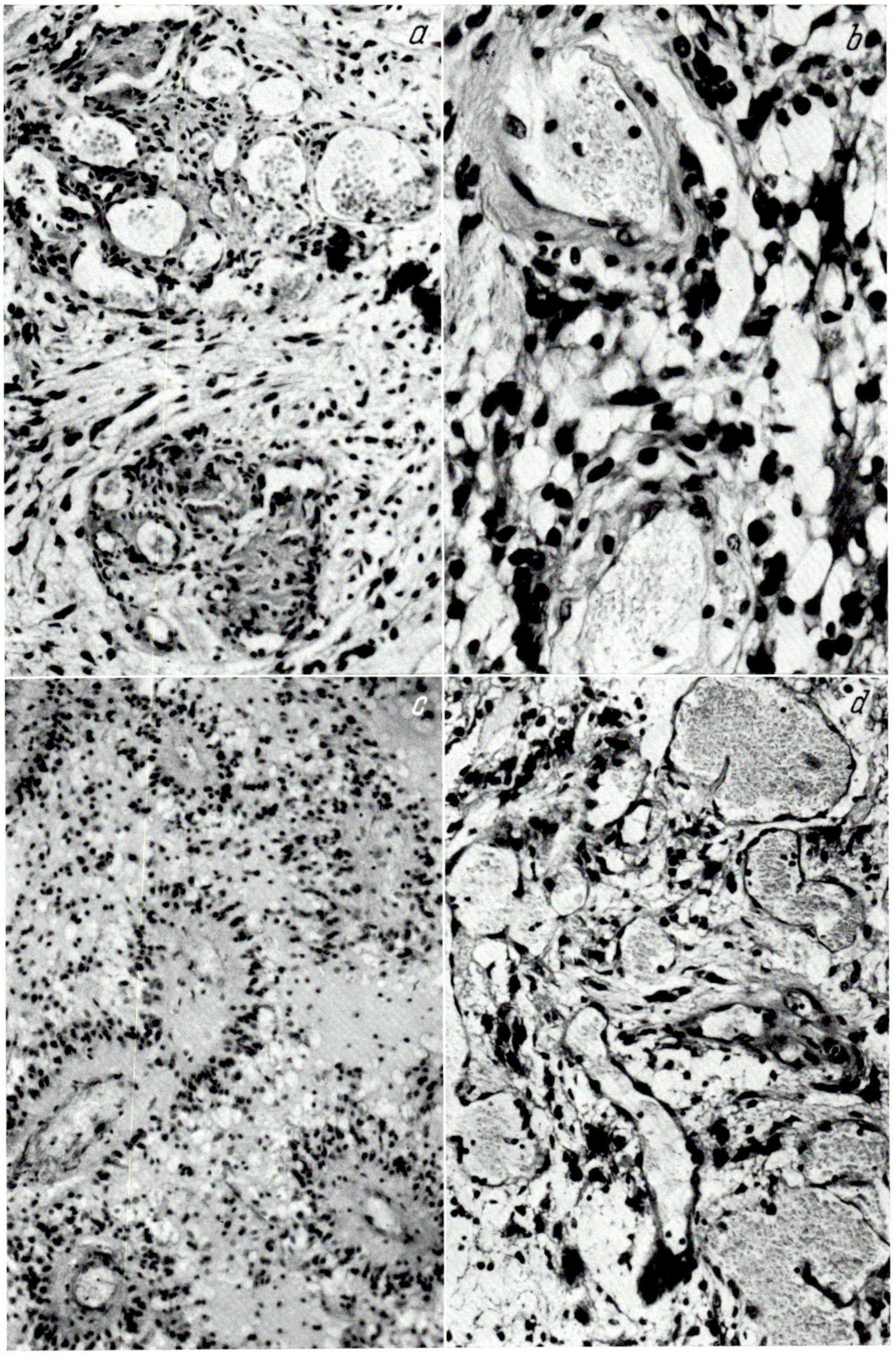

Fig. 56a—d: a ×136, b and d ×272, c ×104
Cresyl violet stain

Fig. 57 — Spongioblastomas, Polar

a) Formation of vascular loops and marked proliferation of cells composing the vascular walls at the border of a cyst.
b) Glomerular structures and loop formations at the border of a necrotic area in a spongioblastoma.
c) Hyaline degeneration of vessels in a spongioblastoma.
d) Angiomatous-like formations produced by vascular convolutions in a spongioblastoma.

a) Gefäßschlingenbildung mit reichlicher Wucherung der Gefäßwandzellen am Rande einer Cyste.
b) Gefäßknäuel- und Schlingenbildung in einem Spongioblastom am Rand einer Nekrose.
c) Hyaline Verquellung der Gefäße in einem Spongioblastom.
d) Angiomartige Bildung von Gefäßkonvoluten in einem Spongioblastom.

a) Formation d'un réseau vasculaire et importante prolifération cellulaire des parois vasculaires au bord d'un kyste.
b) Pelotons et réseaux vasculaires en bordure d'une nécrose dans un spongioblastome.
c) Gonflement hyalin des parois vasculaires dans un spongioblastome.
d) Amas vasculaires d'aspect angiomateux dans un spongioblastome.

a) Entrelazamiento de vasos intensamente proliferados en la pared de un quiste.
b) Ovillo vascular y entrelazamiento en un espongioblastoma en la periferia de una necrosis.
c) Degeneración hialina de los vasos en un espongioblastoma.
d) Aspecto angiomatoso de los vasos en un espongioblastoma.

a) Стенки сосуда по краям кисты.
b) Образование сосудистых клубочков и петель в спонгиобластоме по краю некроза.
c) Гиалиновое набухание сосудов в спонгиобластоме.
d) Ангиоподобное образование сосудистых конгломератов в спонгиобластоме.

a) 嚢胞の辺縁における、血管壁細胞の増殖をともなった血管係蹄形成。
b) 海綿芽細胞腫の壊死辺縁部にみられた血管糸球体ならびに係蹄形成。
c) 海綿芽細胞腫にみられた血管の硝子様膨大。
d) 海綿芽細胞腫内の、血管糸球体による血管腫様形成。

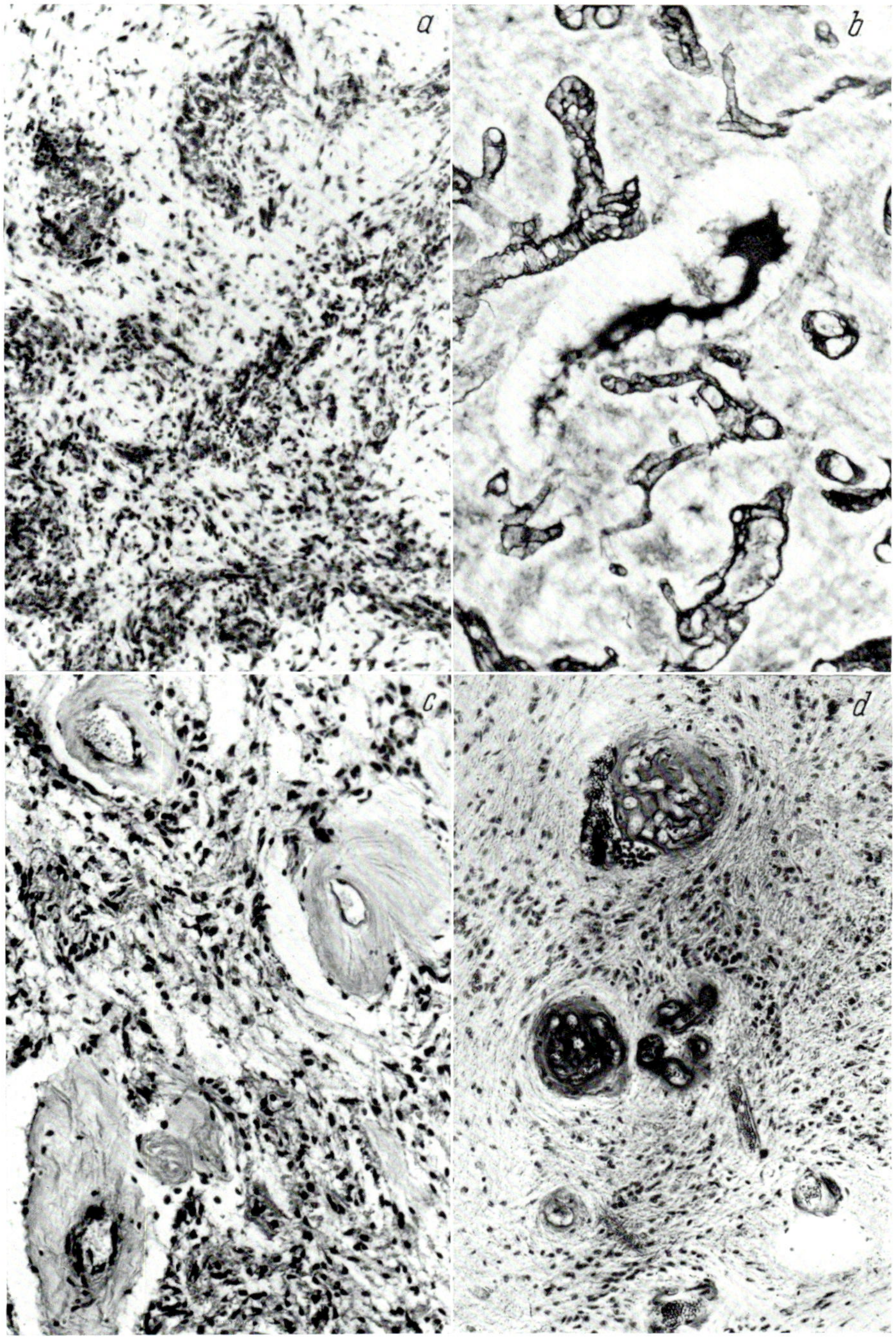

Fig. 57a—d: a ×96. Nissl stain
b ×96, Perdrau's method
c ×104. Cresyl violet stain
d ×72. Van Gieson stain

Fig. 58 — Spongioblastomas, Polar

a) Rosenthal fibers in an impregnation pattern: Here the long, wavy glial fibers become clearly visible.
b) and c) By using Heidenhain's stain, one can clearly discern the sausage-shaped formations, which occasionally consist of single fragments, tapering off like tails.
d) In the staining of glial fibers, one sees that Rosenthal fibers are formed inside the glial fibers by the deposition of special substances: A normal glial fiber is being transformed into a Rosenthal fiber.

a) Rosenthalsche Fasern in einem Imprägnationsbild: Hier werden die langen, gewellt verlaufenden Gliafasern besonders deutlich.
b) u. c) Bei Heidenhain-Färbung erkennt man deutlich die wurstförmige, gelegentlich auch aus einzelnen Bruchstücken bestehenden Bildungen, die sich schwanzartig verjüngen.
d) Bei Gliafaserfärbung sieht man, daß die Rosenthalschen Fasern sich innerhalb der Gliafasern durch Einlagerung besonderer Substanzen bilden: eine normale Gliafaser geht in die Rosenthalsche Faser über.

a) Une imprégnation métallique met bien en évidence les fibres de Rosenthal ainsi que l'aspect ondulant des longues fibres gliales.
b) et c) La coloration de Heidenhain montre nettement l'aspect boudiné et parfois fragmenté des fibres de Rosenthal, qui peuvent être réduites à de tout petits fragments.
d) Par la coloration des fibres gliales, on voit que les fibres de Rosenthal sont constituées par le dépôt de substances particulières à l'intérieur des fibres gliales: une fibre gliale normale se prolonge en fibre de Rosenthal.

a) Fibrilla de Rosenthal en una impregnación argéntica. Aquí se ven especialmente claras las largas y onduladas fibrillas gliales.
b) y c) Con la tinción de Heidenhain se reconocen claramente formaciones como salchichas, en ocasiones constitudas por varias fracciones, que se estrechan en forma de cola.
d) Con la tinción para la glía se ve que las fibras de ROSENTHAL se forman en el interior de las fibras gliales por la aparición de una substancia especial; una fibra glial pasa por encima de una fibra de Rosenthal.

a) Волокна Розенталя на импрегнированном препарате: особенно четко видны длинные волнистые глиальные волокна.
b) и c) При окраске по Гейденгайну четко видны сосиско-подобные образования, иногда состоящие из отдельных глыбок, истончающихся в виде хвоста.
d) При окраске на глиальные волокна видно, что глиальные волокна перешли в волокна Розенталя вследствие отложения в последних особых веществ

a) 金昇汞標本における Rosenthal 線維。長い、波状のグリヤ線維が、こゝで特にはっきりみとめられる。
b) および c) Heidenhain 染色によって、Rosenthal 線維は、先端がとがった、腸詰様、あるいは時に、多数の破片から成るものとして、明瞭にみとめられる。
d) グリア線維染色では、Rosenthal 線維は、グリヤ線維内物質沈着によって形成されることがわかる。正常のグリヤ線維が Rosenthal 線維に移行している。

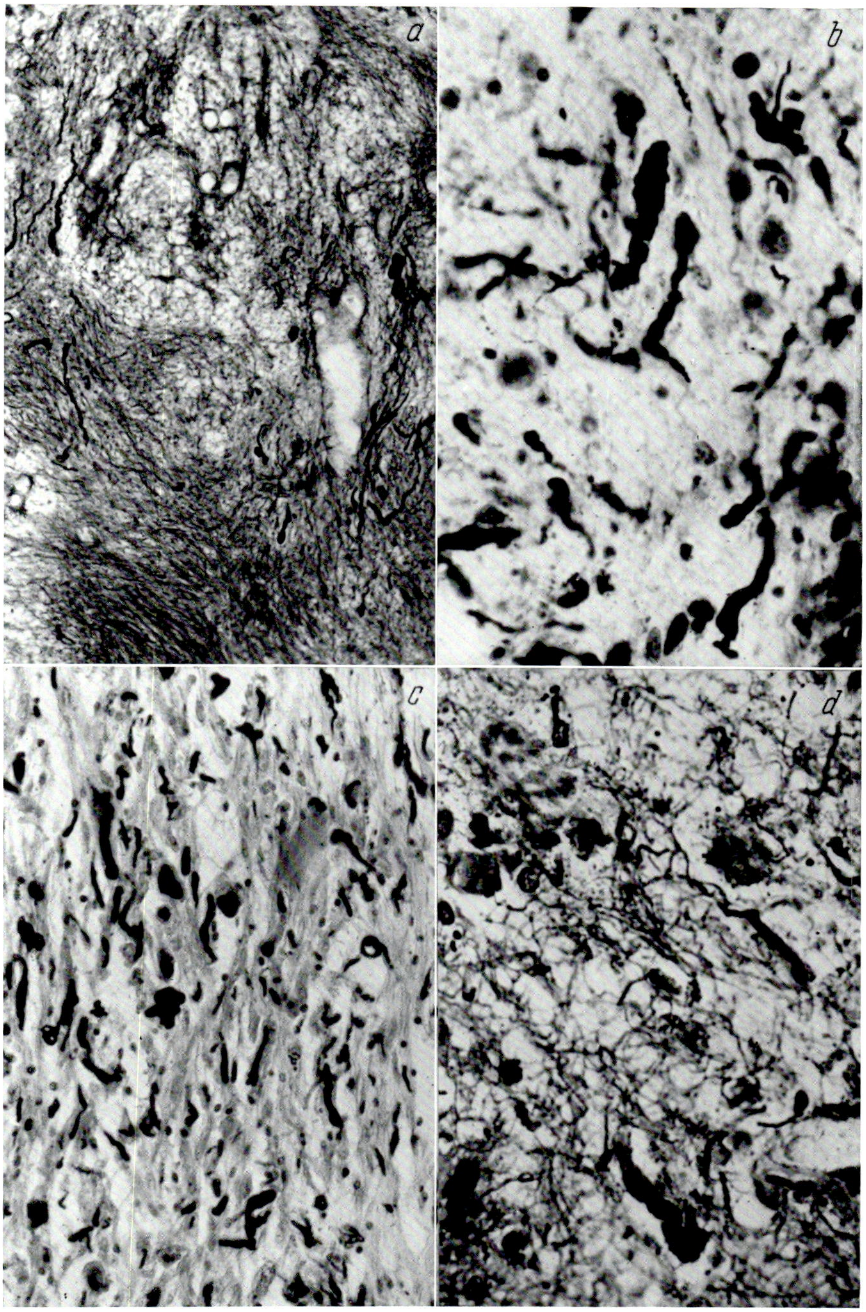

Fig. 58a—d: a ×192. Gold sublimate impregnation
b ×254, c ×122. Heidenhain's stain
d ×108. Holzer's stain

Fig. 59 — Spongioblastomas, Polar

In the *polymorphous* spongioblastoma one finds long fasicles of spindle-shaped cells as well as characteristic features of this tumor group (Rosenthal fibers, granular corpuscles). In addition, there is also evidence of rapid growth i.e. necrosis and an increased cellular polymorphism.

a) Low magnification showing an unusual amount of necrosis as well as giant cells with hyperchromatic nuclei.
b) A similar case showing several mitotic figures.
c) At 500× magnification, one sees a "granular corpuscle" in addition to individual, polymorphic, hyperchromatic, giant cells.
d) Another polymorphous spongioblastoma exhibiting several "granular corpuscles" and polymorphic giant cells.

Beim *polymorphen* Spongioblastom findet man spindelige Zellen in langen Strömen sowie die üblichen Merkmale dieser Tumorgruppe (Rosenthalsche Fasern, granulierte Körperchen), daneben aber auch die Zeichen eines beschleunigten Wachstums (Nekrosen) und einer höheren Zell-Polymorphie.

a) Bei kleiner Vergrößerung sieht man die im Spongioblastom sonst ungewöhnlichen Nekrosen sowie einzelne Riesenzellen mit hyperchromatischen Kernen.
b) In einem ähnlichen Fall findet man auch reichliche Mitosen.
c) Bei 500facher Vergrößerung findet man ein „granuliertes Körperchen" ebenso wie einzelne polymorphe hyperchromatische Riesenzellen.
d) In einem anderen Falle eines polymorphen Spongioblastoms sieht man 500fach vergrößert mehrere „granulierte Körperchen" wie auch polymorphe Riesenzellen.

Dans le spongioblastome *polymorphe*, on observe non seulement des cellules fusiformes, disposées en longs faisceaux, ainsi que des fibres de Rosenthal et des «corpuscules granuleux», qui sont caractéristiques de ce groupe de tumeurs, mais aussi des signes de croissance accélérée (nécroses) et un polymorphisme cellulaire plus marqué.

a) Au faible grossissement, on voit des nécroses inhabituelles dans le spongioblastome ainsi que de rares cellules géantes à noyaux hyperchromatiques.
b) Dans un cas similaire, on trouve également de nombreuses mitoses.
c) A un grossissement de 500×, on reconnaît un «corpuscule granuleux» et quelques cellules géantes, polymorphes et hyperchromatiques.
d) Dans un autre cas de spongioblastome polymorphe, on voit aussi plusieurs «corpuscules granuleux» ainsi que des cellules géantes polymorphes.

En los espongioblastomas *polimorfos* encuéntrase células fusiformes, alargadas con la caracteristica de estos tumores (fibras de Rosenthal y «cuerpos granulosos») pudiendose ver zonas de crecimiento rápido (necrosis) y un alto grado de polimorfismo.

a) Vemos a pequeño aumento necrosis, no común en estos tumores, con células grandes de núcleos hipercromáticos.
b) En otro caso parecido se ven muchas mitosis.
c) Con 500 aumentos vemos «cuerpos granulosos» como también células gigantes, polimorfas hipercromáticas.
d) En otro caso de espongioblastoma polimorfo se ven varios «cuerpos granulosos» así como células gigantes polimorfas.

В полиморфной спонгиобластоме видны расположенные длинными тяжами веретенообразные клетки и характерные для этой группы опухолей волокна Розенталя и зернистые тельца. Кроме того отмечается ускоренный рост (некрозы) и выраженный клеточный полиморфизм.

a) Под малым увеличением в спонгиобластоме обнаруживают необычные некрозы, а также единичные гигантские клетки с гиперхромными ядрами.
b) В аналогичном случае видны многочисленные митозы.
c) Под 500-кратным увеличением видно «зернистое тельце», а также единичные полиморфные гиперхромные гигантские клетки.
d) В другом случае полиморфной спонгиобластомы под увеличением 500× можно увидеть многочисленные «зернистые тельца», а также полиморфные гигантские клетки.

Continued on page 162

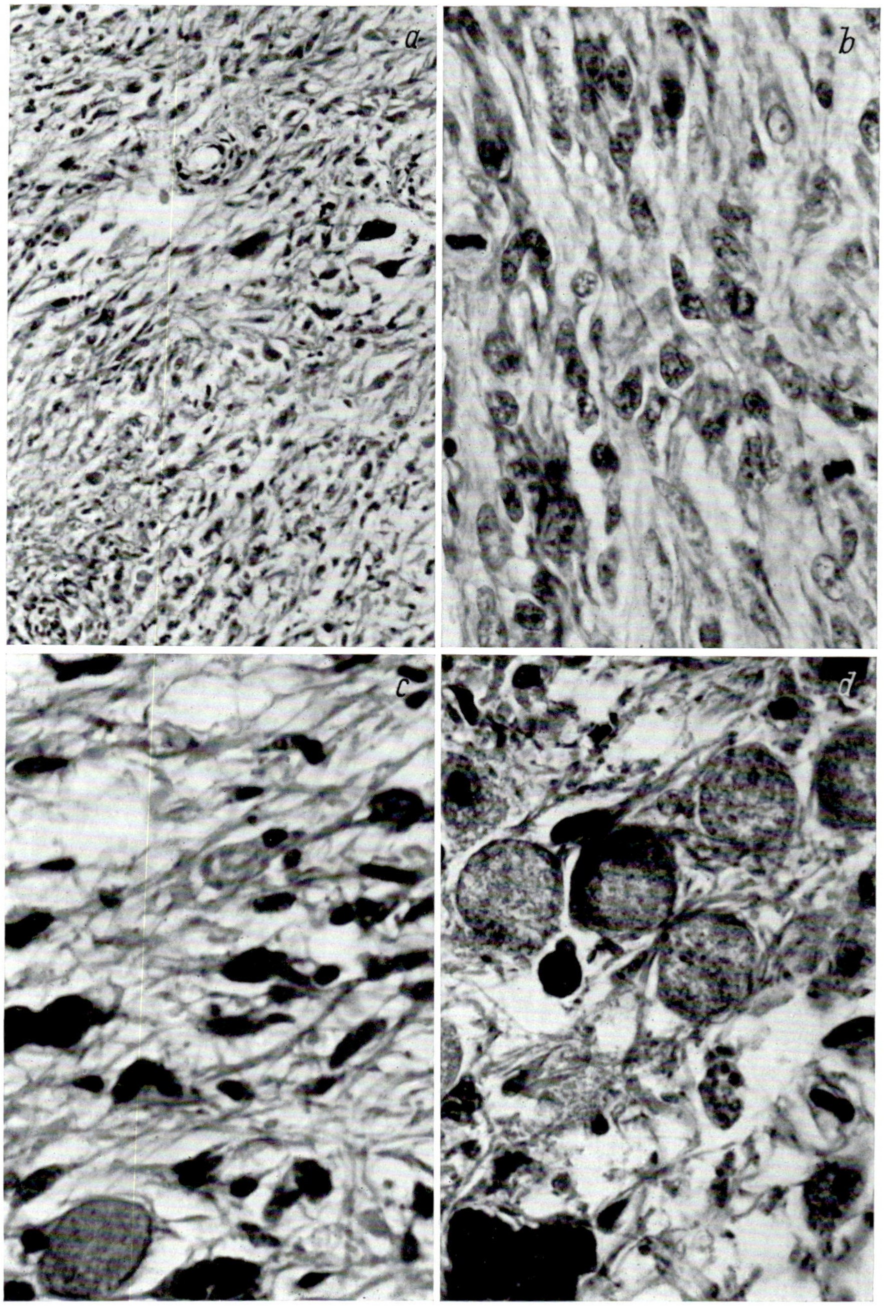

Fig. 59a—d: a ×125. H. & E. stain
b ×500. PAS
c ×500. H. & E. stain
d ×500. H. & E. stain

Fig. 59 — Spongioblastomas, Polar (continued)

多形性の海綿芽細胞腫では、紡錘形の細胞とこの腫瘍群の特徴である Rosenthal 線維および顆粒状小体がみられる。さらに急速に増殖している徴候（壊死）と高度の細胞多形性をみとめる。

a) 弱拡大では、海綿芽細胞腫内に異常な壊死部と濃染核をもった二三の巨細胞をみる。
b) 同じような例での多数の分裂像。
c) 500 倍拡大にて、多形性、濃染性巨細胞と共に顆粒状小体をみとめる。
d) 他の多形性の海綿芽細胞腫の1例にも、多形性巨細胞ならびに多数の顆粒状小体がある。

Medulloblastomas

Neuroblastoma, glioma sarcomatodes, isomorphic glioblastoma, granuloblastoma, embryonic neurogliocytoma, neurospongioma, spheroblastoma. — Medullomyoblastoma, myo-medulloblastoma

Fig. 60 — Medulloblastomas

a) General view of a typical medulloblastoma: The cells lie very densely packed in a typical architecture, in particular, pseudo-rosettes.
b) Magnification of a). Here one discerns the numerous mitoses.
c) The medulloblastoma is characterized by oval or round nuclei with a clear nuclear membrane.
d) One sees many mitoses in this medulloblastoma.

a) Übersichtsbild eines typischen Medulloblastoms: die Zellen liegen sehr dicht und bilden typische Architekturen, insbesondere auch Pseudorosetten.
b) Vergrößerung von a). Hier erkennt man deutlich die zahlreichen Mitosen.
c) Das Medulloblastom ist durch ovale oder rundliche Kerne mit deutlicher Kernmembran charakterisiert.
d) Man sieht in diesem Medulloblastom besonders viele Mitosen.

a) Vue d'ensemble d'un cas typique de médulloblastome: les cellules sont tassées les unes contre les autres et l'architecture est caractérisée notamment par le formation de pseudo-rosettes.
b) Agrandissement de a). On note un grand nombre de mitoses.
c) Les noyaux caractéristiques du médulloblastome sont ovalaires ou arrondis et possèdent une nette membrane nucléaire .
d) Dans ce cas de médulloblastome, les mitoses sont particulièrement abondantes.

a) Vista de conjunto de un meduloblastoma típico: agrupamiento compacto de células configurando una arquitectura típica, especialmente con pseudorosetas.
b) Aumento de a). Aquí se reconocen claramente las numerosas mitosis.
c) El meduloblastoma se caracteriza por núcleos ovales o redondos con una evidente membrana nuclear.
d) En este meduloblastoma se aprecian especialmente muchas mitosis.

a) Обзорный снимок типичной медуллобластомы. Густое расположение опухолевых клеток. Типичная структура с образованием псевдорозеток.
b) Увеличение a). Четко видны многочисленные митозы.
c) Медуллобластома с овальными или округлыми ядрами с отчетливой ядерной мембраной.
d) Медуллобластома с многочисленными митозами.

a) 定型的な髄芽腫の概観像。腫瘍細胞は非常に密で、偽ロゼッテを伴い典型的な組織構造を示す。
b) a)の拡大。こゝには、多数の核分裂がみられる。
c) 髄芽腫の細胞核は楕円ないし円形で明瞭な核膜を有する。
d) この髄芽腫例には核分裂が特に多い。

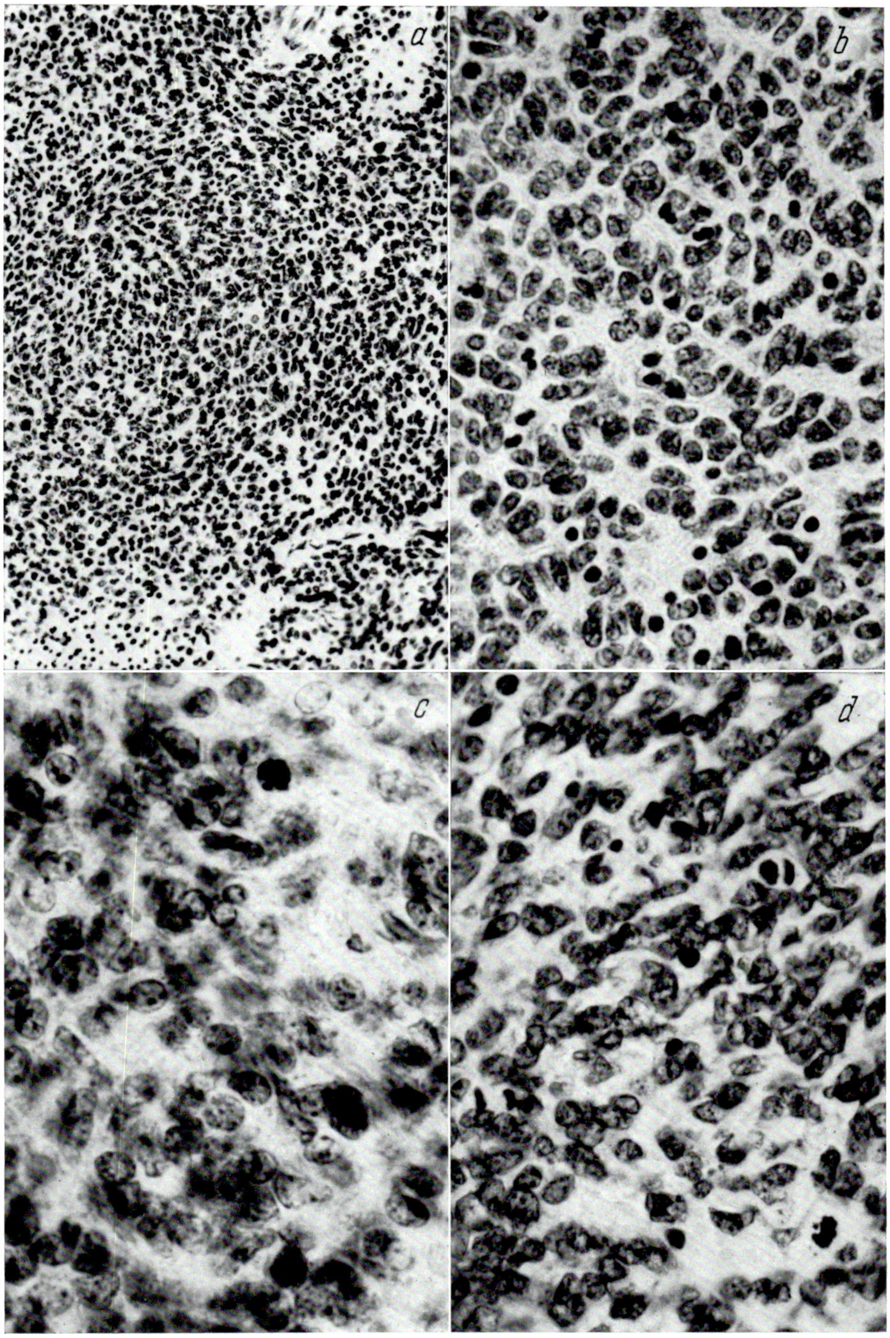

Fig. 60a—d: a ×80. Cresyl violet stain
b ×230. Cresyl violet stain
c ×600. Nissl stain
d ×448. Cresyl violet stain

Fig. 61 — Medulloblastomas

a) Higher magnifications occasionally show more vesicular cell nuclei with delicate chromatin network, clearly visible nuclear membranes and a single dark nucleolus. The cell body can still be recognized as a cap on the top and bottom of the nucleus.
b) A "classical" pseudo-rosette formation is further accentuated by the turnip-shaped appearance of the tumor cells.
c) In other medulloblastomas one sees a symmetrical chromatin network with some rather coarse granules, which frequently lie peripherally. In the center there are often one or two nucleoli.
d) With silver staining, one can demonstrate individual delicate protoplasmic processes in between the nuclei.

a) Höhere Vergrößerungen zeigen gelegentlich mehr bläschenförmige Zellkerne mit zartem Chromatinnetz und deutlicher Kernmembran und einem einzelnen dunklen Nucleolus. Der Zelleib ist als polständige Kappe noch zu erkennen.
b) Eine „klassische" Ausbildung von Pseudorosetten wird noch durch die rübenförmige Gestalt der Geschwulstzellen betont.
c) In anderen Medulloblastomen sieht man ein gleichmäßiges Chromatinnetz mit einigen gröberen Körnchen, die häufig randständig liegen. In der Mitte oft 1—2 Nucleolen.
d) Bei Versilberung kann man zwischen den Kernen einzelne zarte protoplasmatische Fortsätze darstellen.

a) A un grossissement plus élévé, les noyaux du médulloblastome ont parfois un aspect vésiculaire et présentent un réseau délicat de chromatine, une membrane nucléaire nette et un seul nucléole dense. Le cytoplasme est à peine visible et coiffe l'extrémité du noyau.
b) Les cellules tumorales ont une forme nettement allongée, qui accentue encore l'aspect «classique» des pseudo-rosettes.
c) Dans d'autres cas de médulloblastome, les noyaux contiennent un réseau chromatinien uniforme, au sein duquel on note quelques granules plus volumineux et fréquemment disposés à la périphérie. Un ou deux nucléoles occupent souvent le centre du noyau.
d) Entre les noyaux, quelques fins prolongements cellulaires peuvent être mis en évidence par une imprégnation argentique.

a) A mayores aumentos pueden verse en ocasiones más núcleos vesiculares con una red de cromatina débil, membrana nuclear evidente y ún nucleolo obscuro, único. El cuerpo celular se puede reconocer como un pequeño polo restante.
b) La clásica formación de pseudorosetas se ve todavía acentuada por la forma de nabo de las células tumorales.
c) En otros meduloblastomas se ve una red cromatínica uniforme con algunos gránulos más gruesos que generalmente se sitúan periféricamente. En el medio se encuentran uno o dos nucleolos.
d) Con la tinción de la plata se pueden demostrar algunas débiles prolongaciones protoplasmáticas entre los núcleos.

a) Под большим увеличением видны многочисленные пузырькообразные ядра с нежной хроматиновой сетью, отчетливой ядерной мембраной и темным ядрышком.
b) «Классическое» образование псевдорозеток еще больше подчеркивается свеклообразной формой опухолевых клеток.
c) В других медуллобластомах видны клетки с равномерной хроматиновой сетью с виде отдельных крупных зёрен, расположенных по краям. В центре 1—2 ядрышка.
d) На препарате, импрегнированном серебром, между ядрами отдельные нежные протоплазматические отростки.

a) 強拡大によって、せん細なクロマチン網、明瞭な核膜、1個の濃染核小体をもった小胞状の核が時々みとめられる。胞体は一部核周辺にみとめるのみ。
b) 紡錘状の腫瘍細胞が形作る「古典的」な偽ロゼッテ。
c) 別な髄芽腫例における核の所見。クロマチン網は一様に分布し、おもに辺在する粗大顆粒をともなっている。しばしば1個ないし2個の核小体が、核の中心部にある。
d) 鍍銀によって、いくつかの細い胞体突起が核の間に染出される。

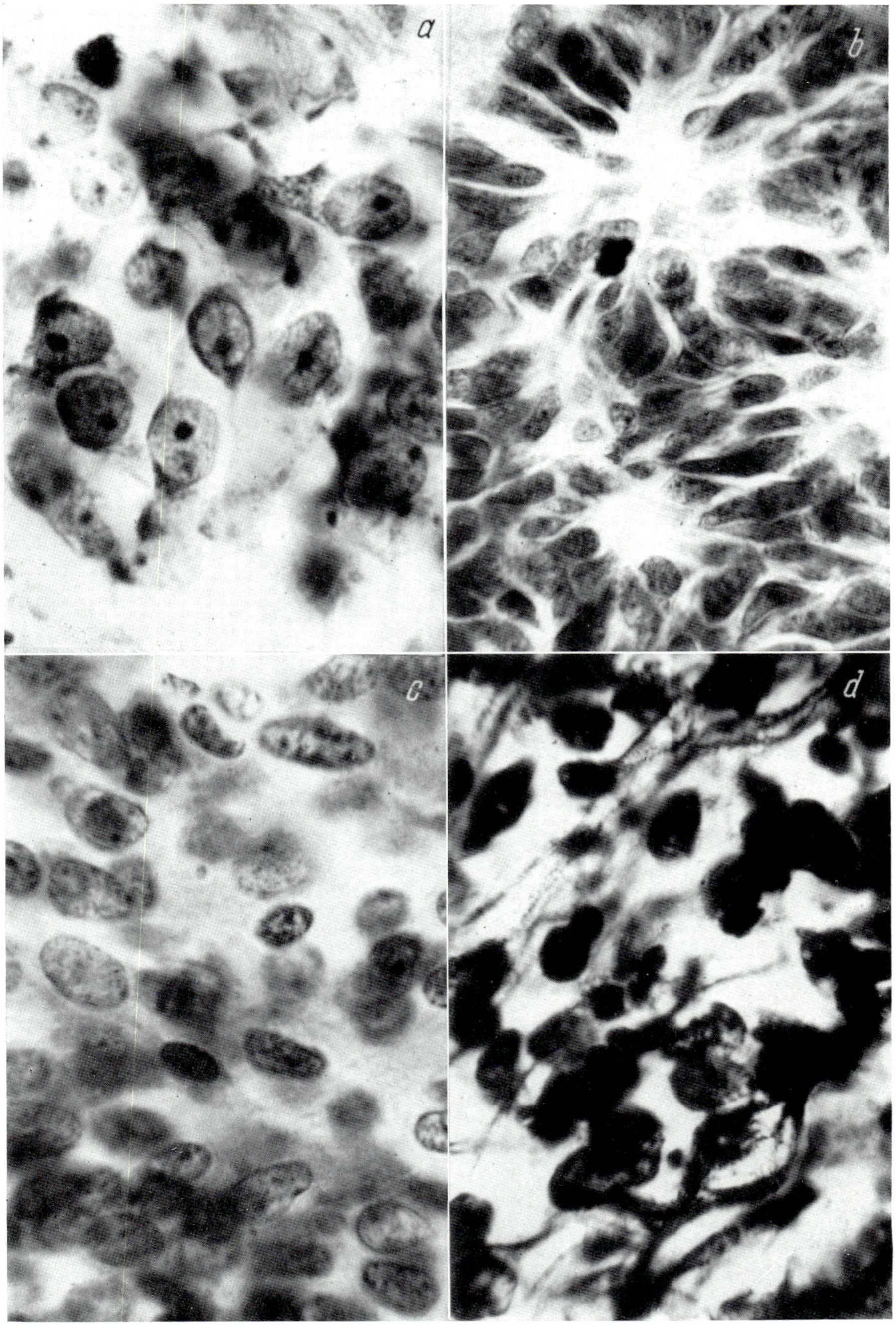

Fig. 61a—d: a ×1,440. Nissl stain
b ×780. c ×948. Cresyl violet stain
d ×1,200. Perdrau's method

Fig. 62 — Medulloblastomas

a) The action of the arachnoidal meshes in shaping the tumor cells of a medulloblastoma can be perceived here in that the cells are all placed in narrow bands.
b) Occasionally, on infiltration of the cerebellar cortex, a "comb" formation occurs between the dendrites of the Purkinje cells.
c) Between the longitudinally oriented cells the fibers of the arachnoidal meshwork are still clearly recognizable.
d) On infiltration of the arachnoidea one occasionally sees, an island-shaped architecture, in addition to an orientation in to narrow bands.

a) Die formende Wirkung der arachnoidalen Maschen auf die Geschwulstzellen eines Medulloblastoms kann man daran erkennen, daß hier die Zellen alle in schmalen Bändern gelagert sind.
b) Gelegentlich entsteht bei Infiltration der Kleinhirnrinde zwischen den Dendriten der Purkinjezellen eine ,,Kamm"-Bildung.
c) Zwischen den längsausgerichteten Zellen sind die Fasern des arachnoidalen Maschenwerks noch deutlich erkennbar.
d) Bei Infiltration der Arachnoidea sieht man außer einer Ausrichtung in schmalen Bändern auch gelegentlich eine inselförmige Architektur.

a) Les cellules tumorales d'un médulloblastome sont moulées dans les espaces sous-arachnoïdiens, ce qui explique leur disposition en petits rubans.
b) Image en «peigne» due à l'invasion de l'écorce cérébelleuse par les cellules tumorales, qui s'infiltrent entre les dendrites des cellules de Purkinje.
c) Les travées sous-arachnoïdiennes sont encore bien visibles entre les colonnes de cellules alignées.
d) Dans les espaces sous-arachnoïdiens envahis par la tumeur, les cellules se disposent en petites rangées et se groupent parfois en îlots.

a) La acción modeladora de las mallas aracnoidales sobre las células tumorales de un meduloblastoma se reconoce en que aquí las células se disponen todas en estrechas bandas.
b) Ocasionalmente se encuentra una formación en peine por la infiltración de la corteza cerebelosa a través de las dendritas de las células de Purkinje.
c) A través de las células alineadas pueden reconocerse todavía claramente los fascículos de las mallas aracnoidales.
d) Debido a la infiltración de la aracnoides ocasionalmente se ve, además de la disposición en estrechas bandas, una arquitectura insular.

a) Формирующее воздействие арахноидальных петель на опухолевые клетки медуллобластомы явствует из того, что в ней все клетки расположены в виде узких тяжей.
b) Иногда при инфильтрации коры мозжечка между дендритами клеток Пуркинье возникают образования в виде «гребешка».
c) Между удлиненными клетками еще четко видны волокна арахноидальной сети.
d) При инфильтрации паутинной оболочки кроме узких тяжей также видны островкоподобные структуры.

a) 髄芽腫浸潤に際して、クモ膜線維網は腫瘍構築の形成にあづかる。その結果、腫瘍細胞はここにみられるように、すべて細索状にならんでいる。
b) 小脳皮質浸潤の場合、腫瘍細胞は、時々、Purkinje 細胞樹状突起間にならんで「櫛状」の配列を示す。
c) 長い列をなした腫瘍細胞間に、クモ膜の線維がまだはっきりみとめられる。
d) クモ膜浸潤巣には、索状のならびのほかに、島状の構造もまた存在している。

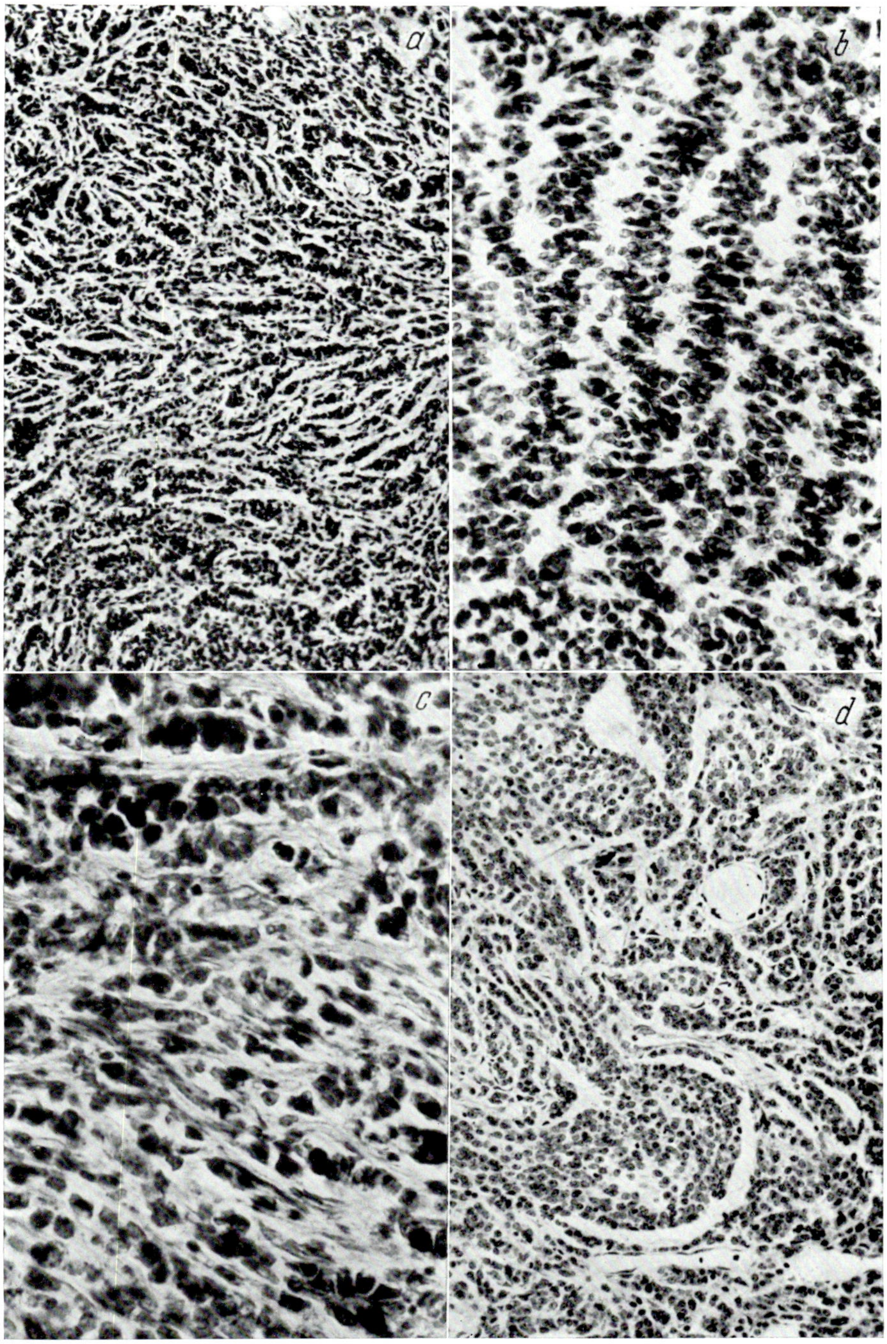

Fig. 62a—d: a ×84. Nissl stain
b ×272, c ×370, d ×136. Cresyl violet stain

Fig. 63 — Medulloblastomas

a) Between light, barely visible, tumor cells lay foci of very dark, perhaps smaller, cells.
b) Fresh, diffuse necrosis: remaining cells are barely recognizable; in contrast one sees numerous chromatin clumps resulting from nuclear fragmentation.
c) Foci of small, dark, "lymphoid" cells in a medulloblastoma.
d) Necrosis in a linear form in a medulloblastoma. At the border there is, characteristically, a wall of hyperchromatic cells showing degenerative changes.

a) Zwischen den hellen, kaum sichtbaren Geschwulstzellen liegen Herde von besonders dunkel gefärbten, etwas kleineren Zellen.
b) Frische, diffuse Nekrose: Die noch verschonten Zellen sind kaum zu erkennen, dagegen sieht man reichlich grobe Chromatinbrocken als Reste des Kernzerfalls.
c) Herd kleiner, dunkler „lymphoider" Zellen in einem Medulloblastom.
d) Strichförmige Nekrose in einem Medulloblastom. Am Rande liegt typisch ein Wall von hyperchromatischen Zellen in regressiver Veränderung.

a) Entre les cellules tumorales claires, à peine visibles, on voit des amas de cellules un peu plus petites et de coloration nettement plus foncée.
b) Nécrose récente et diffuse: à côté de cellules qui sont encore épargnées et qui se reconnaissent difficilement, de nombreux blocs grossiers de chromatine sont les restes de noyaux détruits.
c) Foyer de petites cellules «lymphoïdes» dans un médulloblastome.
d) Dans un médulloblastome, nécrose linéaire, entourée par une rangée typique de cellules devenues hyperchromatiques par suite des altérations régressives.

a) Entre células claras, hinchadas, encuentranse otras pequeñas obscuras.
b) Necrosis difusa reciente; células apenas reconocibles junto con granulaciones cromatínicas, restos de núcleos.
c) Grupos de pequeñas células de tipo linfoide en un meduloblastoma.
d) Necrosis en forma linear en un meduloblastoma. En el límite aparece, de forma típica, una secuencia de células hipercromáticas en regresiôn.

a) Между светлыми, едва различимыми, опухолевыми клетками находятся очаги темно-окрашенных мелких клеток.
b) Свежий диффузный некроз: едва различимы еще сохранившиеся клетки. Зато видны многочисленные грубые глыбки хроматина — остатки разрушенных ядер.
c) Очаг мелких, темных «лимфоидных» клеток в медуллобластоме.
d) Полосы некроза в медуллобластоме. По краю типичный вал из гиперхромных регрессивно измененных клеток.

a) 明るく、輪郭の不明な腫瘍細胞の間に、特に濃染したやゝ小形の細胞群がある。
b) 新鮮なびまん性壊死。大部分の細胞が変化をうけている。他方、核崩壊の遺残として、粗大なクロマチン塊がみられる。
c) 髄芽腫内にみられた小型、濃染性リンパ球様細胞の集団。
d) 髄芽細胞腫内の索状壊死。壊死辺縁部に退行変化を示す濃染核をもった細胞の壁がある。

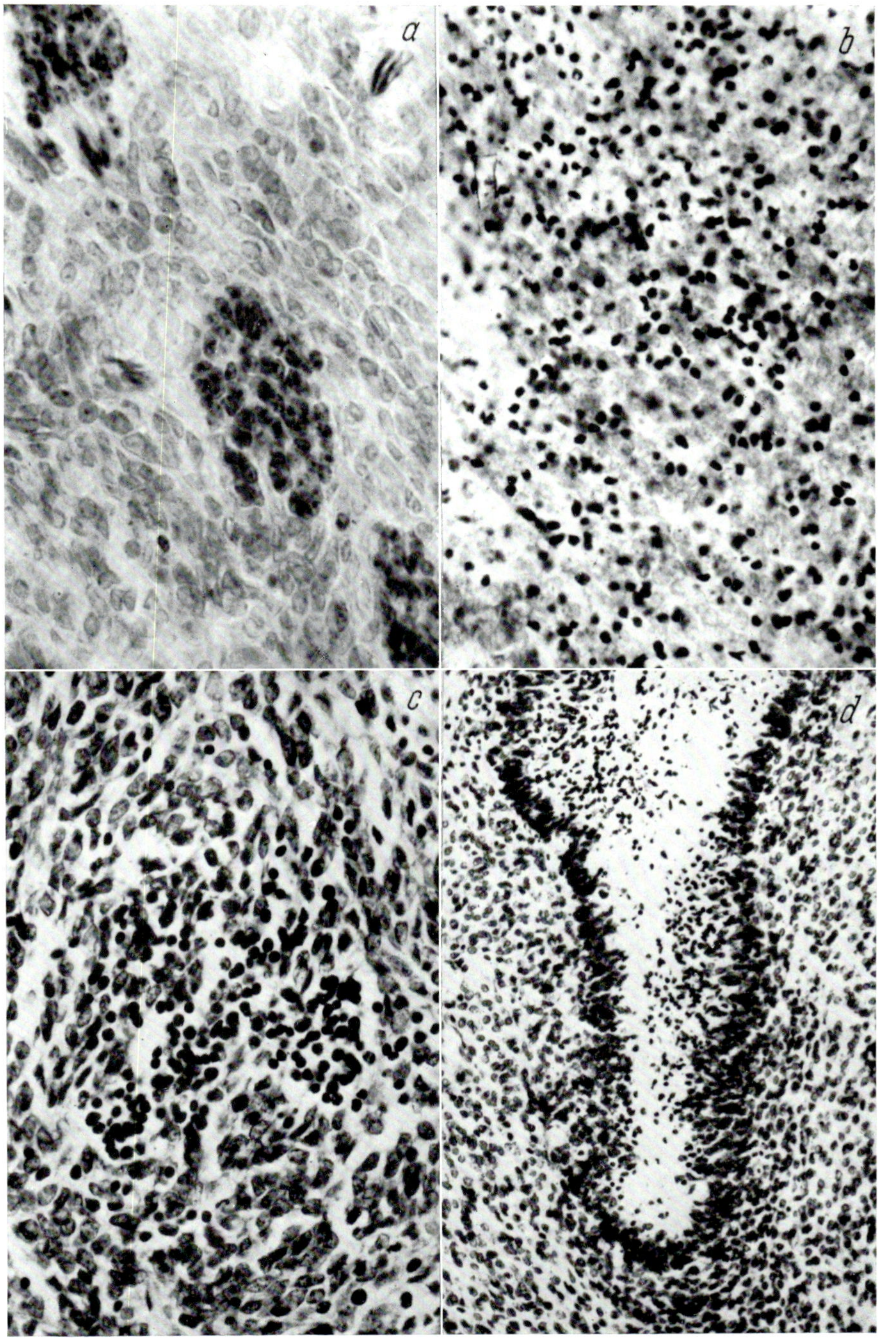

Fig. 63a—d: a ×405. Perdrau's method
b ×405, c ×272, d ×136. Cresyl violet stain

Fig. 64 — Medulloblastomas

a) Smooth muscle cells along the vessels of a medulloblastoma.
b) Progressive enlargement of the fibrous net of the arachnoid and increase in the size of individual fibers associated with an infiltrating medulloblastoma.
c) Pronounced accumulation of small and large vessels in a medulloblastoma: the plexus became overgrown and included within the tumor. Plexus epithelium is still recognizable within the tumor.
d) Glomerular-like growth of vessels along a necrotic border (rare).

a) Glatte Muskelzellen entlang den Gefäßen eines Medulloblastoms.
b) Progressiv verstärktes und vermehrtes Maschennetz der Arachnoidea bei Infiltration durch ein Medulloblastom.
c) Ausgesprochene Häufung von kleineren und größeren Gefäßen in einem Medulloblastom: Hier wurde der Plexus umwachsen und in die Geschwulst miteinbezogen. Man erkennt noch einzelne Plexusepithelien.
d) Glomerulusartige Wucherung von Gefäßen am Rande einer Nekrose (selten!).

a) Cellules musculaires lisses le long d'un vaisseau dans un médulloblastome.
b) Epaississement et prolifération des trabécules des espaces sous-arachnoïdiens envahis par un médulloblastome.
c) Accumulation importante de petits et de grands vaisseaux dans un médulloblastome, par suite de l'infiltration des plexus choroïdes, qui sont englobés dans la tumeur. On reconnaît encore quelques fragments épithéliaux des plexus.
d) Prolifération de vaisseaux en forme de glomérules au bord d'une nécrose (rare!).

a) Células musculares lisas a lo largo de vasos en un meduloblastoma.
b) Progresivo aumento de la malla aracnoidea por infiltración de un meduloblastoma.
c) Conglomerados de vasos grandes y pequeños en un meduloblastoma. Aqui infiltran plexos y tumor, viéndose todavía el epitelio de los plexos.
d) Crecimiento en forma glomerular de los vasos alrededor de una necrosis (raro!).

a) Гладкие мышечные клетки вдоль сосудов медуллобластомы.
b) Усиленное разрастание петель паутинной оболочки при инфильтрации ее медуллобластомой.
c) Выраженное скопление мелких и крупных сосудов в медуллобластоме: прорастание плексуса опухолью. Еще распознаются единичные эпителиальные клетки плексуса.
d) Клубочковидное разрастание сосудов по краю некроза (редкое явление!).

a) 髄芽腫内の血管に沿って散在する平滑筋細胞。
b) 髄芽腫の浸潤にみられたクモ膜の網状構造の進行性増強。
c) 髄芽腫の大小さまざまな血管の著明な充血。こゝでは脉絡叢は増殖し、腫瘍内に含まれている。まだ二三の脉絡叢上皮をみとめる。
d) 壊死辺縁部における血管の糸球体状増殖(稀である！)。

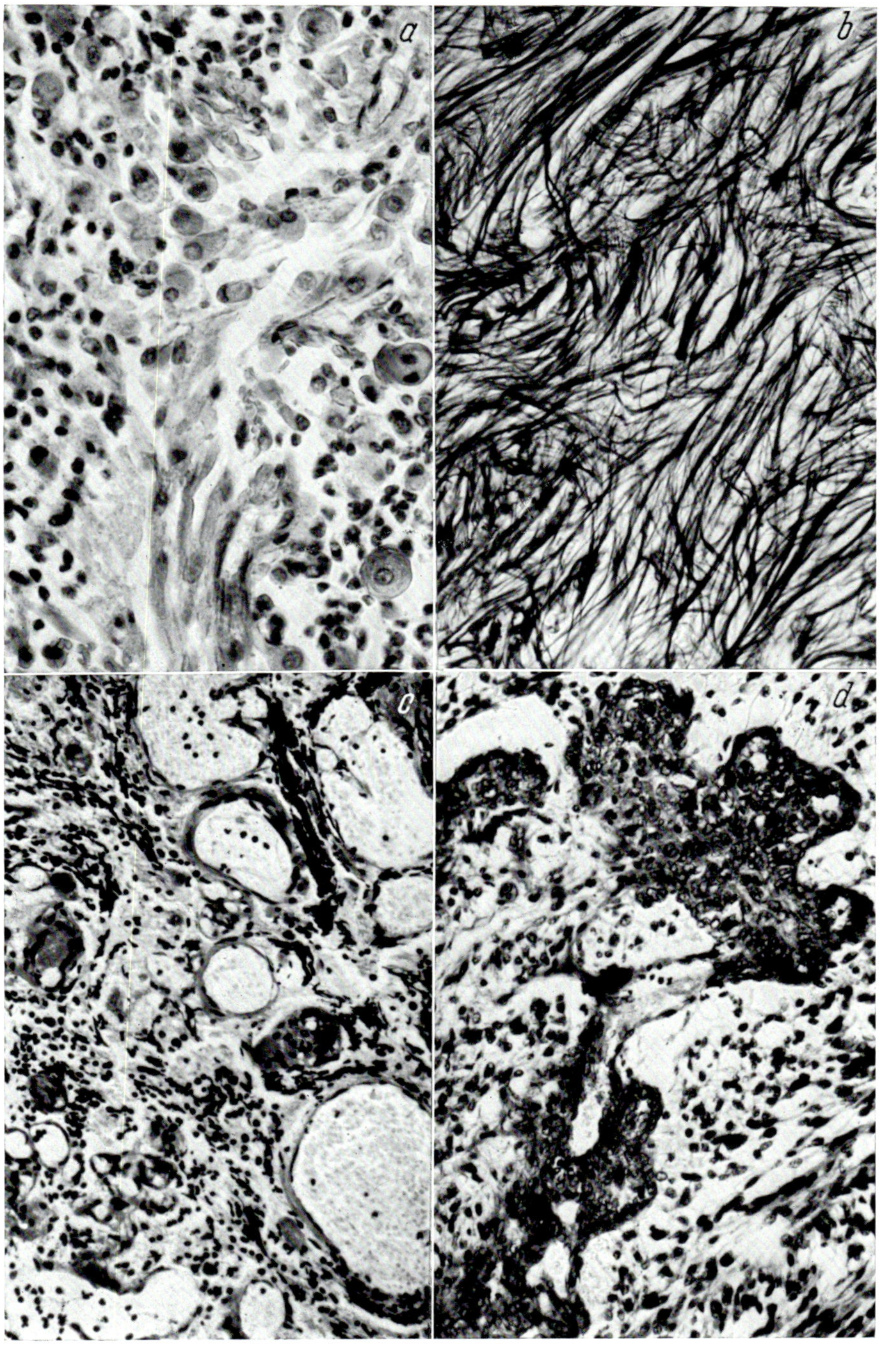

Fig. 64a—d: a ×288. H. & E. stain
b ×136. Perdrau's method
c and d ×136. Cresyl violet stain

Fig. 65 — Medulloblastomas

a) On low magnification the infiltration of the arachnoidea is demonstrated (bottom), while one recognizes a cerebellar lobule still containing some Purkinje cells (*top*). The molecular layer is thinly infiltrated and the granular layer densely permeated.
b) The darkly stained portions in the tumor tissue are still easy to recognize as infiltrated lobes which are swollen by proliferation and are being turned into a uniform tumor mass. At the cerebellar lobule in the midline, one discerns the individual stages of infiltration: The subpial zone is expanded, the molecular layer densely permeated, as well as the granular layer.
c) Here one perceives the dense infiltration in the subpial layer of two lobes adjoining one another: From the arachnoidea the tumor cells advance in narrow rows against the granular layer (*bottom right*).
d) Pronounced perivascular growth of a medulloblastoma.

a) Bei kleiner Vergrößerung stellt sich hier die Infiltration der Arachnoidea (unten) dar, während man oben ein Kleinhirnläppchen noch mit einigen Purkinjezellen erkennt. Die Molekularschicht ist dünn infiltriert, die Körnerschicht dicht durchsetzt.
b) Die dunkel gefärbten Partien im Geschwulstgewebe sind unschwer noch als infiltrierte und durch Infiltration aufgetriebene Läppchen zu erkennen, die gerade zu einer einheitlichen Geschwulstmasse verbacken werden. An den Kleinhirnläppchen in der Mitte erkennt man die einzelnen Stadien der Infiltration: die subpiale Zone ist verbreitert, die Molekularschicht stark durchsetzt, ebenso die Körnerschicht.
c) Hier erkennt man in der subpialen Schicht zweier aneinander grenzender Läppchen die dichte Infiltration: von der Arachnoidea dringen die Geschwulstzellen in schmalen Reihen gegen die Körnerschicht (rechts unten) vor.
d) Ausgesprochen perivasculäres Wachstum eines Medulloblastoms.

a) A un plus faible grossissement, on voit bien l'infiltration des espaces sous-arachnoïdiens (en bas). Dans la partie supérieure de la figure, on reconnaît une lamelle cérébelleuse contenant encore des cellules de Purkinje. Il existe une infiltration modérée de la couche moléculaire et un envahissement dense de la couche granulaire par la tumeur.
b) On peut facilement reconnaître que les parties foncées du tissu tumoral sont constituées par les lamelles cérébelleuses infiltrées et refoulées, qui se sont agglutinées entre elles pour former une seule masse tumorale. Dans une petite lamelle située au milieu de la figure, on reconnaît les différents stades de l'infiltration: propagation importante dans la zone sous-piale, envahissement diffus des couches moléculaire et granulaire.
c) Au niveau de deux lamelles contiguës, la tumeur infiltre fortement la couche sous-piale, à partir de laquelle de petites rangées de cellules tumorales s'enfonçent vers la couche granulaire à la partie inférieure droite de la figure.
d) Forte croissance périvasculaire des cellules d'un médulloblastome.

a) A pequeño aumento podemos ver (abajo) la infiltración de la aracnoides; en cambio arriba puede verse un lobulillo cerebeloso todavía con algunas células de Purkinje. La capa molecular está escasamente infiltrada, la granular en cambio, fuertemente invadida.
b) Las partes obscuras del tejido tumoral son fácilmente reconocibles como lobulillos infiltrados y desplazados, que acaban de aglutinarse en una única masa tumoral. En el lobulillo cerebeloso se reconocen, en el medio, los diversos estadíos de la infiltración: la zona subpial está ensanchada, la molecular fuertemente ocupada lo mismo que la granular.
c) En la capa subpial de estos dos lobulillos fronterizos se reconoce la fuerte infiltración: las células tumorales penetran desde la aracnoides en finas hileras hacia la capa de los granos (derecha, abajo).
d) Pronunciado crecimiento perivascular de un meduloblastoma.

Continued on page 176

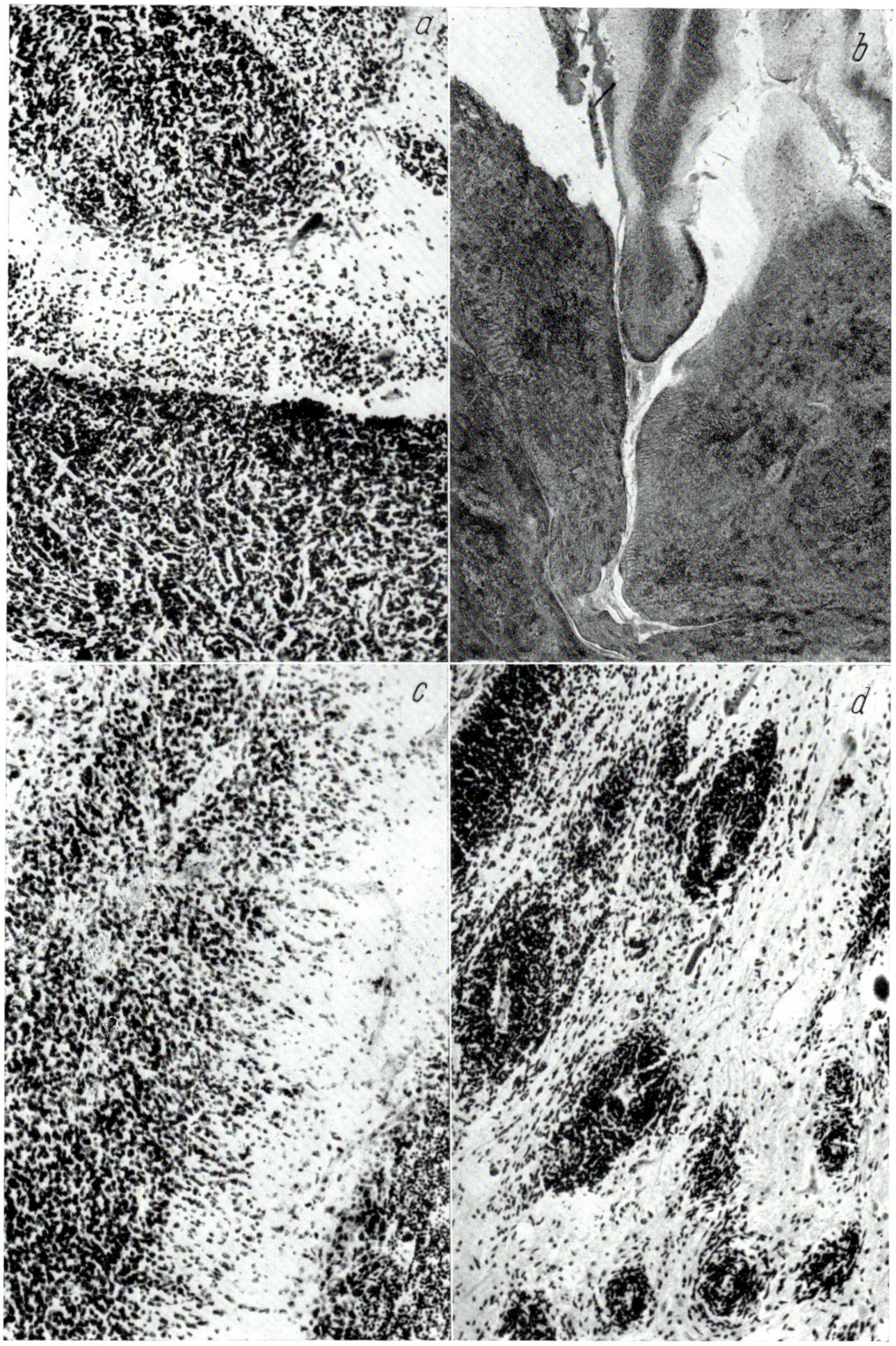

Fig. 65a—d: a ×78, b ×10. Nissl stain
c ×90, d ×84. Cresyl violet stain

Fig. 65 — Medulloblastomas (continued)

a) Под малым увеличением прослеживается инфильтрация паутинной оболочки (внизу), а вверху еще видна долька мозжечка с клетками Пуркинье. Редкая инфильтрация молекулярного слоя и густая инфильтрация зернистого слоя.
b) В тёмно-окрашенных участках единой опухолевой массы еще легко распознаются инфильтрированные опухолевыми клетками дольки мозжечка. В центре долек мозжечка видны отдельные стадии инфильтрации: расширение субпиальной зоны, прорастание молекулярного, а также зернистого слоев мозжечка.
c) Густая инфильтрация опухолевыми клетками двух граничащих долек субпиального слоя, распространяющейся узкими рядами в зернистый слой мозга (справа внизу).
d) Выраженный периваскулярный рост медуллобластомы.

a) クモ膜浸潤（図下）の弱拡大像。図の上半に、まだいくらかの Purkinje 細胞の残存した小脳小葉がある。分子層には疎な、顆粒層には密な腫瘍浸潤をみとめる。
b) 腫瘍組織の濃染した部分は、浸潤と増殖によって腫大した小葉であることがまだ判別できる。これらはたがいに融合をはじめる。浸潤の各時期、すなわち軟膜下層の拡張、分子層顆粒層内のびまん性浸潤が図の中央の小葉にみられる。
c) むかいあった２小葉間に、密な軟膜下腫瘍浸潤がある。腫瘍細胞は、クモ膜から細い列をなして、顆粒層に浸入している。
d) 髄芽腫にみられた、著明な血管周囲増殖。

Neurinomas

Schwannoma, neurilemoma, perineurial fibroblastoma, neurofibroma, lemmoma, lemmoblastoma, chitoneuroma, gliofibroma, peripheral glioma

Fig. 66 — Neurinomas

Various architectures in the fibrillary portions of a neurinoma:
a) and b) Very pronounced palisading of the nuclei in a spinal neurinoma.
c) Arrangement of the tumor cells in long streams.
d) Retroversion and whorl formation.

Verschiedene Architekturen in den fibrillären Partien eines Neurinoms:
a) u. b) Besonders ausgeprägte Palisadenstellung der Kerne in einem spinalen Neurinom.
c) Anordnung der Geschwulstzellen in langen Strömen.
d) Umbiegungsstellen und Strudelbildung.

Différents aspects architecturaux dans les zones fibrillaires d'un neurinome.
a) et b) Arrangement très prononcé des noyaux en palissades dans un neurinome spinal.
c) Disposition des cellules tumorales en longs faisceaux.
d) Disposition sinueuse et tourbillonnante.

Diferentes arquitecturas en las zonas fibrilares de un neurinoma.
a) y b) Zonas especialmente extensas con nucleos dispuestos en empalizada en un caso de neurinoma espinal.
c) Disposición de las células tumorales en largas corrientes.
d) Zonas con acodaduras y formación de remolinos.

Различное строение фибриллярных участков невриномы:
a) и b) Невринома спинного мозга. Выраженное расположение ядер в виде палисадов.
c) Расположение опухолевых клеток в виде длинных пучков.
d) Образование завитков и завихрений.

神経鞘腫の線維性部の種々な組織像。
a) および b) 脊椎内神経鞘腫にみられた著明な核の柵状配列。
c) 腫瘍細胞の流線状配列。
d) 腫瘍細胞束の折れ返りと渦状配列。

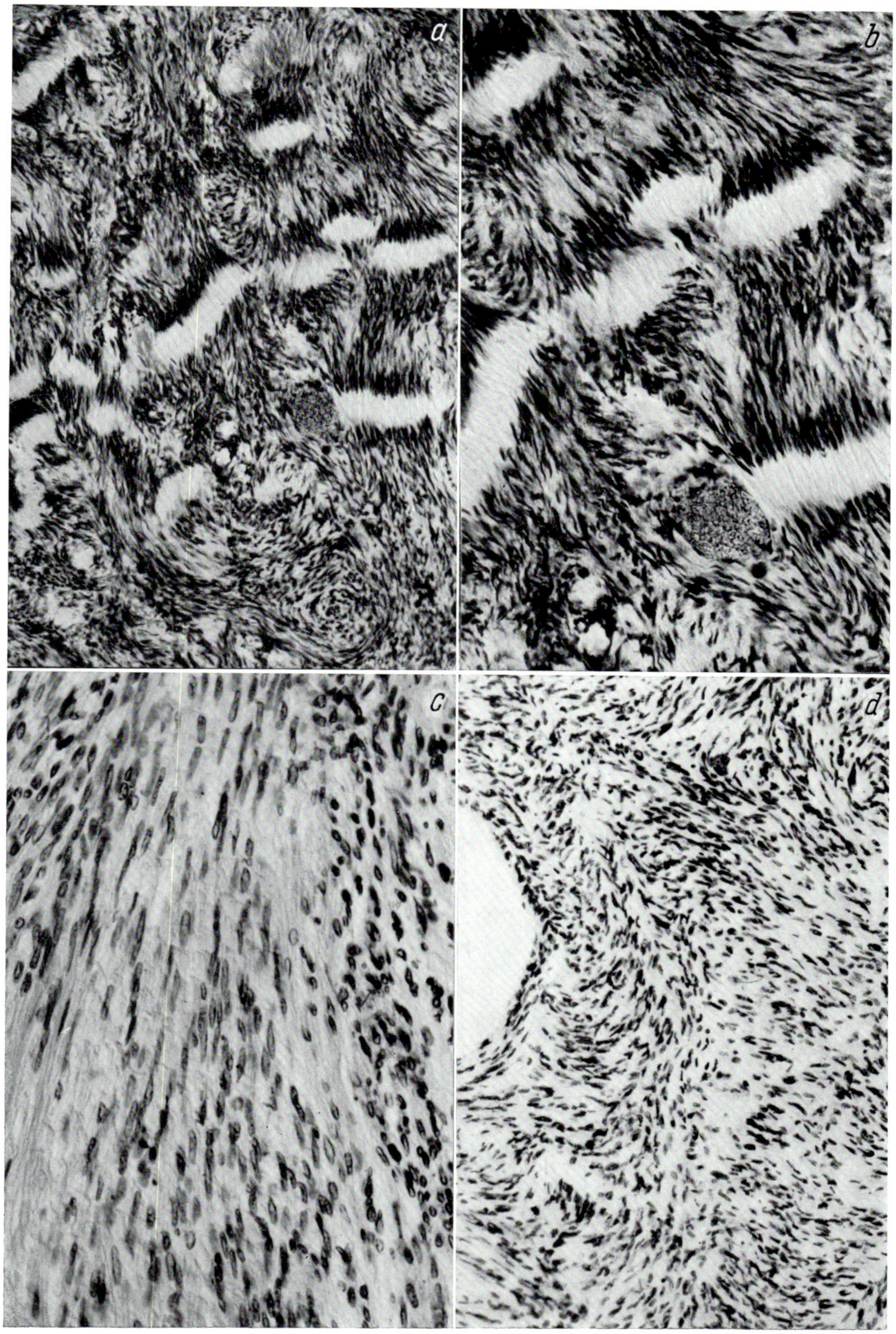

Fig: 66a—d: a and d ×86, b ×134, c ×285
Cresyl violet stain

Fig. 67 — Neurinomas

a) Large oval nuclei in an otherwise typical neurinoma.
b) Typical rod-shaped nuclei; otherwise like a).
c) A giant cell with a chromatin-rich nucleus.
d) Accumulation of large "ganglioid" cells in a small neurinoma of the cauda (accidental finding).

a) Große ovale Kerne in einem sonst typischen Neurinom.
b) Typische stäbchenförmige Kerne, sonst wie a).
c) Eine Riesenzelle mit chromatinreichem Kern.
d) Ansammlung großer ,,ganglioider" Zellen in einem kleinen Neurinom der Cauda (Zufallsbefund).

a) Volumineux noyau ovalaire au sein d'un neurinome par ailleurs typique.
b) Noyaux typiques en bâtonnets.
c) Présence d'une cellule géante avec noyaux riche en chromatine.
d) Accumulation de grandes cellules «ganglioïdes» dans un petit neurinome de la queue de cheval (découverte occasionnelle).

a) Nucleos grandes y ovales en un neurinoma por lo demás típico.
b) Típicos núcleos en maza; por lo demás como a).
c) Una célula gigante con núcleo rico en cromatina.
d) Acúmulo de grandes células ganglioides en un pequeño neurinoma de la cola (encuentro fortuito).

a) Типичная невринома с крупными овальными ядрами.
b) Типичные палочковидные ядра в том же случае.
c) Гигантская клетка с ядром, богатым хроматином.
d) Небольшая невринома конского хвоста (обнаруженная случайно). Скопление крупных «ганглиоидных» клеток.

a) 大きな楕円形核。その他の構造は定型的な神経鞘腫の特徴をそなえている。
b) 神経鞘腫に特有な、小桿状の核。ほかは a) に同じ。
c) 濃染核をもった巨細胞。
d) 馬尾神経の神経鞘腫の１例にみられた、神経細胞様の細胞群。

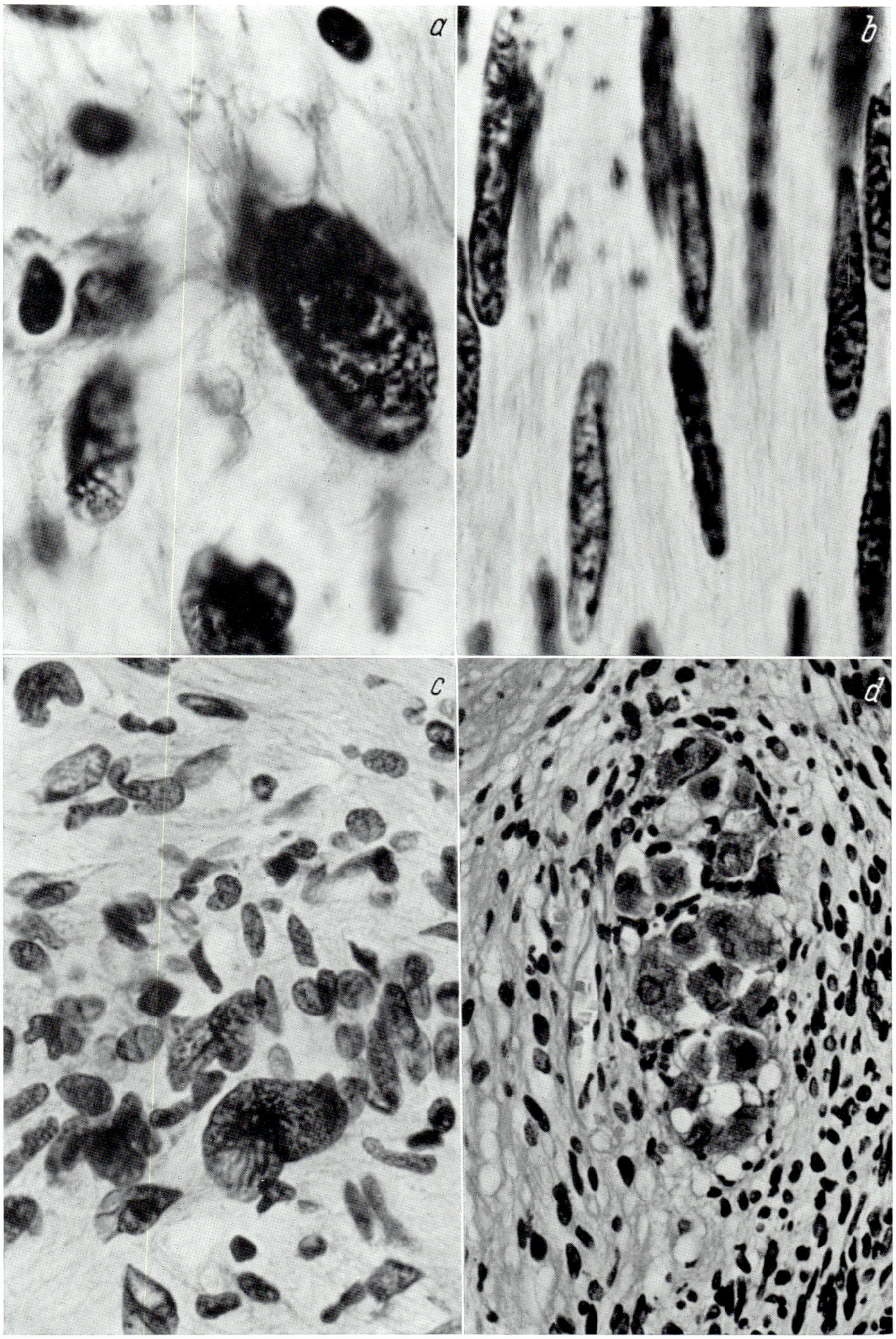

Fig. 67a—d: a and b ×1,100, c ×540, d ×262
Cresyl violet stain

Fig. 68 — Neurinomas

Types of fatty degeneration in the neurinoma:

a) Fatty degeneration in a fibrillary section: One sees the drops of fat lying parallel in long pathways.
b) Cells with fatty degeneration at higher magnification: One can discern clearly the foamy structure of the cells.
c) Region with total fatty degeneration of the cells, where, in the cell body (demonstrated in the positive), the clear vacuole of the nucleus is spared.
d) An aniline stain forms the negative of c). Here the nuclei are stained, with the fat appearing as a clear vacuole, whereby the architecture of an oligodendroglioma can be simulated.

Typen der Verfettung im Neurinom:

a) Verfettung in einer fibrillären Partie, man sieht die Fetttropfen parallel in langen Straßen.
b) Verfettete Zellen bei hoher Vergrößerung: man erkennt deutlich die schaumige Struktur der Zellen.
c) Gebiet mit totaler Verfettung der Zellen, wo in dem positiv dargestellten Zelleib die helle Vacuole des Kerns ausgespart bleibt.
d) Eine Anilinfärbung bildet ein Negativ zu c). Hier sind die Kerne gefärbt, das Fett erscheint dagegen als eine helle Vacuole, wodurch die Architektur eines Oligodendroglioms vorgetäuscht werden kann.

Types de dégénérescence graisseuse dans le neurinome.

a) Dégénérescence graisseuse dans une région fibrillaire: les gouttelettes graisseuses se disposent en longues colonnes parallèles.
b) Dégénérescence graisseuse des cellules à un plus fort grossissement: on reconnaît bien la structure spumeuse des cellules.
c) Dans cette région, toutes les cellules sont en dégénérescence graisseuse: les noyaux apparaissent comme des vacuoles au milieu des cytoplasmes colorés positivement.
d) La coloration à l'aniline donne une image négative de la figure précédente: les noyaux sont colorés tandis que la graisse apparaît comme des vacuoles claires, ce qui peut ainsi simuler l'architecture d'un oligodendrogliome.

Tipos de degeneración grasa en un neurinoma:

a) Adiposis en una zona fibrilar; se ven las gotas de grasa en largos regueros, paralelas.
b) Células en degeneración grasa a mayor aumento; se ve claramente la estructura mucosa de las células.
c) Territorio con adiposis total de las células en cuyo cuerpo, en el cliche positivo, permanece visible la clara vacuola del núcleo.
d) Con la tinción de la anilina queda un negativo de c): los núcleos se tiñen, apareciendo por lo contrario la grasa como una clara vacuola, por lo que se puede confundir con la arquitectura de un oligodendroglioma.

Типы отложения липидов в невриноме:

a) Отложение липидов в фибриллярном участке. Жировые капли расположены длинными параллельными рядами.
b) Клетки с липидными включениями под большим увеличением. Четко видна пенистая структура клеток.
c) Участок тотального жирового перерождения клеток. В позитиве тело клетки со светлой вакуолей ядра.
d) Негатив к с) при окраске анилином. Ядра окрашены, а липиды представлены светлой вакуоли, симулируя строение олигодендроглиомы.

神経鞘腫の脂肪変性の各型。

a) 線維性部分の脂肪変性。脂肪滴が索状にならんでいる。
b) 脂肪変性した細胞の強拡大。細胞の泡沫状構造が明瞭である。
c) 脂肪変性の高度な部分。脂肪陽性の細胞体の中に核が不染のまま残っている。
d) アニリン染色では、c)図の逆の所見（陰画像）がみられる。すなわち、核は染色され、脂質は明るい空胞としてみられる。この結果、稀突起膠腫の構造と誤認されることがある。

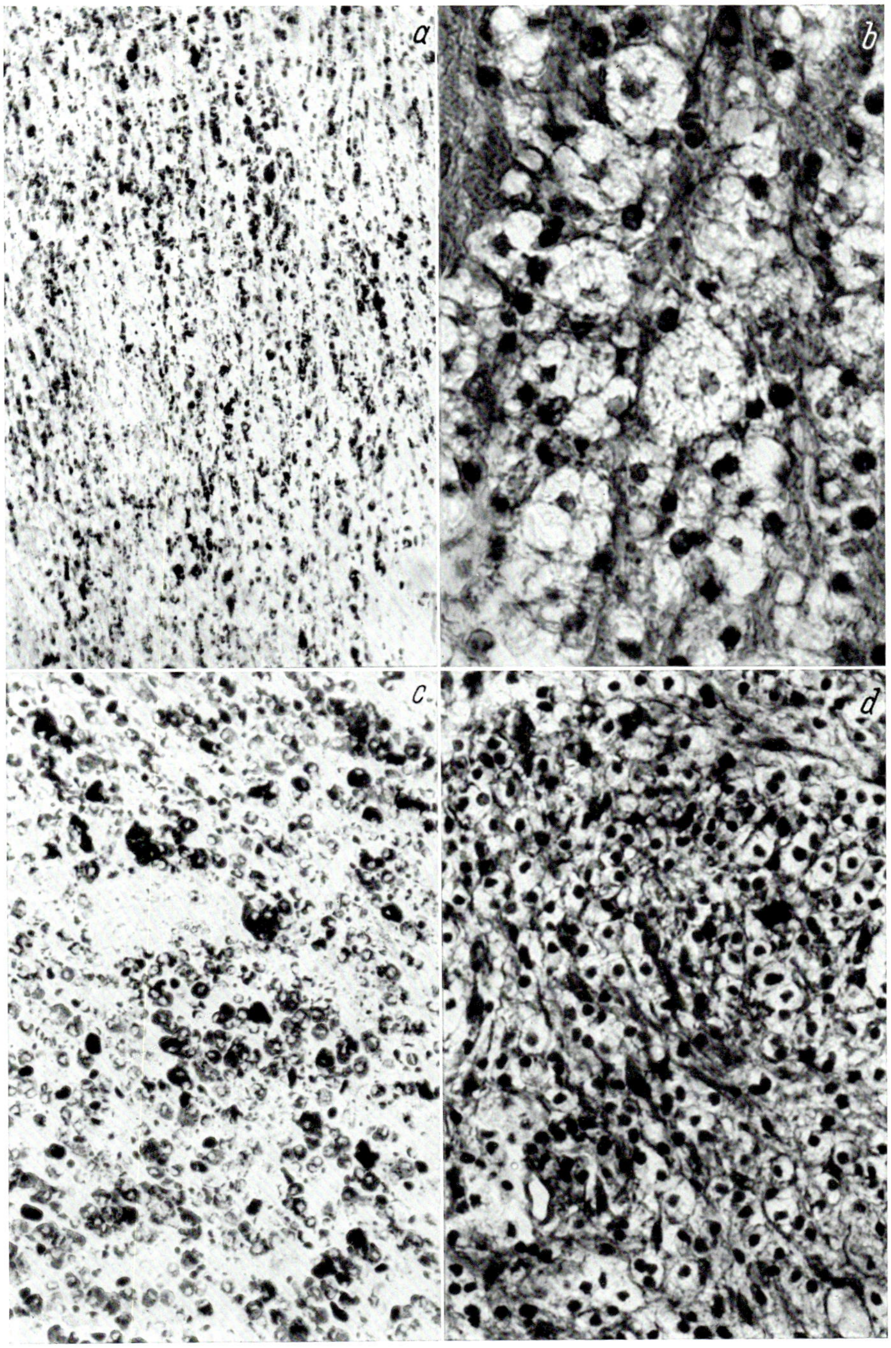

Fig. 68a—d: a ×86. Sudan stain
b ×540, Mallory's stain
c ×220. Fat-Ponceau stain
d ×220. H. & E. stain

Fig. 69 — Neurinomas

Various forms of the regressive processes:
a) Predominantly fibrous, cell-poor sections.
b) Predominantly hyaline transformation of the tissue with slight liquefaction. Only a few cells can be recognized in the amorphous mass.
c) Partly hyalinization, partly fatty degeneration of fibrillary sections.
d) A section that has undergone fatty degeneration and containing chromatin-rich spindle cells with a large plasma-rich cell body, which appears here as a clear vacuole.

Verschiedene Formen der regressiven Vorgänge:
a) Vorwiegend faserige, zellarme Partie.
b) Vorwiegend hyaline Umänderung des Gewebes mit leichter Verflüssigung. Nur wenige Zellen sind in der amorphen Masse zu erkennen.
c) Teils Hyalinisierung, teils Verfettung von fibrillären Partien.
d) Verfettete Partie mit einzelnen chromatinreichen, spindeligen Zellen mit großem plasmareichem Zelleib, der hier als helle Vacuole erscheint.

Différents aspects de phénomènes régressifs.
a) Zone pauvre en cellules et riche en fibres.
b) Début de liquéfaction et surtout transformation hyaline du tissu. On ne reconnaît plus que quelques cellules au sein d'une masse amorphe.
c) Hyalinisation et dégénérescence graisseuse d'une région fibrillaire.
d) Dans une région en dégénérescence graisseuse, on observe quelques cellules fusiformes à noyau riche en chromatine et à cytoplasme abondant, qui contient de grandes vacuoles claires.

Distintas formas de los procesos regresivos.
a) Zona predominante fibrosa, pobre en células.
b) Transformación predominantemente hialina del tejido con ligera fluidificación. En la masa amorfa sólo se reconocen escasas células.
c) En parte hialinización, en parte degeneración grasa, de una zona fibrilar.
d) Zonas de degeneración grasa, con algunas células fusiformes, ricas en cromatina, con protoplasma grande, que aquí aparece como una vacuola clara.

Различные формы регрессивных процессов:
a) Преимущественно волокнистый бедный клетками участок.
b) Преимущественно гиалиновые перерождения ткани с явлениями разжижения. В аморфной массе лишь немногие сохранившиеся клетки.
c) Частичная гиалинизация, частичное жировое перерождение фибриллярных участков.
d) Участок жирового перерождения с отдельными, богатыми хроматином, веретенообразными клетками, с цитоплазмой, представленной в виде светлой вакуоли.

種々の退行変性像。
a) 大部分線維で占められ、細胞の少い部分。
b) 軽度の液化を伴った、広汎な硝子様変性。わずかの細胞が無構造な組織内に見られるにすぎない。
c) 線維性腫瘍部にみられた部分的な硝子様変性と脂肪変性。
d) 脂肪変性を示す部分。濃染核をもった紡錘形細胞は明るい空胞状の胞体をもつ。

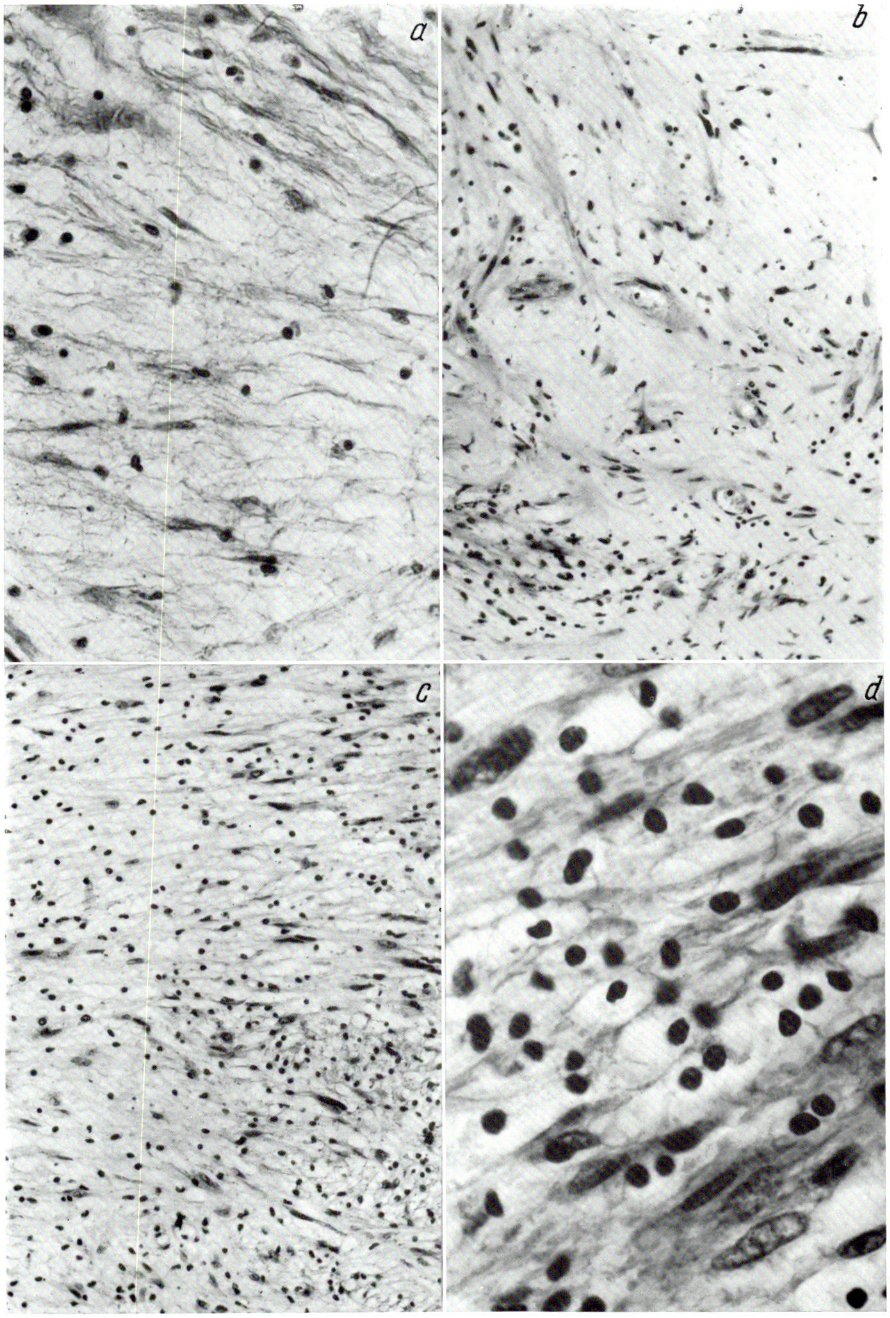

Fig. 69a—d: a ×348. Van Gieson's stain
b ×142, c ×120, d ×648. Cresyl violet stain

Fig. 70 — Neurinomas

a) Typical palisading in a trigeminal neurinoma.
b) Rare variants of peripheral neurinomas: The cells are longer and twisted or kinked.
c) Lattice-fiber network in the capsule zone of an acoustic neurinoma (bottom).
d) Delicate silver fibrils between and at the margin of the neurinoma cells.

a) Typische Palisadenstellung in einem Trigeminusneurinom.
b) Seltene Variante peripherer Neurinome: Die Zellen sind länger und gewunden bzw. geknickt.
c) Gitterfasernetz in der Kapselzone eines Acusticusneurinoms (unten).
d) Zarte Silberfibrillen zwischen und am Rande der Neurinomzellen.

a) Disposition palissadique typique dans un neurinome du trijumeau.
b) Variété rare de neurinome périphérique; les cellules sont très longues et spiralées ou fragmentées.
c) Réseau de fibres réticuliniques dans la capsule d'un neurinome de l'acoustique (au-dessous).
d) Fibrilles argentophiles délicates qui séparent et longent les cellules du neurinome.

a) Típica disposición en empalizada en un neurinoma del trigémino.
b) Variante extraña de un neurinoma periférico: las células son más largas, torcidas o bien rotas.
c) Enrejado de fibras en la zona capsular de un neurinoma del acústico (abajo).
d) Delicadas fibrillas argénticas en los bordes y entre las células neurinomatosas.

a) Невринома тройничного нерва. Типическое образование палисадов.
b) Редкий вариант невриномы периферического нерва. Клетки удлинены, извиты, с изгибами.
c) Протоплазматическая сеточка в зоне капсулы невриномы слухового нерва (внизу).
d) Невринома. Расположенные по краям и между клетками, импрегнируемые серебром нежные волокна.

a) 三叉神経の神経鞘腫にみられた、定型的柵状配列。
b) 末梢の神経鞘腫が示すまれな像：細胞は長く、うねりあるいは屈曲している。
c) 聴神経の神経鞘腫の被膜部（図下）にみられた好銀線維網。
d) 神経鞘腫細胞間や、細胞に接している微細な好銀線維。

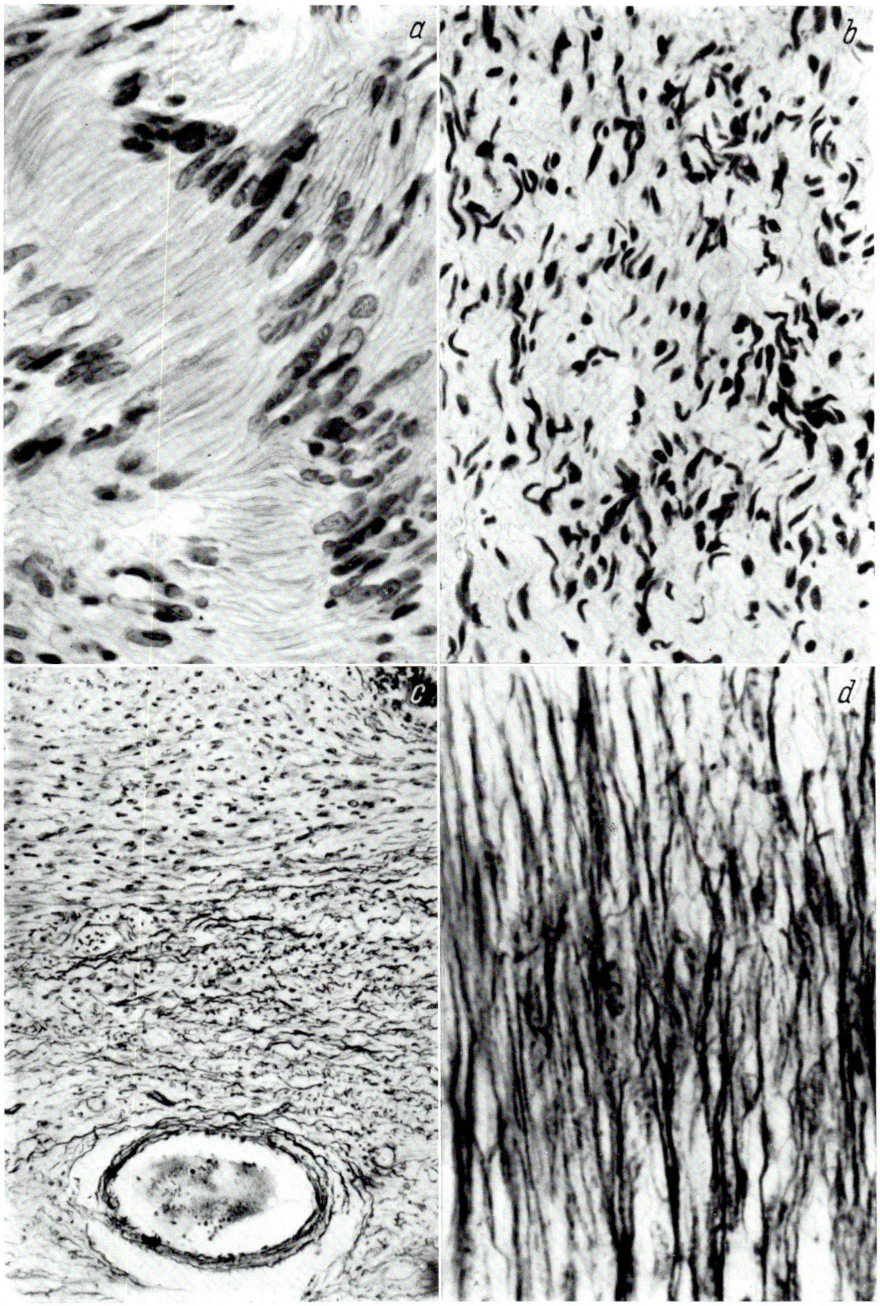

Fig. 70a—d: a ×524. H. & E. stain
b ×336. Cresyl violet stain
c ×84, d ×540. Perdrau's method

Fig. 71 — Neurinomas

a) Single, large blood vessels from the marginal zone of a neurinoma: They have a wide, hyalinized wall; sometimes they lie cavernoma-like next to one another.
b) Mitoses in an acoustic neurinoma (rarity).
c) Fine silver fibers at the margin of the cells of a neurinoma.
d) Small, zig-zag silver fibers; the cells are encased by these fibers.

a) Einzelne große Gefäße aus der Randzone eines Neurinoms: Sie haben eine breite hyalinisierte Wand, manchmal liegen sie kavernomartig beieinander.
b) Mitosen in einem Neurinom des Acusticus (Rarität).
c) Feine Silberfasern am Rande der Zellen eines Neurinoms.
d) Kleine gezackte Silberfasern, die die Zellen umspinnen.

a) Dans la zone périphérique d'un neurinome, présence de quelques larges vaisseaux, qui présentent un épaississement hyalin de leur paroi et qui se rassemblent souvent comme dans un cavernome.
b) Mitoses dans un neurinome de l'acoustique (rareté).
c) Fines fibres argentophiles longeant les cellules d'un neurinome.
d) Les cellules sont enserrées par ces minces fibres argentophiles de forme crénelée.

a) Algunos vasos grandes en la perifería de un neurinoma: tienen una ancha pared hialinizada; a veces se disponen uno con otro en forma cavernosa.
b) Mitosis en un neurinoma del acústico (rareza).
c) Finas fibrillas argénticas al borde de las células de un neurinoma.
d) Pequeñas fibrillas argénticas zigzageantes que contornean las células.

a) Единичные крупные сосуды с толстой гиалинизированной стенкой в краевой зоне. В некоторых участках сосуды образуют каверноматозные полости.
b) Редкий случай появления митозов в невриноме слухового нерва.
c) Невринома. Тонкие, импрегнируемые серебром волокна по краям клеток.
d) Мелкие, импрегнированные серебром волокна.

a) 神経鞘腫辺縁部の大きな血管。壁は厚く硝子様を呈している。このような血管は、しばしば、海綿腫状に相接して存在する。
b) 聴神経鞘腫内の核分裂像（稀な所見）。
c) 神経鞘腫の細胞に接する微細な好銀線維。
d) 小さくうねる好銀線維。腫瘍細胞をてんらくしているのが明瞭にみとめられる。

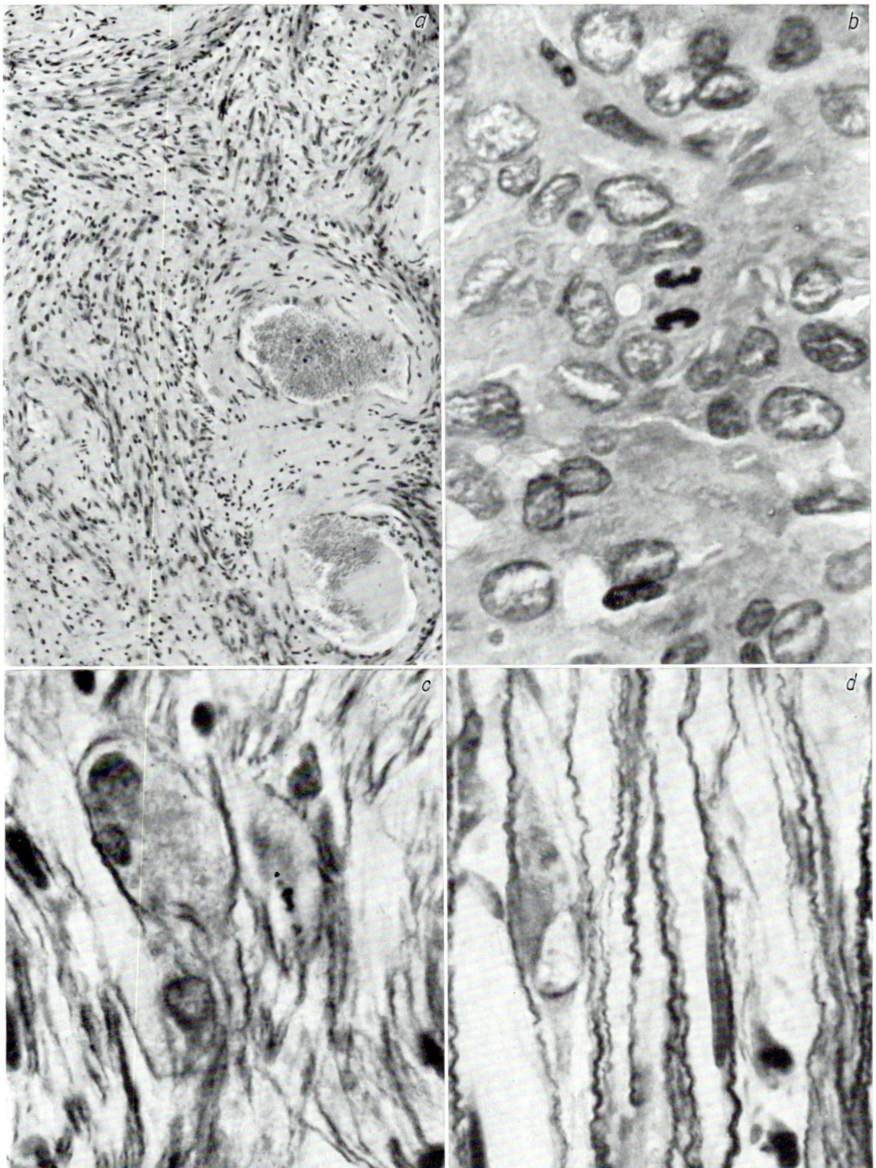

Fig. 71 a—d: a ×112. Cresyl violet stain
b ×1,076. H. & E. stain
c ×648, d ×1,100. Perdrau's impregnation

Fig. 72 — Neurinomas

a) Characteristic of peripheral neurofibroma is the presence of long bands of Schwann cells admixed with considerable quantities of collagen fibers. Abundant collagen fibers are noted along the Schwann cells in Von Recklinghausen's neurofibromas, as well as in single neurofibromas of peripheral nerves. The clear rhythmic architecture of the neurinoma is nevertheless still recognisable.

b) The malignant neurinoma has an architecture similar to the benign form, but in addition shows mitoses and giant hyperchromatic cells. The tumors are more cellular and richer in cell processes.

c) Although the cigarette-like appearance of the Schwann cells in the cellular types is clearly visible, there are marked variations in size and shape. Single mitoses are apparent.

d) In this polymorphic neurinoma the loss of architecture is obvious although some individual cells are of the Schwann cell type. Mitoses are apparent. The polymorphism has increased.

a) Beim Neurofibrom der von Recklinghausenschen Krankheit bzw. einzelnen Neurofibromen der peripheren Nerven ist das kollagene Element neben den Schwannschen Zellen sehr stark verbreitet. Man erkennt aber noch die rhythmische Architektur der Neurinome. Das Vorkommen von langen Zügen Schwannscher Zellen und eine starke Durchmischung mit kollagener Faserung ist charakteristisch für die peripheren Neurofibrome.

b) Die malignen Neurinome haben eine ähnliche Architektur wie die benignen Formen, nur treten Mitosen und hyperchromatische Riesenzellen auf. Sie sind teils mehr faserig, teils mehr zellig.

c) Bei den zelligen Formen erkennt man noch deutlich die typische Zigarettenform der Schwannschen Zellen, doch gibt es starke Variationen in Größe und Form. Einzelne Mitosen sind deutlich sichtbar.

d) In diesem polymorphen Neurinom ist der Verlust der Architektur deutlich, wenn auch einzelne Zellen dem Schwannschen Typus gleichen. Die Polymorphie hat zugenommen, Mitosen sind sichtbar.

a) Dans la maladie de von Recklinghausen, les neurofibromes des nerfs périphériques contiennent beaucoup de fibres collagènes parmi les cellules de Schwann. La présence de longues traînées de cellules de Schwann et l'abondance des fibres collagènes interstitielles sont typiques des neurofibromes périphériques. Cependant, on reconnaît l'architecture rythmique du neurinome.

b) Les neurinomes malins présentent la même architecture que dans les formes bénignes, mais on y trouve des mitoses et des cellules géantes hyperchromatiques. Ils sont soit plus fibreux, soit plus cellulaires.

c) Dans les formes cellulaires, on reconnaît nettement l'aspect en cigarette, typique de la cellule de Schwann, mais il existe des variations importantes de volume et de forme. Quelques mitoses sont nettement visibles.

d) Dans ce neurinome polymorphe, on ne reconnaît plus du tout l'architecture bien que certains éléments ressemblent aux cellules de Schwann. Le polymorphisme s'est accentué et des mitoses sont visibles.

a) En el neurofibroma de la enfermedad de von Recklinghausen, o bien particular neurofibroma de los nervios perifericos verse elementos colagenos junto con celulas de Schwann. La presencia de largas estructuras de tipo de células de Schwann mezcladas con fibras colagenas, es característico de los neurofibromas perifericos. Puede verse también la arquitectura rítmica del neurinoma.

b) Los neurinomas malignos tienen una arquitectura parecida a las formas benignas, sólo que encontramos mitosis y células grandes hipercromáticas. Unas veces aparecen más fibrosos otras más celulares.

c) En los ricos en celulas se reconocen las tipicas disposiciones en cigarillos de las celulas de Schwann pues se trata de variaciones en tamaño y forma. Son visibles algunas mitosis.

d) En este neurinoma polimorfo la perdida de la arquitectura es clara pero pueden verse algunas células del tipo de Schwann. El polimorfismo es patente, son visibles mitosis.

Continued on page 192

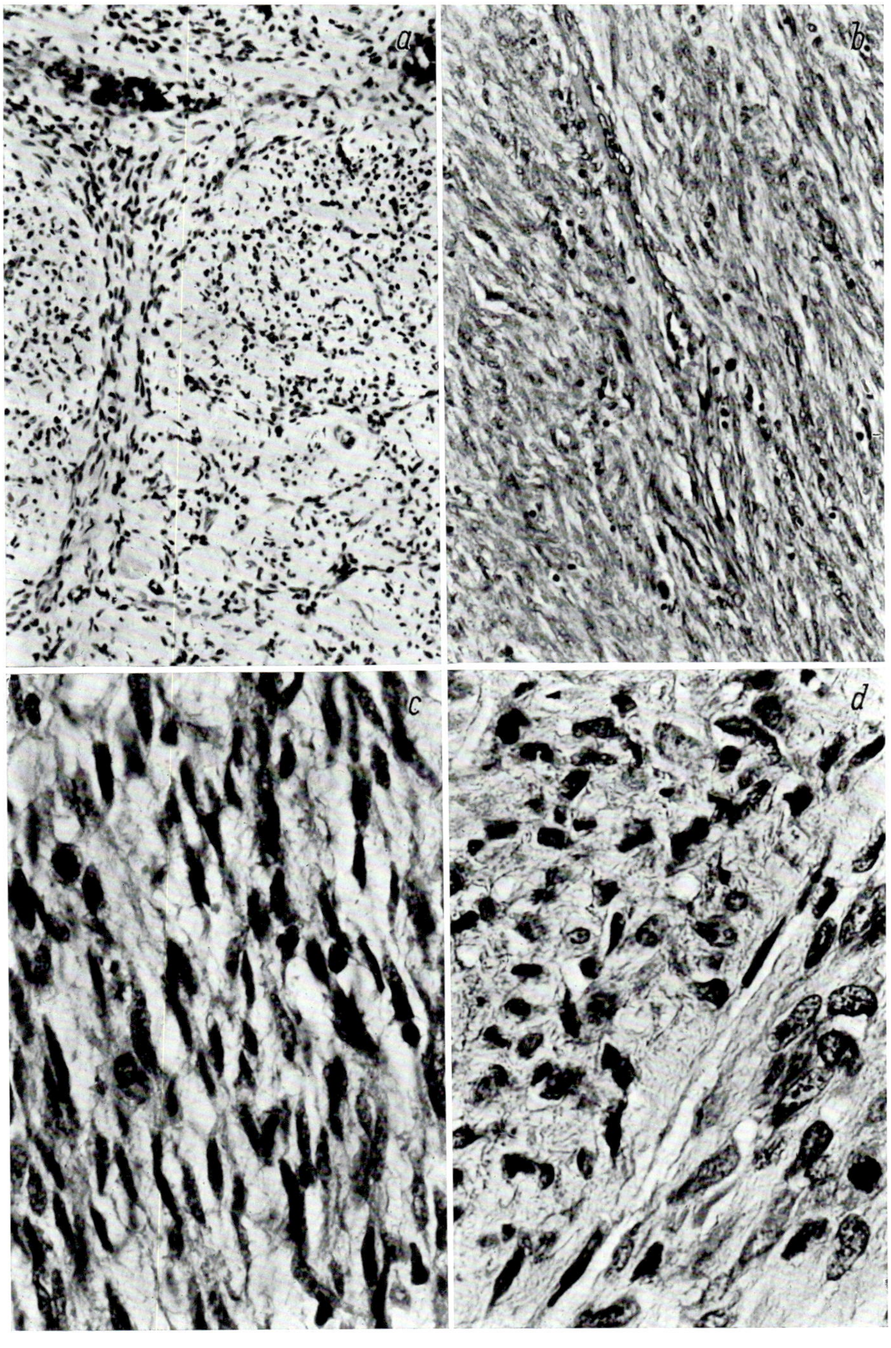

Fig. 72a—d: a and b ×125, c and d ×500
H. & E. stain

Fig. 72 — Neurinomas (continued)

a) При нейрофиброме (болезнь Реклингаузена) и соответственно при нейрофибромах периферических нервов отмечается обилие коллагеновых волокон вокруг шванновских клеток, однако ритмическая структура невриномы еще различима. Характерные для нейрофибромы периферических нервов длинные тяжи шванновских клеток наряду с большим количеством коллагеновых волокон.

b) Злокачественные невриномы имеют структуру, подобную доброкачественным формам этих опухолей с появлением в нервах митозов и гиперхромных гигантских клеток. В них преобладают то волокнистые, то клеточные элементы.

c) В клеточных формах все еще четко виден типичный сигаретоподобный вид шванновских клеток, форма и величина которых однако значительно вариирует. Четко видны отдельные митозы.

d) Эта полиморфная невринома явно утратила свою структуру, хотя отдельные клетки похожи на шванновские. Полиморфизм увеличился, видны митозы. Аденома гипофиза. Крупные базофильные полиморфные эпителиальные клетки базофильной аденомы гипофиза.

a) Recklinghausen 病の際、あるいは単独に末梢神経に生ずる神経線維腫では、Schwann 細胞の近くに膠原線維性成分が多くみられる。Schwann 細胞の細長い突起と膠原線維が混在することが末梢性の神経線維腫の特徴である。これに対し神経鞘腫には律動的な構造がある。

b) 悪性神経鞘腫は良性の神経鞘腫に似た構造をもつ。ただ悪性神経鞘腫では分裂像と濃染性巨細胞が現われる。悪性神経鞘腫には線維に富むものと、細胞に富むものとがある。

c) 細胞に富む悪性神経鞘腫ではタバコ型の構造をもったSchwann細胞をみとめる。この細胞の大きさ、形は多様である。分裂像をみる。

d) 多形性の神経鞘腫の細胞は、Schwann 型の腫瘍細胞と比較すると、構造の乱れが明らかである。多形性は増し、分裂像が出現する。

Meningiomas

Endotheliomatous, fibroblastic, psammomatous, angioblastic meningiomas, psammoma, fibroma, sarcoma, endothelioma, exothelioma or mesothelioma of the dura mater; meningeal fibroendothelioma, meningeal or arachnoidal fibroblastoma, meningothelioma; meningocytoma or-blastoma, pachymeningioma, arachnothelioma, leptomeningioma, fungus durae matris, etc.

Fig. 73 — Meningiomas

The architecture of an endotheliomatous meningioma:

a) In cell staining, one recognizes the islands, which are divided by only a small amount of connective tissue. The islands themselves are subdivided into smaller concentric cell nests. Top: Capsule zone.

b) Silver impregnation shows the stroma between the islands of cells.

c) and d) The interstitial tissue here is somewhat more strongly developed.

Die Architektur des endotheliomatösen Meningeoms:

a) Man erkennt bei Zellfärbung die Inseln, die nur durch wenig Bindegewebe unterteilt werden. Die Inseln selbst sind in kleinere konzentrische Zellnester unterteilt. Oben: Kapselzone.

b) Die Silberimprägnation zeigt das Stroma zwischen den Zellinseln.

c) und d) Das Zwischengewebe ist hier etwas stärker ausgebildet.

L'architecture du méningiome endothéliomateux.

a) Par une coloration cytologique, on reconnaît les îlots cellulaires, qui ne sont séparés les uns des autres que par un peu de tissu conjonctif. Les îlots eux-mêmes sont subdivisés en petits nids cellulaires concentriques. La capsule est visible dans la partie supérieure.

b) L'imprégnation argentique met en évidence le stroma entre les îlots cellulaires.

c) et d) Le tissu interstitiel est ici un peu plus abondant.

La arquitectura de los meningiomas endoteliomatosos.

a) Con las coloraciones celulares se reconocen islas divididas solo por escaso tejido conectivo. Las islas mismas estan subdivididas en nidos celulares concéntricos más pequeños. Arriba: zona capsular.

b) La impregnación pone de manifiesto estroma entre las islas de células.

c) y d) El tejido celular intersticial tiene aquí mas consistencia.

Строение эндотелиоматозной менингиомы:

a) При окраске клеток видны островки, разделенные скудной соединительной тканью. Сами островки образуют мелкие концентрические клеточные гнезда. Вверху: зона капсулы.

b) При импрегнации серебром видна строма между островками клеток.

c) и d) Межуточная ткань несколько лучше выражена.

内皮腫性脳膜腫の組織構造。

a) 少量の結合組織で分けられた細胞集団（島）。この島の中に小さな細胞小群がある。図の上部は被膜部。

b) 鍍銀によって島の間の結合組織が染出される。

c) および d) 間質はここではやゝ多い。

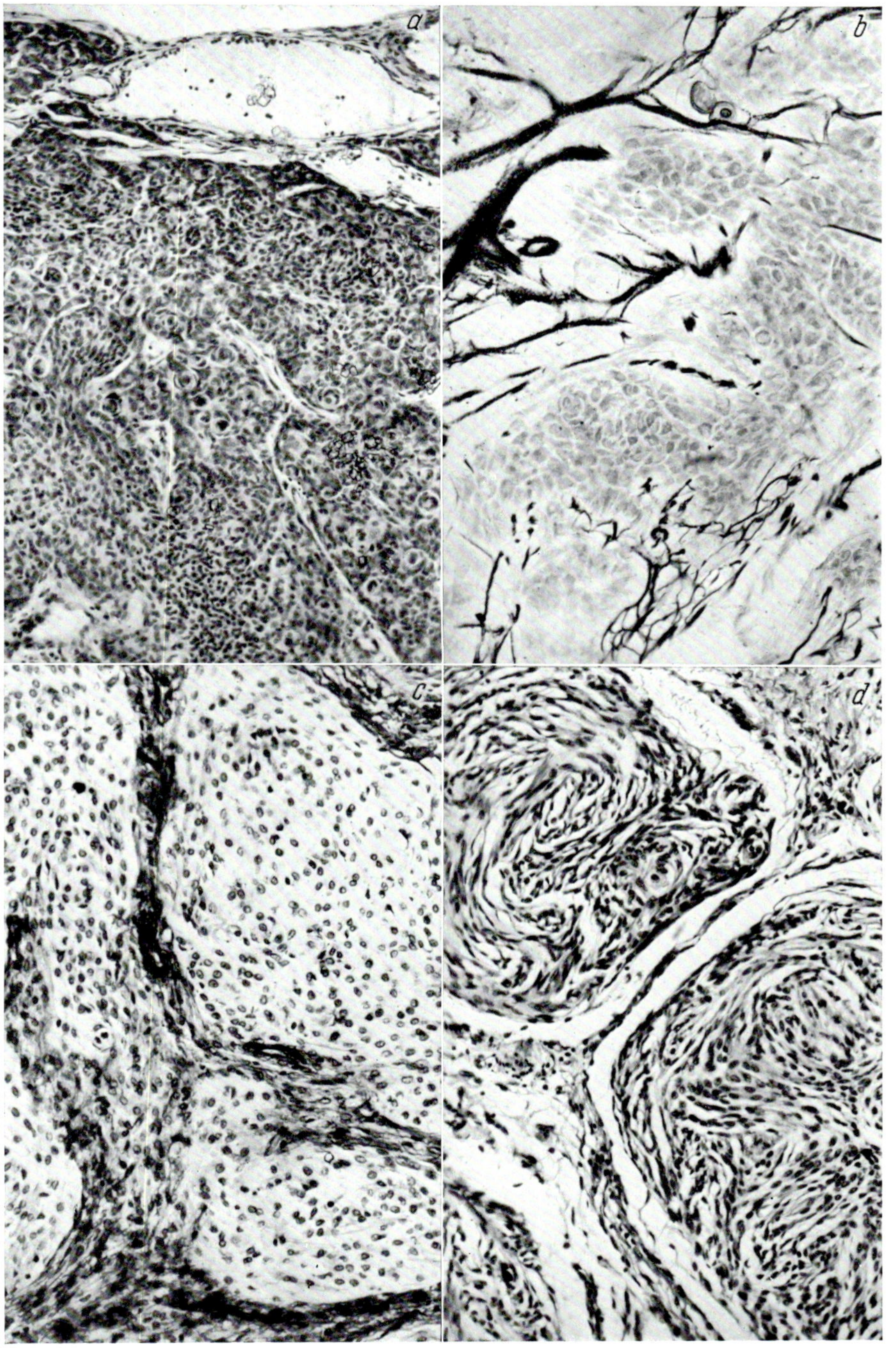

Fig. 73a—d: a ×120, c and d ×136. Cresyl violet stain
b ×136. Perdrau's method

Fig. 74 — Meningiomas

Endotheliomatous meningioma with a pronounced tendency towards the formation of concentric whorls, hyalinization and calcium deposit (psammona bodies). One finds this extreme calcification especially frequently in spinal meningiomas of the thoracic region.

Endotheliomatöse Meningeome mit ausgesprochener Neigung zur Bildung von konzentrischen Wirbeln, Hyalinisierung und Kalkeinlagerung (Psammomkörner). Man findet diese hochgradige Verkalkung besonders häufig bei spinalen Meningeomen im Thorakalbereich.

Méningiome endothéliomateux présentant une tendance très marquée à la formation de tourbillons concentriques, avec hyalinisation et calcification (psammomes). Cette tendance prononcée à la calcification s'observe principalement dans les méningiomes spinaux au niveau thoracique.

Meningioma endoteliomatoso, con marcada tendencia a la formación de remolinos, a la hialinización y depósito de calcio (corpúsculos psamomatosos). Esta acusada calcificación se encuentra con especial frecuencia en los meningiomas espinales de la región torácica.

Эндотелиоматозная менингеома с выраженной тенденцией к образованию концентрических завихрений, гиалинизации и обызвествлению (псаммомные тельца). Такое яркое обызвествление особенно часто наблюдается при менингеомах спинного мозга в грудном отделе.

渦状構造化、硝子化、石灰化（砂粒腫小体）の傾向の強い内皮腫性脳膜腫。石灰化は胸椎部の脳膜腫に特に多い。

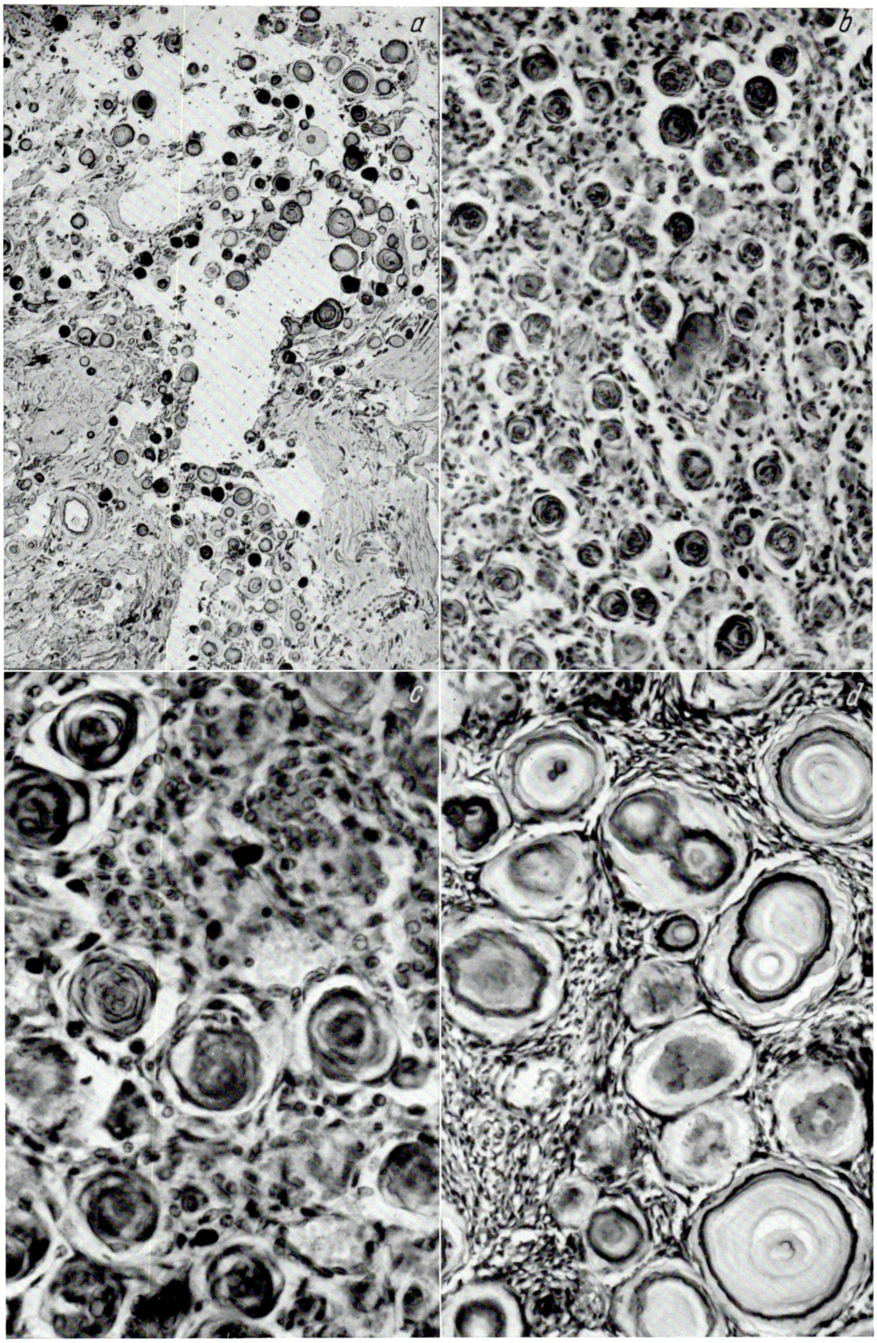

Fig. 74a—d: a ×18, d ×136. H. & E. stain
b ×118, c ×544. Cresyl violet stain

Fig. 75 — Meningiomas

Fibromatous meningioma:

a) The capsule zone consists of dense, hyalinized, cell-poor connective tissue.
b) Silver fibers between the cells.
c) Predominantly cellular form with few fibers.
d) Peculiar meningioma consisting of two sections: *Bottom right:* endotheliomatous marginal zone; *top left:* fibromatous center of the tumor.

Fibromatöses Meningeom:

a) Die Kapselzone besteht aus einem dichten, hyalinisierten zellarmen Bindegewebe.
b) Silberfasern zwischen den Zellen.
c) Vorwiegend zellige Form mit wenig Fasern.
d) Eigenartiges Meningeom aus zwei Anteilen: unten rechts endotheliomatöse Randzone, oben links fibromatöses Zentrum der Geschwulst.

Méningiome fibromateux.

a) La zone capsulaire est constituée par du tissu conjonctif dense, hyalinisé et pauvre en cellules.
b) Fibres argentophiles entre les cellules.
c) Forme surtout cellulaire, contenant peu de fibres.
d) Cas particulier de méningiome constitué de deux parties: la zone périphérique est du type endothéliomateux (en bas et à droite), le centre de la tumeur est du type fibromateux (en haut et à gauche).

Meningioma fibromatoso.

a) La zona capsular consiste en un grueso tejido conectivo hialinizado, pobre en células.
b) Fibras argentófilas entre las células.
c) Forma predominantemente celular con pocas fibras.
d) Meningioma especial, con dos partes: abajo y a la derecha borde endoteliomatoso, arriba y a la izquierda, centro fibromatoso del tejido.

Фиброматозная менингеома:

a) Зона капсулы состоит из плотной, гиалинизированной бедной клетками соединительной ткани.
b) Между клетками видны импрегнированные серебром волокна (по методу Пердро).
c) Преимущественно клеточная форма с немногочисленными волокнами.
d) Своеобразная менингеома, состоящая из двух участков: внизу справа — эндотелиоматозная краевая зона, вверху слева — фиброматозный центр опухоли.

線維腫性脳膜腫。

a) 被膜部は細胞が少なく、硝子化した厚い結合組織からなっている。
b) 細胞間の好銀線維。
c) 細胞に富み線維の少ない部分。
d) ふたつの成分からなる脳膜腫。右下に内皮腫性、左上に線維腫性腫瘍がみられる。

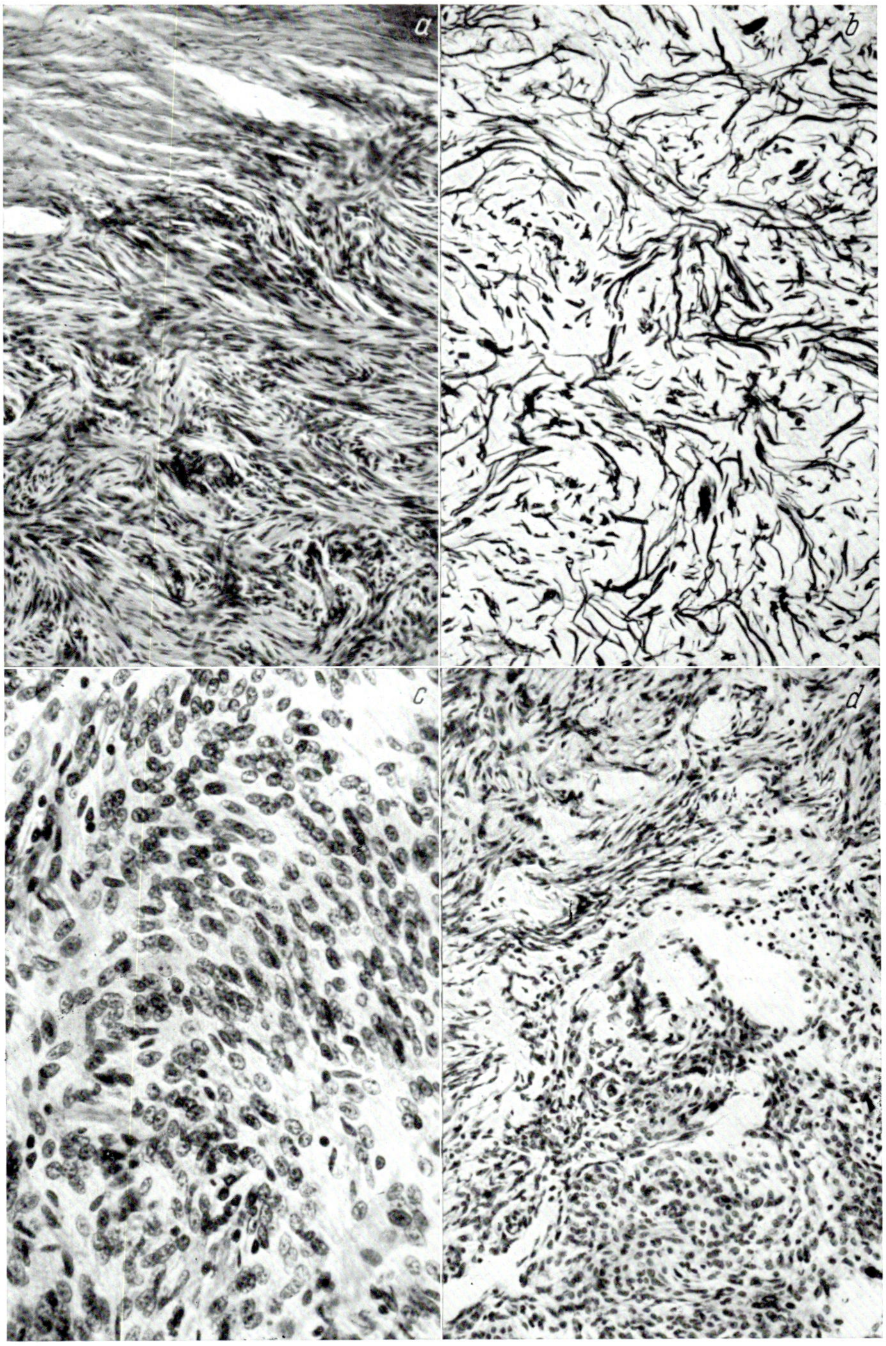

Fig. 75a—d: a ×120, c ×272. H. & E. stain
b ×120. Perdrau's method
d ×136. Cresyl violet stain

Fig. 76 — Meningiomas

Regressive processes in a meningioma:

a) Focal, fine-drop fatty degeneration in the center of the island of an endotheliomatous meningioma (“foam cells”).
b) Diffuse fatty degeneration in a fibromatous meningioma.
c) Liquefaction as a preliminary stage in cyst formation.
d) Fairly small cysts in a meningioma. In their vicinity, macrophages with old blood pigment; likewise in the interior, macrophage-like cells.

Regressive Vorgänge in einem Meningeom:

a) Herdförmige feintropfige Verfettung im Zentrum der Inseln eines endotheliomatösen Meningeoms („Schaumzellen“).
b) Diffuse Verfettung in einem fibromatösen Meningeom.
c) Verflüssigung als Vorstufe der Cystenbildung.
d) Kleinere Cysten in einem Meningeom. In ihrer Umgebung Makrophagen mit altem Blutpigment, ebenso im Inneren makrophagenartige Zellen.

Phénomènes régressifs dans un méningiome.

a) Au centre d'un îlot cellulaire de méningiome endothéliomateux, on observe un petit foyer de dégénérescence graisseuse à petites vacuoles (cellules «spumeuses»).
b) Dégénérescence graisseuse diffuse dans un méningiome fibromateux.
c) La liquéfaction précède la formation de kystes.
d) Dans un méningiome, présence de petits kystes autour desquels des macrophages contiennent du vieux pigment sanguin et dans lesquels il existe également des cellules ressemblant à des macrophages.

Procesos regresivos en un meningioma:

a) Focos de degeneración grasa en pequeñas gotas en el centro de la isla de un meningioma endoteliomatoso (células espumosas).
b) Degeneración grasa difusa en un meningioma fibromatoso.
c) Liquefacción, como etapa preliminar de la formación de quistes.
d) Pequeños quistes en un meningioma. A su alrededor se encuentran macrófagos con pigmento sanguíneo antiguo, lo mismo que en el interior de sus células de tipo macrofágico.

Регрессивные процессы в менингеоме:

a) Очаговое мелкокапельное липидное перерождение в центре островков эндотелиоматозной менингеомы («пенистые клетки»).
b) Диффузное липидное перерождение в фиброматозной менингеоме.
c) Разжижение как предпосылка для кистообразования.
d) Мелкие кисты в менингеоме, в окружности которых видны макрофаги со старым кровяным пигментом. Внутри макрофагоподобные клетки.

脳膜腫の退行変性。

a) 内皮腫性脳膜腫の島中央部におこった小滴状脂肪変性 (泡沫細胞)。
b) 線維腫性脳膜腫にみられたびまん性脂肪変性。
c) 嚢胞形成の前段階としての腫瘍組織液化。
d) 脳膜腫内の小嚢胞。周囲にヘモジデリンを摂取した喰細胞がある。

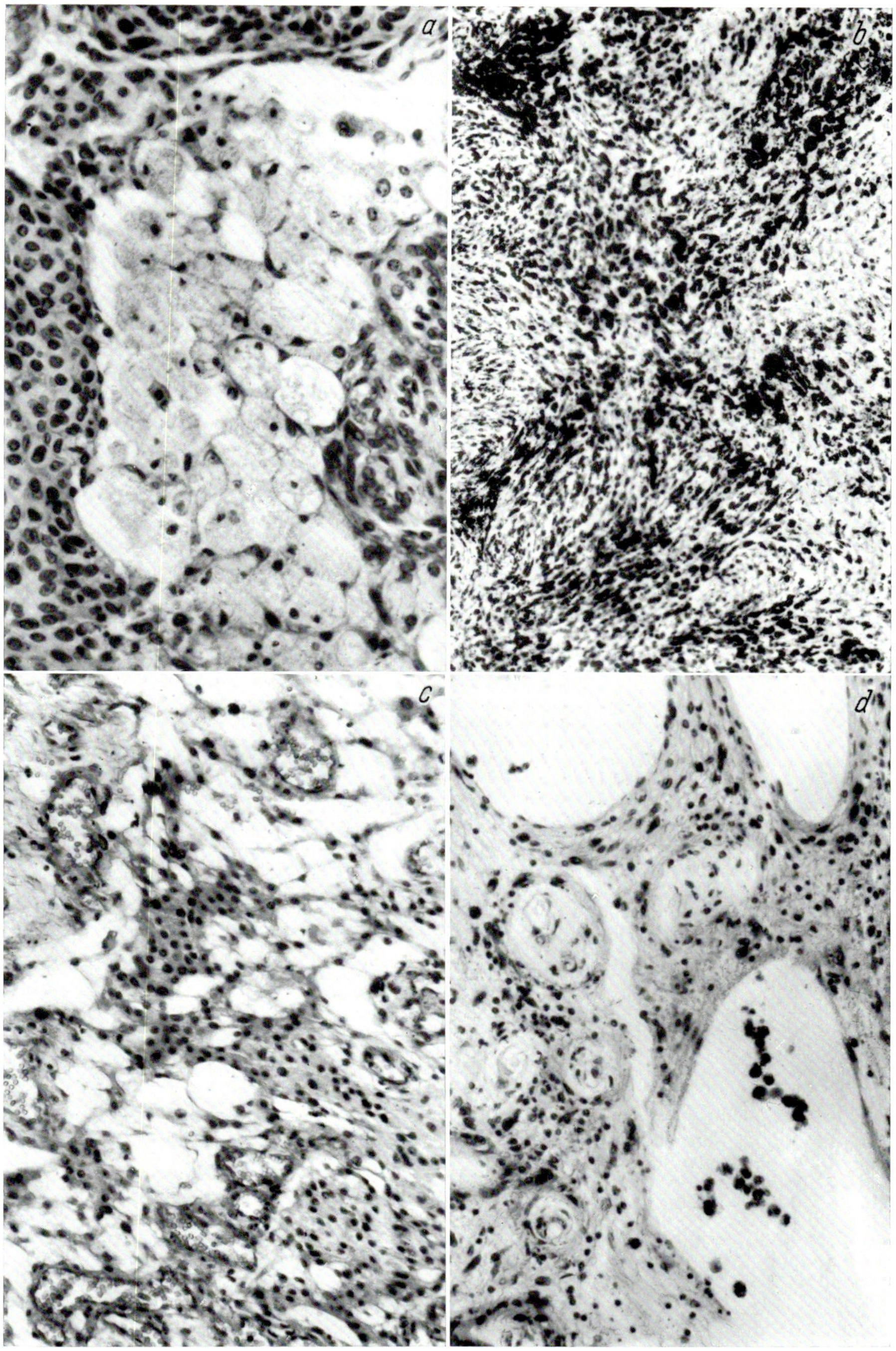

Fig. 76a—d: a ×174, d ×136. Cresyl violet stain
b ×120. Fat-Ponceau stain
c ×136. H. & E. stain

Fig. 77 — Meningiomas

a) Malignant meningioma with metastasis to the lung and various organs after a total of 22 years of growth.
b)—d) Rapidly growing meningiomas with mitoses. They are usually of the fibroma-like type. One can clearly discern cell columns and whorls; the nuclei are quite vesicular and have large nucleoli, and one sees numerous mitoses.

a) Malignes Meningeom mit Metastasierung in Lunge und verschiedene Organe nach insgesamt 22jährigem Wachstum.
b)—d) Rasch wachsende Meningeome mit Mitosen. Sie sind meist vom fibromartigen Typ. Man erkennt deutlich Zellzüge und Wirbel, die Kerne sind recht bläschenförmig, haben große Nucleolen und man sieht zahlreiche Mitosen.

a) Méningiome malin, qui a métastasé dans les poumons et divers organes après une évolution d'une durée de 22 ans.
b)—d) Méningiome à croissance rapide et contenant des mitoses. Ces méningiomes sont généralement du type fibromateux. On reconnaît bien les courants cellulaires et les tourbillons. Les noyaux sont très gonflés et contiennent de gros nucléoles. Les mitoses sont nombreuses.

a) Meningioma maligno con metástasis pulmonares y en diferentes órganos, después de 22 años de crecimiento.
b)—d) Meningioma de crecimiento rápido con mitosis. La mayoría de estos meningiomas son de tipo fibromatoso. Se reconocen fácilmente corrientes y remolinos celulares; los núcleos son francamente vesiculosos, tienen grandes nucleolos y presentan numerosas mitosis.

a) Злокачественная менингеома, с метастазами в легкое и другие органы после 22-летнего роста.
b)—d) Быстрорастущая менингеома с митозами фибромоподобного типа. Четко видны тяжи и завихрения, ядра пузырьковидные с большими ядрышками и многочисленными митозами.

a) 22年の経過の後、肺および多種の臓器に転移した悪性脳膜腫。
b) —d) 核分裂をみる、増殖の速い脳膜腫。この種の脳膜腫は、多くは線維腫性である。細胞の束状、渦状配列が著明である。核は空胞状で大きな核小体をもち、核分裂像が多い。

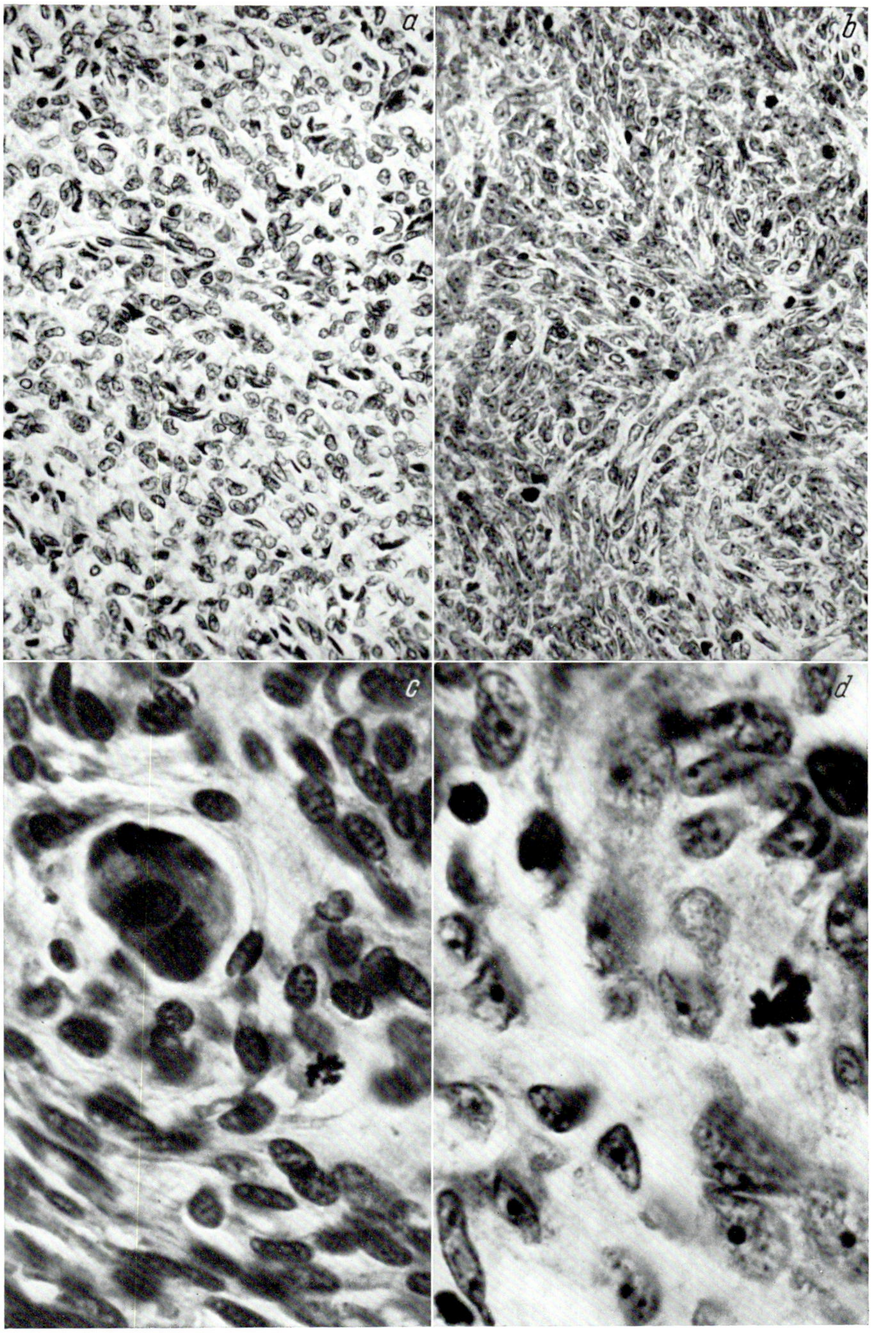

Fig. 77a—d: a × 272, Cresyl violet stain
b × 272, H. & E. stain
c × 469, Cresyl violet stain
d × 1072, Cresyl violet stain

Special Meningiomas

Fig. 78a, b

Angioblastomas

Fig. 78c, d, Fig. 79—80

Hemangioblastoma, capillary hemangioblastoma, Lindau's cyst, disease or tumor, angiomatosis of the central nervous system, cerebellar angioma, epithelial angioma, angioreticuloma, cerebellar hemangioendothelioma

Fig. 78 Meningiomas — Angioblastomas (continued on page 206)

a) *Angiomatous meningioma:* Characteristic of this tumor is the large number of blood vessels in an angioma-like arrangement. Between the blood vessels however, there are nests of cells showing the typical structure of an endotheliomatous meningioma.
b) *Malignant meningioma:* This picture shows throughout a number of gigantic multinucleated cells, which however in part still maintain the genuine onion bulb like architecture, characteristic of this tumor.
c) The *hemangioblastoma* (Lindau's disease) is characterized by a network of capillaries, larger blood-vessels and in between the so-called intermediate cells. Occasionally these cells may show a hyperchromatic nucleus. The "Zwischenzellen" are frequently loaded with lipoid substances.
d) In some areas the "intermediate-cells" of the hemangioblastoma appear arranged in a syncitial fashion. Although the nuclei are hyperchromatic the benign character of the growth is not altered.

a) *Angiomatöses Meningeom:* Die große Zahl der Gefäße, die fast angiomartig zu nennen ist, gibt diesem Typus das entscheidende Merkmal. Zwischen den Gefäßen aber liegen noch Zellnester, die die charakteristische Struktur des endotheliomatösen Meningeoms aufweisen.
b) *Malignes Meningeom:* Das vorliegende Bild zeigt überall die Bildung hyperchromatischer mehrkerniger Riesenzellen, die sich aber z.T. noch an die genuine Zwiebelschalen-Architektur dieser Tumoren halten.
c) Das *Hämangioblastom* (Lindau) ist charakterisiert durch eine netzartige Architektur von Capillaren und etwas größeren Gefäßen, zwischen denen die sog. ,,Zwischenzellen" liegen. Diese können gelegentlich hyperchromatische Kerne haben. Außerdem ist eine Lipoidspeicherung an den Zwischenzellen oft sehr deutlich.
d) An einzelnen Stellen können die Zwischenzellen des Hämangioblastoms wie in einem Syncytium miteinander vereinigt sein, gleichzeitig werden die Kerne hyperchromatisch, ohne daß dadurch aber die gutartige Wachstumsform sich ändert.

Fig. 78 Meningiomas — Angioblastomas (continued)

a) *Méningiome angiomateux.* Le grand nombre de vaisseaux, qu'on pourrait presque appeler angiomateux, constitue la caractéristique la plus marquante de ce type. Cependant, entre les vaisseaux, on retrouve encore des nids cellulaires, dans lesquels on reconnaît la structure typique du méningiome endothéliomateux.

b) *Méningiome malin.* Sur cette image, on note la présence de nombreuses cellules géantes, multinucléées et hyperchromatiques, qui cependant respectent en partie l'architecture en pelure d'oignons, propre à cette tumeur.

c) *L'hémangioblastome* (Lindau) est caractérisé par une architecture réticulée, formée par des capillaires et des vaisseaux légèrement plus volumineux, entre lesquels se trouvent des cellules appelées «intermédiaires». Celles-ci peuvent occasionnellement contenir un noyau hyperchromatique. En outre, ces cellules interstitielles présentent souvent une nette surcharge lipoïdique.

d) En quelques endroits, les cellules «intermédiaires» de l'hémangioblastome peuvent confluer en un syncytium, tandis que les noyaux deviennent hyperchromatiques, sans que la nature bénigne de la tumeur ne soit modifiée pour autant.

a) *Meningioma angiomatoso:* La gran cantidad de vasos, casi verdadero angioma, es la característica de este tipo. Entre los vasos existen grupos de celulas de estructura característica de los meningiomas endoteliomatosos.

b) *Meningioma maligno:* En este cuadro vemos principalmente células multinucleadas, gigantes, pero todavía se conserva la forma característica en bulbo de cebolla de estos tumores.

c) El *hemangioblastoma* (Lindau) se caracteriza por la arquitectura reticular de los capilares y los vasos un poco mayores existiendo entre ellos las llamadas «células intersticialles». Estas pueden tener ocasionalmente núcleos hipercromáticos. Por otro lado el acúmulo lipoideo en las células intersticiales es muy claro.

d) A veces las células intersticiales en el hemangioblastoma pueden presentarse como un sincicio, incluso con núcleos hipercromáticos que, sin embargo, permanecen como células maduras benignas.

a) Ангиоматозная менингеома: Отличительная черта этой опухоли — большое количество почти ангиомоподобных сосудов. Однако между сосудами имеются участки клеток, характерных для эндотелиоматозной менингеомы.

b) Злокачественная менингеома: Повсеместно видны гиперхромные многоядерные гигантские клетки, которые однако еще частично сохранили луковицеподобную структуру этих опухолей.

c) Гемангиобластома (Линдау) характеризуется сетевидным строением капилляров и несколько увеличенными сосудами, между которыми расположены так называемые «промежуточные клетки», содержащие в ряде случаев гиперхромные ядра. Кроме этого в промежуточных клетках довольно часто отмечается накопление липоидов.

d) В отдельных местах промежуточные клетки соединяются как в синцитии. Одновременно ядра становятся гиперхромными, но при этом доброкачественная форма роста не меняется.

a) 血管腫性脳膜腫。血管腫様とよびうるほど多くの血管があり、この腫瘍の特徴となっている。しかし、まだ血管の間には内皮腫性脳膜腫に特徴的な細胞巣をみとめる。

b) 悪性脳膜腫。この組織像は、おもに濃染性、多核巨細胞の形成を示すものである。しかしまだこの腫瘍はたまねぎ様の渦状配列を保っている。

c) 血管芽細胞腫（Lindau）では、毛細血管とそれよりやゝ大きい血管がつくる網状構造が特徴的である。これら血管の間にはいわゆる間細胞が存在する。この細胞はときに濃染核をもつ。さらに間細胞はしばしばリポイドをとりこむ。

d) 二三の部位で間細胞が合胞体のように融合している。核は濃染しているが、腫瘍は良性である。

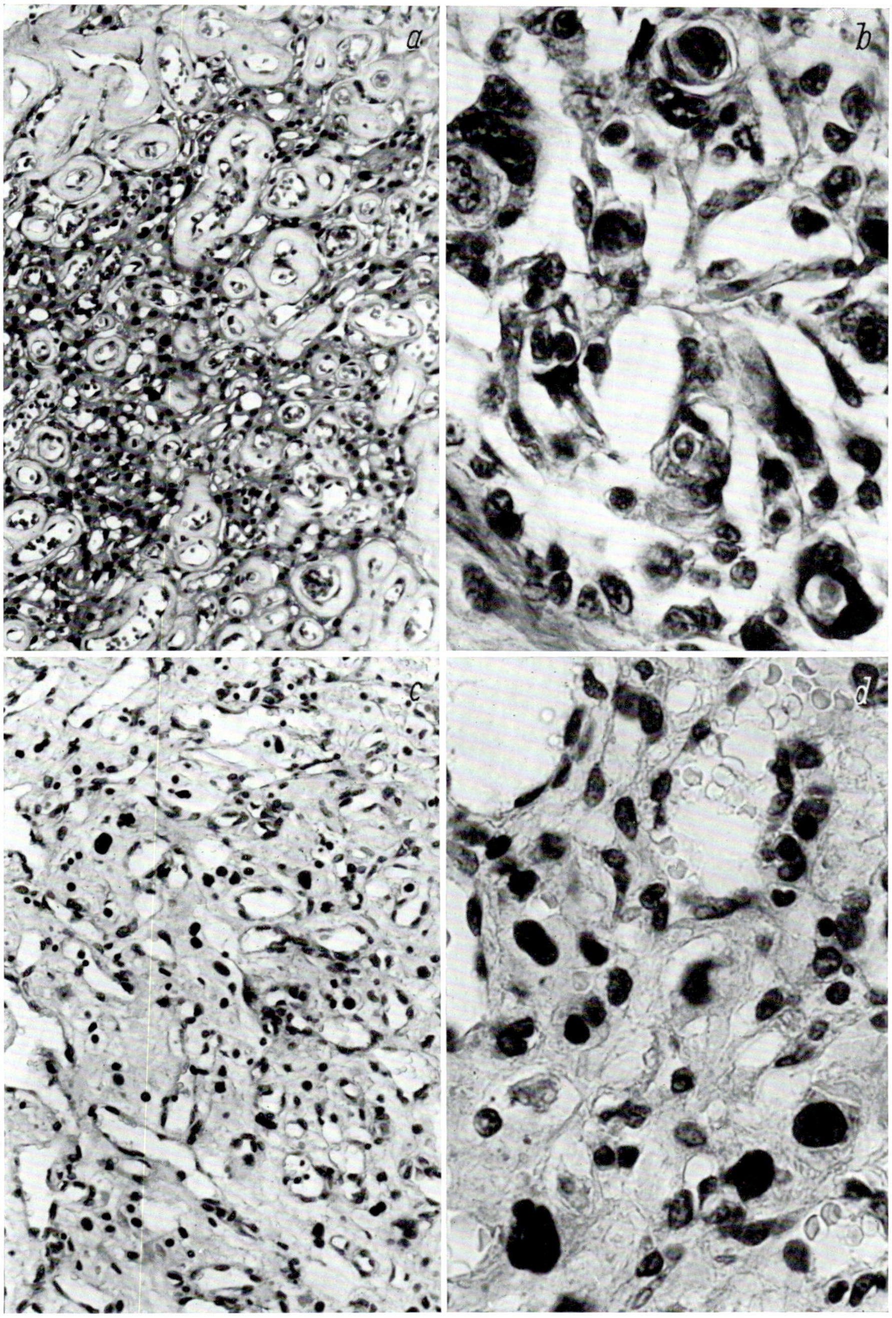

Fig. 78a—d: a ×150, b ×500. H. & E. stain
c ×175, d ×500. Cresyl violet stain

Fig. 79 — Angioblastomas

Concerning the architecture of the hemangioblastoma:

a) Total fatty degeneration of the interstitial cells.
b) Hyaline change of numerous capillaries.
c) Capillary network, well demonstrated by impregnation: One recognizes small cysts, which are occasionally lined with connective tissue.
d) In the dense capillary network of the hemangioblastoma lie single, fairly large blood vessels.

Zur Architektur des Hämangioblastoms:

a) Totale Verfettung der Zwischenzellen.
b) Hyaline Veränderung zahlreicher Capillaren.
c) Capillarnetz, durch Imprägnation gut dargestellt, man erkennt kleine Cysten, die jeweils mit Bindegewebe ausgekleidet sind.
d) In dem dichten Capillarnetz des Hämangioblastoms liegen einzelne größere Gefäße.

Architecture de l'hémangioblastome.

a) Dégénérescence graisseuse complète des cellules interstitielles.
b) Transformation hyaline de nombreux capillaires.
c) Réseau capillaire bien mis en évidence par une imprégnation argentique. On reconnaît de petits kystes qui sont également entourés par du tissu conjonctif.
d) Dans l'angioblastome, il existe quelques vaisseaux plus volumineux au sein du réseau capillaire dense.

Arquitectura del hemangioblastoma:

a) Degeneración grasa total de las células intersticiales.
b) Signos de hialinización en numerosos capilares.
c) Red capilar puesta claramente de manifiesto por la impregnación; se reconocen pequeños quistes, que a veces están recubiertos de tejido conectivo.
d) En la densa red capilar del angioblastoma hay algunos vasos grandes.

Строение ангиобластомы:

a) Тотальное липидное перерождение.
b) Гиалиновое перерождение многочисленных капилляров.
c) Выявленная импрегнацией капиллярная сеть; видны мелкие кисты, которые выстланы соединительной тканью.
d) Отдельные крупные сосуды в густой капиллярной сети ангиобластомы.

血管芽細胞腫の組織構造。

a) 間細胞の完全な脂肪変性。
b) 多数の毛細血管の硝子様変性。
c) 鍍銀で明瞭に示された毛細血管網。結合組織性線維でおおわれた小嚢胞をみとめる。
d) 密な毛細血管網のなかに若干の大きな血管をみとめる。

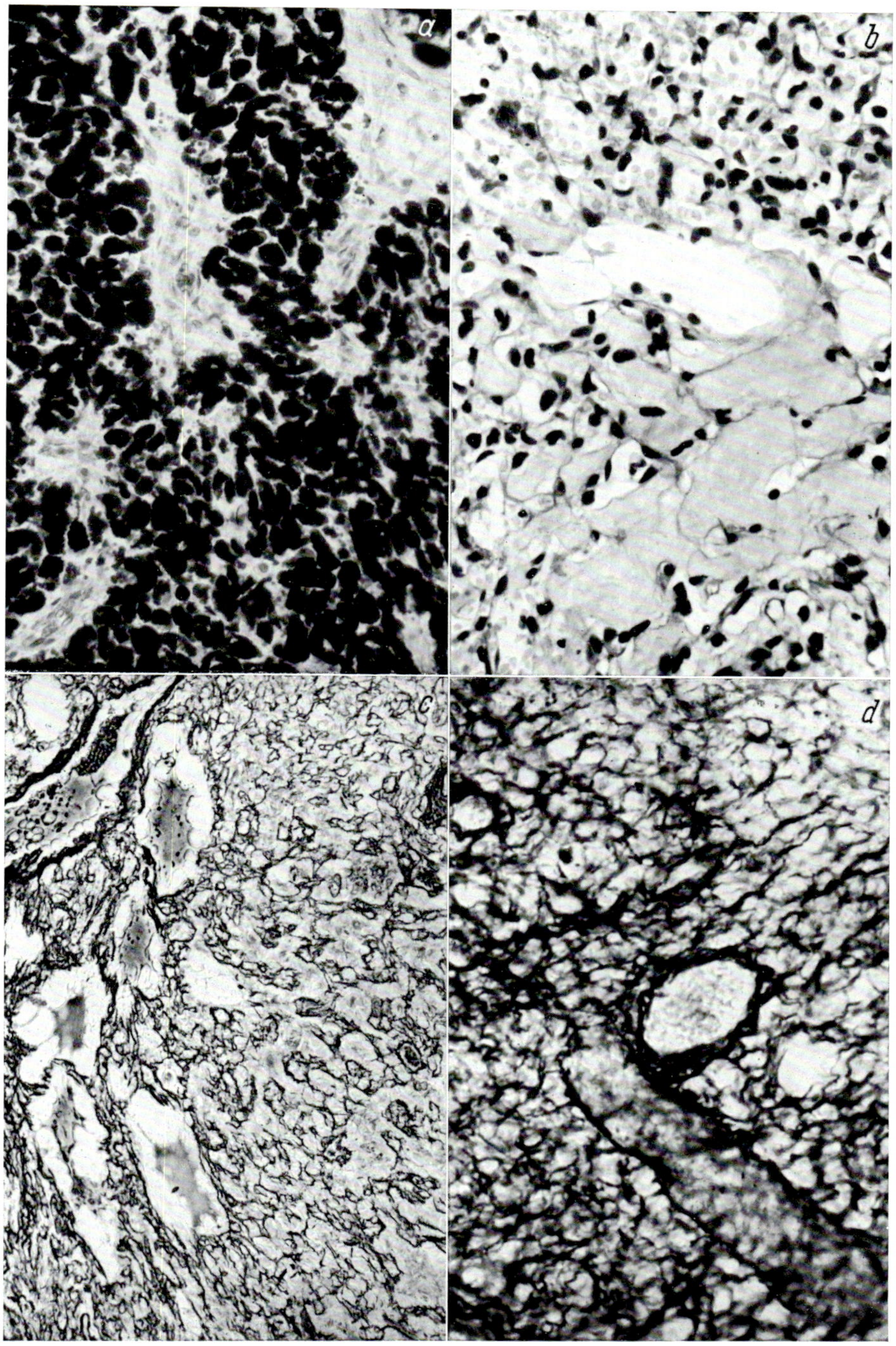

Fig. 79a—d: a ×84. Sudan stain
b ×272. H. & E. stain
c and d ×84, Perdrau's method

Fig. 80 — Angioblastomas

a) and b) Capillary nets or larger vessels and cells composing the vascular wall. One can recognize a few larger "interstitial cells", see c) and d).
c) Typical architecture: many capillaries and lipoid-filled interstitial cells.
d) Higher magnification of c) one sees large "epithelioid" cells possessing abundant cytoplasm lying between fine fibers. The cells contain a fine dust-like accumulation of lipoid material.

a) u. b) Netz von Capillaren oder größeren Gefäßen und Gefäßwandzellen. Man erkennt auch einige größere „Zwischenzellen", s. c) und d).
c) Typisches Bild einer Architektur mit vielen Capillaren und lipoidbeladenen Zwischenzellen.
d) Vergrößerung von c). Man sieht die großen „pseudoepithelialen" cytoplasmareichen Zellen zwischen der feinen Faserung. Die Zellkörper enthalten reichlich feinstaubiges Lipoid.

a) et b) Réseau de capillaires, de vaisseaux de plus grande taille et de cellules endothéliales. On reconnaît aussi quelques «cellules interstitielles» plus volumineuses: voir c) et d).
c) Image architecturale typique avec nombreux capillaires et cellules interstitielles chargées de lipides.
d) Agrandissement de c); on reconnaît les grandes cellules «pseudo-épithéliales» riches en cytoplasme dans un feutrage à fines fibrilles. Les corps cellulaires sont riches en lipoïdes répartis en fines gouttelettes.

a) y b) Redes de capilares o de vasos mayores y células de la pared vascular. Puede verse también alguna «célula intersticial» de mayor tamaño, ver. c) y d).
c) Imagen tipica de la arquitectura, con muchos capilares y células intersticiales con lipoide.
d) Aumento de c): Pueden verse las células pseudoepiteliales, ricas en citoplasma por entre las fibras. Las células poseen finas gótulas.

a) и b) Сеть из капилляров или бóльших сосудов и клеток сосудистой стенки. Видны также отдельные более крупные «Zwischenzellen».
c) Типичная структура: многочисленные капилляры и липоид-содержащие «Zwischenzellen».
d) Увеличение рис. Видны крупные «псевдоэпителиальные», богатые цитоплазмой клетки между тонкими волокнами. В клеточных отростках в изобилии мелкозернистые липоиды.

a) と b) 毛細血管あるいは大きい血管よりなる網状構造、血管壁細胞、さらに二三の大きい間細胞をみとめる。(c)と d)参照)。
c) 定型像：多数の毛細血管とリポイド滴を含んだ間細胞。
d) 例 E 6994 の強拡大。微細な線維の間に胞体に富んだ大きな〝類上皮性〟の細胞をみとめる。細胞体は微細なリポイド滴に富む。

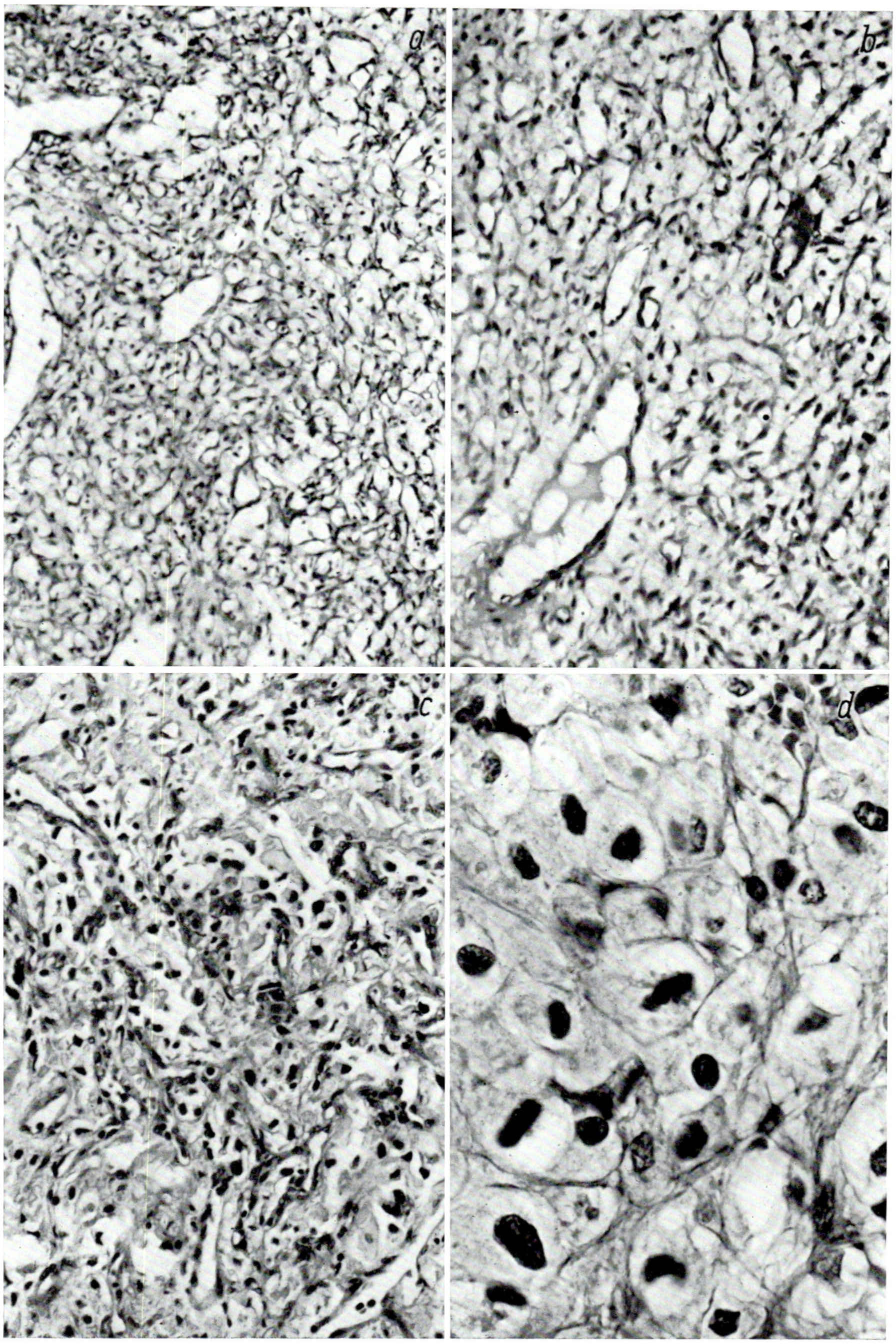

Fig. 80a—d: a $\times$ 125, b $\times$ 250, c $\times$ 175, d $\times$ 500. H. & E. stain

Sturge-Weber's Disease

Fig. 81

Capillary angiomatosis of the leptomeninges

Sarcomas, Various Types

Fig. 82—88

Reticulum cell sarcoma, reticulosarcoma, microglioma, microgliomatosis, retothelial sarcoma
Diffuse sarcomatosis of blood vessels, periadvential diffuse sarcoma.
Sarcomatosis of the meninges, primary meningeal sarcomatosis
Fibrosarcoma (circumscribed), spindle cell sarcoma
Arachnoidal cerebellar sarcoma, circumscribed arachnoidal cerebellar sarcoma

Sarcoma, Monstrocellular

Fig. 84—87

Circumscribed sarcoma of the blood vessels, gigantocellular or giant-cell glioblastoma, spongioblastoma ganglioides

Fig. 81 — Angiomatosis of the meninges

a)—c) Typical pattern of a Sturge-Weber's angiomatosis. The pia is filled with three to four layers of thin-walled (venous and capillary) vessels. The first, second, and third cortical layers are densely permeated by calcium granules and plaques. A second zone of calcification is found in the sixth layer.

d) A peculiar malformation (exencephaly), which has a certain pathogenetic relationship to Sturge-Weber's angiomatosis. The pia was everywhere densely covered by a network of small and medium-sized blood vessels, predominantly of venous structure, which have a certain similarity to Sturge-Weber's angiomatosis.

a)—c) Typisches Bild einer Sturge-Weberschen Angiomatose. Die weichen Häute sind ausgefüllt mit 3—4 Lagen von dünnwandigen (venösen und capillären) Gefäßen. Die 1.—3. Rindenschicht ist dicht von Kalkperlen und Kalkplatten durchsetzt. Eine zweite Verkalkungszone findet sich in der 6. Schicht.

d) Eigenartige Mißbildung (Exencephalie), die in einer gewissen pathogenetischen Beziehung zur Sturge-Weberschen Angiomatose liegt. Die weichen Häute waren überall dicht überzogen von einem Netz von kleineren und mittleren Gefäßen, vorwiegend venösen Baus, die eine gewisse Ähnlichkeit mit der Sturge-Weberschen Angiomatose haben.

a)—c) Image typique d'angiomatose de Sturge-Weber. La leptoméninge est bourrée de 3 ou 4 couches de vaisseaux (veines ou capillaires) à paroi mince. De nombreux grains et plaques calcaires sont concentrés dans les trois premières couches corticales. Une deuxième zone de calcifications occupe la sixième couche.

d) Malformation curieuse (exencéphalie), qui présente un certain rapport pathogénique avec l'angiomatose de Sturge-Weber. La leptoméninge est complètement tapissée par un réseau de petits et moyens vaisseaux, principalement de type veineux, qui présentent une certaine similitude avec l'angiomatose de Sturge-Weber.

a)—c) Típica imagen de una angiomatosis de STURGE-WEBER. Las leptomeninges están ocupadas por tres o cuatro capas de vasos (venosos y capilares) de fina pared. Las capas 1—3 del cortex están densamente ocupadas por perlas y placas calcáreas. Una segunda zona de calcificación se encuentra en la sexta capa.

d) Especial malformación (exencefalia) que tiene una indudable relación patogenética con la angiomatosis de STURGE-WEBER. Por todas partes las leptomeninges se encuentran revestidas por una red de pequeños y medianos vasos, de conformación predominantemente venosa, los cuales tienen un determinado parecido con la angiomatosis de STURGE-WEBER.

a)—c) Типичная картина ангиоматоза Штурге-Вебера. В мягких мозговых оболочках 3—4 слоя тонкостенных венозных и капиллярных сосудов. В 1—3 корковых слоях обилие глыбок и пластинок кальция. Вторая зона обызвествления имеется в 6-м слое.

d) Своеобразное уродство (экзоэнцефалия), в известной мере генетически связанное с ангиоматозом Штурге-Вебера. На мягких мозговых оболочках как бы натянута густая сеть из мелких и средней величины преимущественно венозных сосудов, имеющие определенное сходство с ангиоматозом Штурге-Вебера.

a) —c) Sturge-Weber 血管腫症の定型像。軟膜には壁の薄い血管（静脈性および毛細管性）が層状に並んでいる。大脳皮質第１層から第３層にかけて、密な小石灰化巣がみられる。第６層にも石灰化巣をみとめる。

d) Sturge-Weber 血管腫瘍と関係があると思われる、特有な血管奇型。（脳露出頭蓋に合併したもの）。軟膜は種々の大きさの血管網によっておおわれている。その血管は大部分静脈性で、Sturge-Weber 血管腫瘍のそれと似ている。

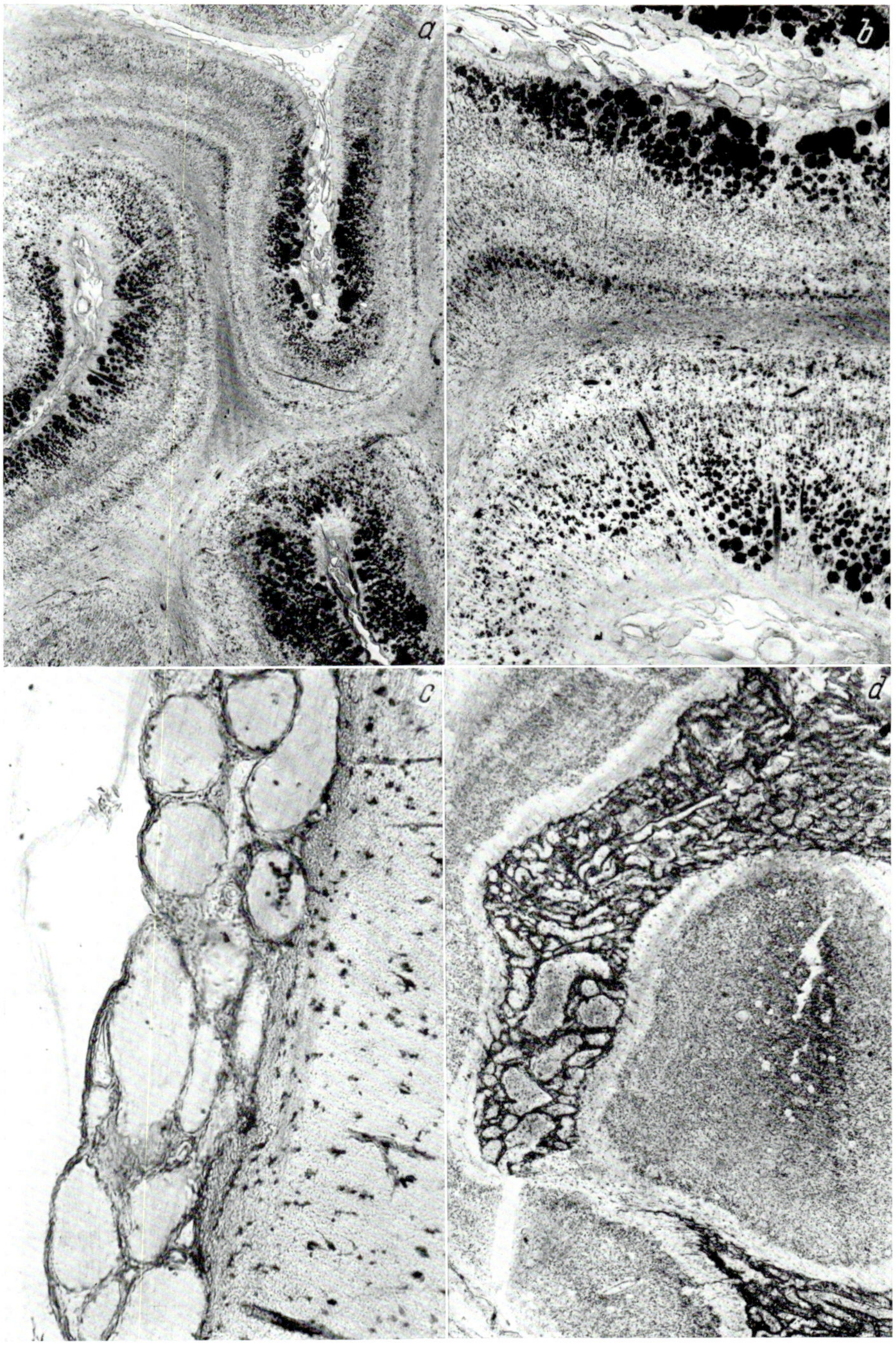

Fig. 81a—d: a ×4, b and d ×8, c ×172
Nissl stain

Fig. 82 — Sarcomas, Various Types

a) Diffuse retothelial sarcoma of various organs of the body: From the meningeal infiltrations the tumor cells advance along the blood vessels into the brain.
b) A "periadventitially" growing blastoma, which is closely related to the retothelial tumors.
c) Sarcomatosis of the *meninges:* The cells advance from the arachnoidea (*left*) along the blood vessels, or in a diffuse form, toward the brain.
d) Diffuse sarcomatosis of the *blood vessels.* The cells lie partly within the adventitial space and partly outside as a wide tunic. Macrogliosis in the vicinity.

a) Diffuses Retothelsarkom verschiedener Körperorgane. Von den meningealen Infiltraten aus dringen die Geschwulstzellen entlang den Gefäßen ins Hirn.
b) „Periadventitiell" wachsendes Blastom, das den retothelialen Tumoren nahesteht.
c) Sarkomatose der *Meningen:* Die Zellen dringen von der Arachnoidea (links) entlang den Gefäßen bzw. in diffuser Form gegen das Hirn vor.
d) Diffuse Sarkomatose der *Gefäße.* Die Zellen liegen teils im Adventitialraum, teils als breiter Mantel außerhalb desselben. Makrogliose der Nachbarschaft.

a) Sarcome rétothélial diffus de divers organes du corps; à partir des infiltrats méningés, les cellules tumorales pénètrent dans le cerveau le long des vaisseaux.
b) Néoplasme à prolifération «péri-adventitielle», qui correspond bien aux tumeurs rétothéliales.
c) Sarcomatose *méningée:* à partir de l'arachnoïde (à gauche), les cellules pénètrent dans le cerveau soit le long des vaisseaux, soit de façon diffuse.
d) Sarcomatose diffuse *des vaisseaux:* des manchons de cellules occupent les espaces adventitiels et infiltrent plus largement le parenchyme environnant. Gliose astrocytaire dans le voisinage.

a) Sarcoma retotelial difuso de diferentes órganos corporales. A partir de los infiltrados meníngeos las células tumorales invaden el cerebro a lo largo de los vasos.
b) Blastoma «periadventicial», que se parece a los tumores retoteliales.
c) Sarcomatosis de las *Meninges:* Las células, a partir de la aracnoides, se abren paso hacía el cerebro, a lo largo de los vasos o bien de forma difusa.
d) Sarcomatosis difusa de los *Vasos.* Las células están por una parte en el espacio adventicial, por otra se extienden fuera de éste como un aplio manto. Macrogliosis de los alrededores.

a) Диффузная ретикулярная саркома разных органов: Из менингеальных инфильтратов опухолевые клетки вдоль сосудов проникают в мозг.
b) «Периадвентициально» растущая бластома, сходная с ретикулярными опухолями.
c) Саркоматоз оболочек: из паутинной оболочки (слева) клетки вдоль сосудов диффузно проникают в мозг.
d) Диффузный саркоматоз сосудов. Частично клетки находятся в адвентициальном пространстве и частично в виде широкого плаща вне его пределов. Макроглиоз соседних участков.

a) 種々の部位に発生したびまん性細網肉腫。腫瘍細胞は、脳膜浸潤巣から血管にそって脳内に浸入している。
b) 血管周囲に増殖した腫瘍。これは細網肉腫と思われる症例。
c) 脳膜にびまん性に広がった肉腫。腫瘍細胞はクモ膜 (左) から血管ぞいに、あるいはびまん性に脳に浸潤している。
d) 血管周囲にびまん性に広がった肉腫。細胞は血管外膜腔に、一部はすでにその外側に厚い外套として存在している。周囲にマクログリアの増殖がみられる。

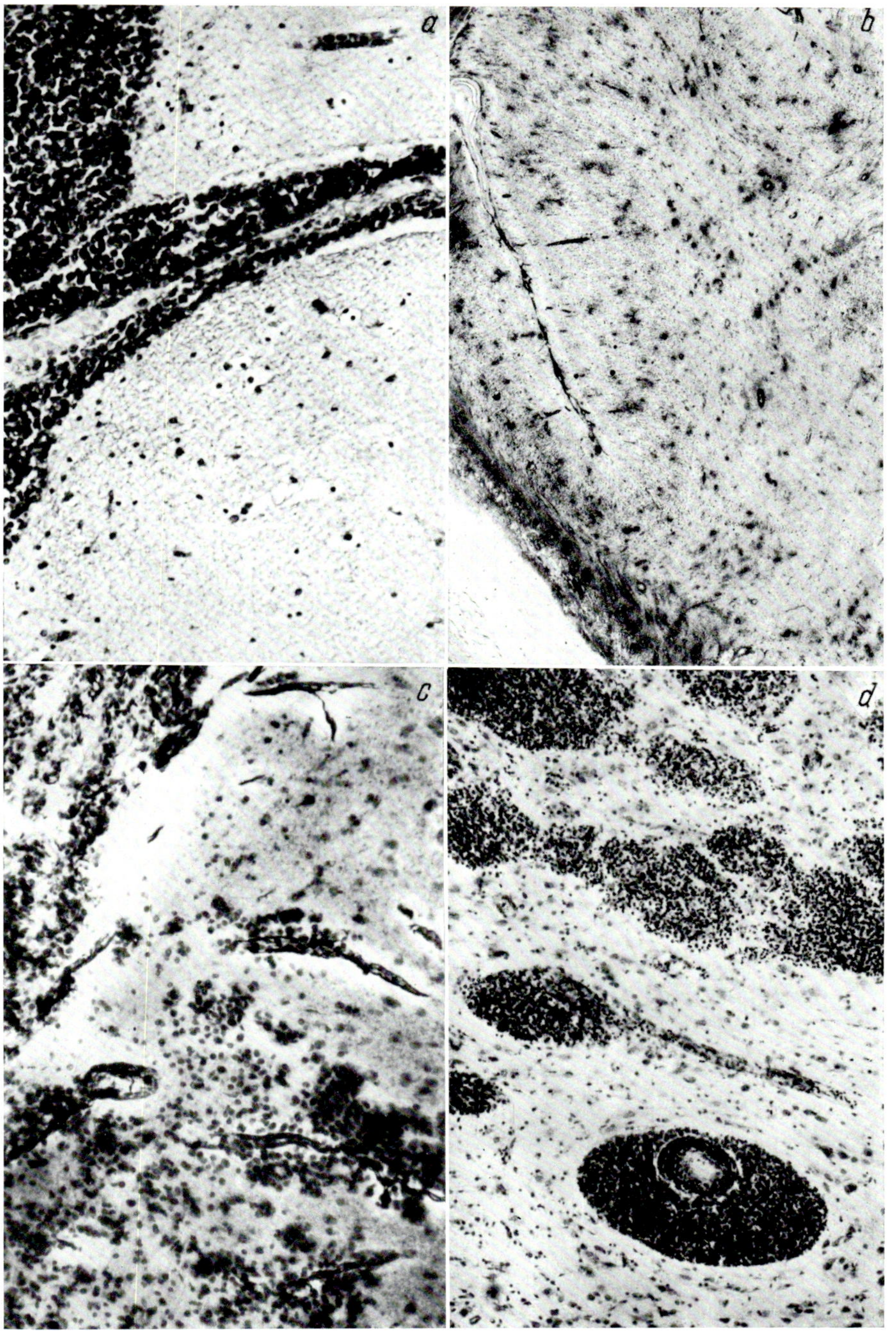

Fig. 82a—d: a ×168. H. & E. stain
b ×22. Nissl stain
c ×378. Perdrau's impregnation with nuclear fast red stain
d ×78. Cresyl violet stain

Fig. 83 — Sarcomas, Various Types

a) Infiltrating, but well-circumscribed growth of a spindle-cell sarcoma of the dura.
b) Higher magnification of a spindle-cell sarcoma of the dura with numerous mitoses.
c) Sarcomatous disintegrated neurofibroma in von Recklinghausen's disease.
d) Fibrosarcoma the Gasserian ganglion (in a elephant).

a) Infiltrierendes, aber doch recht gut begrenztes Vorwachsen eines spindelzelligen Sarkoms der Dura.
b) Höhere Vergrößerung eines Spindelzellsarkoms der Dura mit zahlreichen Mitosen.
c) Sarkomatös entartetes Neurofibrom bei Recklinghausenscher Krankheit.
d) Fibrosarkom am Ganglion Gasseri (bei einem Elefanten).

a) Sarcome fuso-cellulaire de la dure-mère, qui, malgré son caractère infiltrant, reste encore bien délimité.
b) Sarcome fuso-cellulaire de la dure-mères, vu à un plus fort grossissement. Les mitoses sont nombreuses.
c) Dégénérescence sarcomateuse d'un neurofibrome en cas de maladie de von Recklinghausen.
d) Fibrosarcome du ganglion de Gasser (chez un éléphant).

a) Crecimiento infiltrante aún bastante bien delimitado de un sarcoma de la dura.
b) Mayor aumento de un sarcoma fusocelular de la dura con numerosas mitosis.
c) Degeneración sarcomatosa de un neurofibroma en la enfermedad de Recklinghausen.
d) Fibrosarcoma del ganglio de Gasser (en un elefante).

a) Инфильтрирующий, но четко ограниченный рост веретеноклеточной саркомы твердой мозговой оболочки.
b) Бóльшее увеличение веретеноклеточной саркомы твердой мозговой оболочки с многочисленными митозами.
c) Саркоматозно-перерожденная нейрофиброма при болезни Реклингаузена.
d) Фибросаркома гассерова узла у слона.

a) 脳内に浸潤しているものの、境界はまだ鮮明な硬膜紡錘細胞肉腫。
b) 硬膜紡錘細胞肉腫の強拡大。多数の核分裂をみる。
c) Recklinghausen 病にみられた神経線維腫の肉腫化。
d) Gasser 神経節の線維肉腫 (象)。

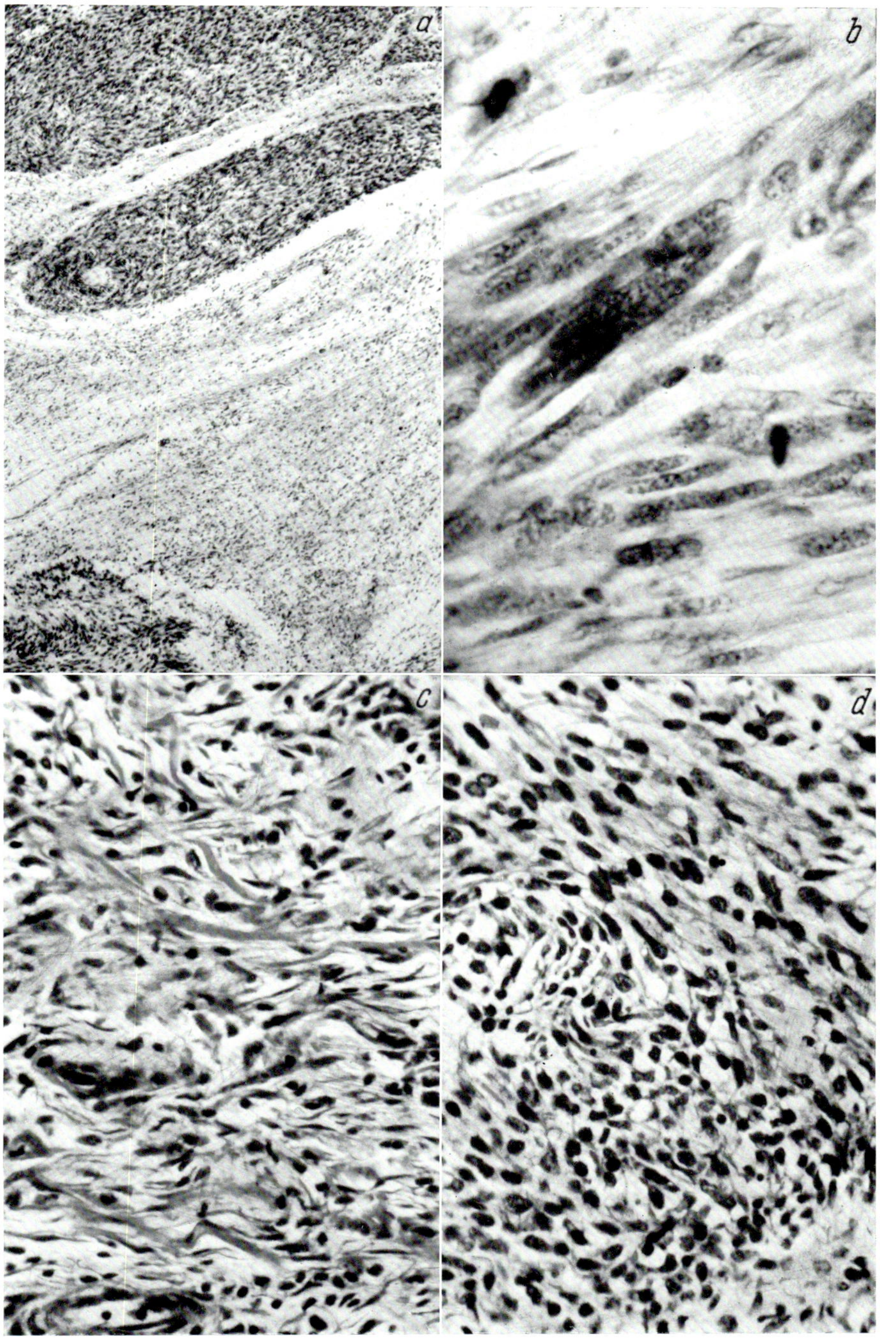

Fig. 83a—d: a ×72, b ×576. Nissl stain
c ×336, d ×172. H. & E. stain

Fig. 84 — Sarcoma, Monstrocellular

Polymorphic cells of a monstrocellular sarcoma. Some cells clearly resemble ganglion cells in their external shape (*top right*) or in their construction (*bottom left*) or at least in their nuclear structure (*bottom right*).

Polymorphe Zellen eines monstrocellulären Sarkoms. Einige Zellen ähneln deutlich in der Außenform (rechts oben) oder im Bau (links unten) oder zumindest in der Kernstruktur (rechts unten) den Ganglienzellen.

Cellules polymorphes dans un sarcome monstrocellulaire. Certaines cellules ressemblent nettement aux cellules nerveuses soit par leur forme extérieure (au-dessus et à droite), soit par leur structure (au-dessous et à gauche), soit au moins par l'aspect de leur noyau (au-dessous et à droite).

Células polimorfas de un sarcoma monstrocelular. Algunas células se parecen en su forma exterior (arriba y a la derecha), o en su construcción (abajo, a la izquierda) o como mínimo en su estructura nuclear (derecha, abajo) a las células ganglionares.

Полиморфные клетки уродливоклеточной саркомы. Некоторые клетки по форме (вверху справа) или строению (внизу слева) или по меньшей мере по структуре ядра сходны с ганглиозными клетками.

Monstrozelluläres Sarkom にみられる多形な腫瘍細胞。いくつかの細胞は、その外形（右上)、構造（左下)、あるいは少くともその核構造（右下）の点で神経細胞によく似ている。

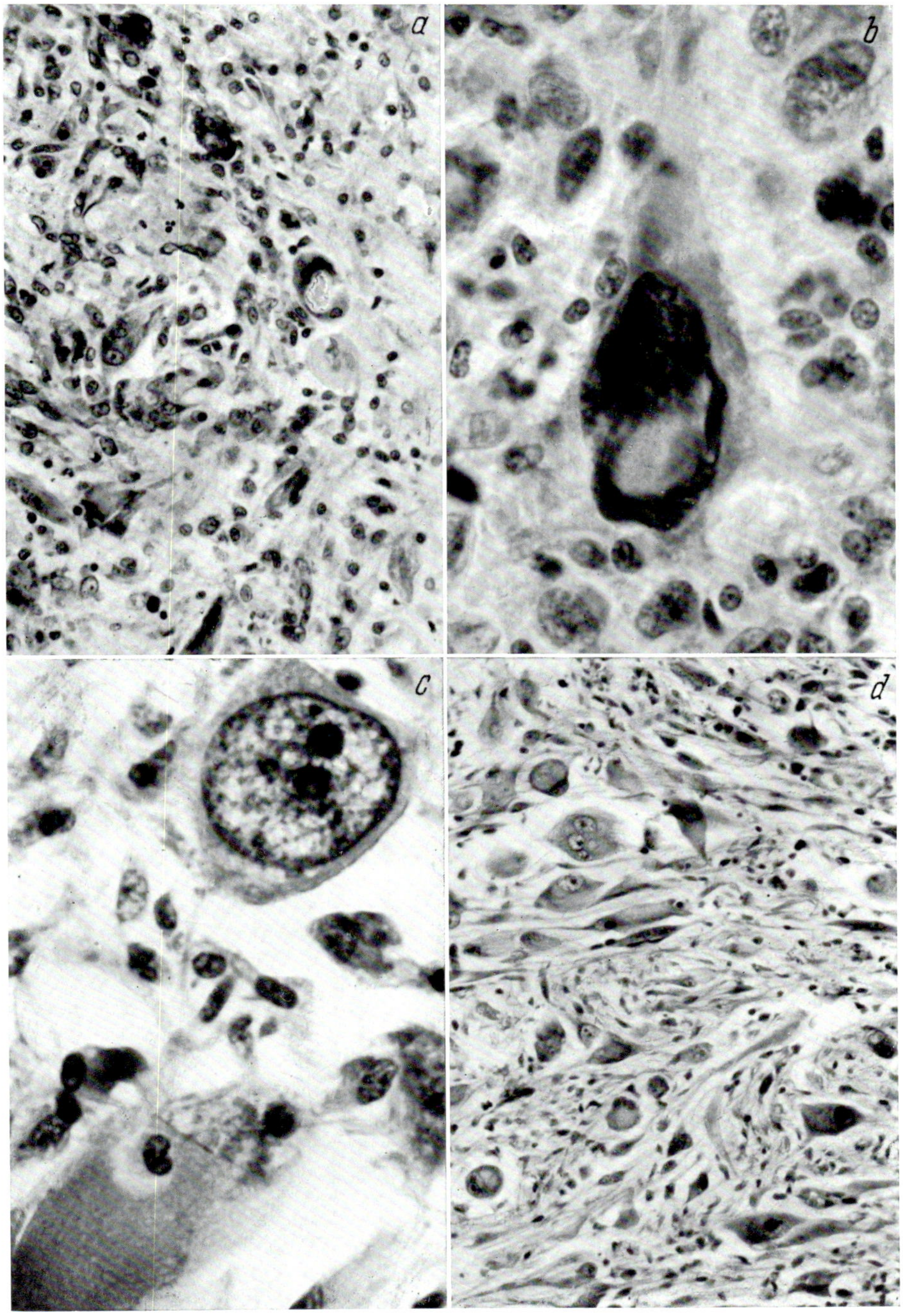

Fig. 84a—d: a ×112, b ×540, c ×372, d ×114
Cresyl violet stain

Fig. 85 — Sarcoma, Monstrocellular

a) Dysmorphic giant cells in the vicinity of a glomerulus formation of vascular coils.
b) Numerous atypically constructed giant mitoses.
c) Two monster cells and other cells of all sizes. The number of the cell nuclei is enormous.
d) A monster cell with countless nuclear components of all sizes. These components were formerly described as "inclusion bodies", "bird's-eye inclusions", etc. Some nuclei have distinct nuclear vacuoles.

a) Dysmorphe Riesenzellen in der Nähe einer Gefäßschlingen- und Glomerulusbildung.
b) Zahlreiche atypisch gebaute Riesenmitosen.
c) Zwei Zellmonstra und weitere Zellen aller Größen. Die Zahl der Zellkerne ist enorm.
d) Zellmonstrum mit unzähligen Kernbestandteilen aller Größen, die früher als „Einschlußkörperchen", „Vogelaugeneinschlüsse", usw. bezeichnet wurden. Einige Kerne haben deutliche Kernvacuolen.

a) Cellules géantes anormales au voisinage d'un amas de vaisseaux enlacés et à disposition glomérulaire.
b) Nombreuses mitoses géantes et atypiques.
c) Parmi des cellules de toutes tailles, on note deux cellules monstrueuses contenant un nombre énorme de noyaux.
d) Cellule monstrueuse contenant une quantité innombrable de particules nucléaires de toutes dimensions, que l'on appelait autrefois «inclusions», «inclusions en forme d'oeil d'oiseau», etc... Dans certains noyaux, il existe des vacuoles.

a) Células gigantes deformes en las cercanías de lazos vasculares y formaciones glomerulares.
b) Numerosas mitosis gigantes atípicas.
c) Dos células monstruosas y otras células de distintos tamaños. El número de núcleos celulares es enorme.
d) Célula monstruosa con innumerables fragmentos nucleares de distintos tamaños, que anteriormente se consideraban como corpúsculos de inclusión o inclusiones en ojo de pájaro. Algunos núcleos tienen claras vacuolas.

a) Аморфные гигантские клетки вблизи сосудистых петель и гломерулоподобных образований.
b) Многочисленные атипичного строения гигантские митозы.
c) Две уродливые клетки и другие клетки разных величин. Огромное число клеточных ядер.
d) Уродливая клетка с бесчисленными составными частями ядра разных величин, которые ранее обозначались как «тельца включения», «включения типа птичий глаз» и т. д. В ряде ядер имеется четкая вакуоля.

a) 糸球体様血管増殖部附近にみられた異型的な巨細胞。
b) 多数の異型的な、しかも巨大な核分裂像。
c) ２個の異様な形をした巨細胞と、種々の大きさの細胞。核の数は異常に多い。
d) 大小不同で、無数の核をもつ異様な形をした巨細胞。これは以前「封入体」、「鳥の目状封入物」とよばれていたもの。二三の核には明瞭な核空胞がある。

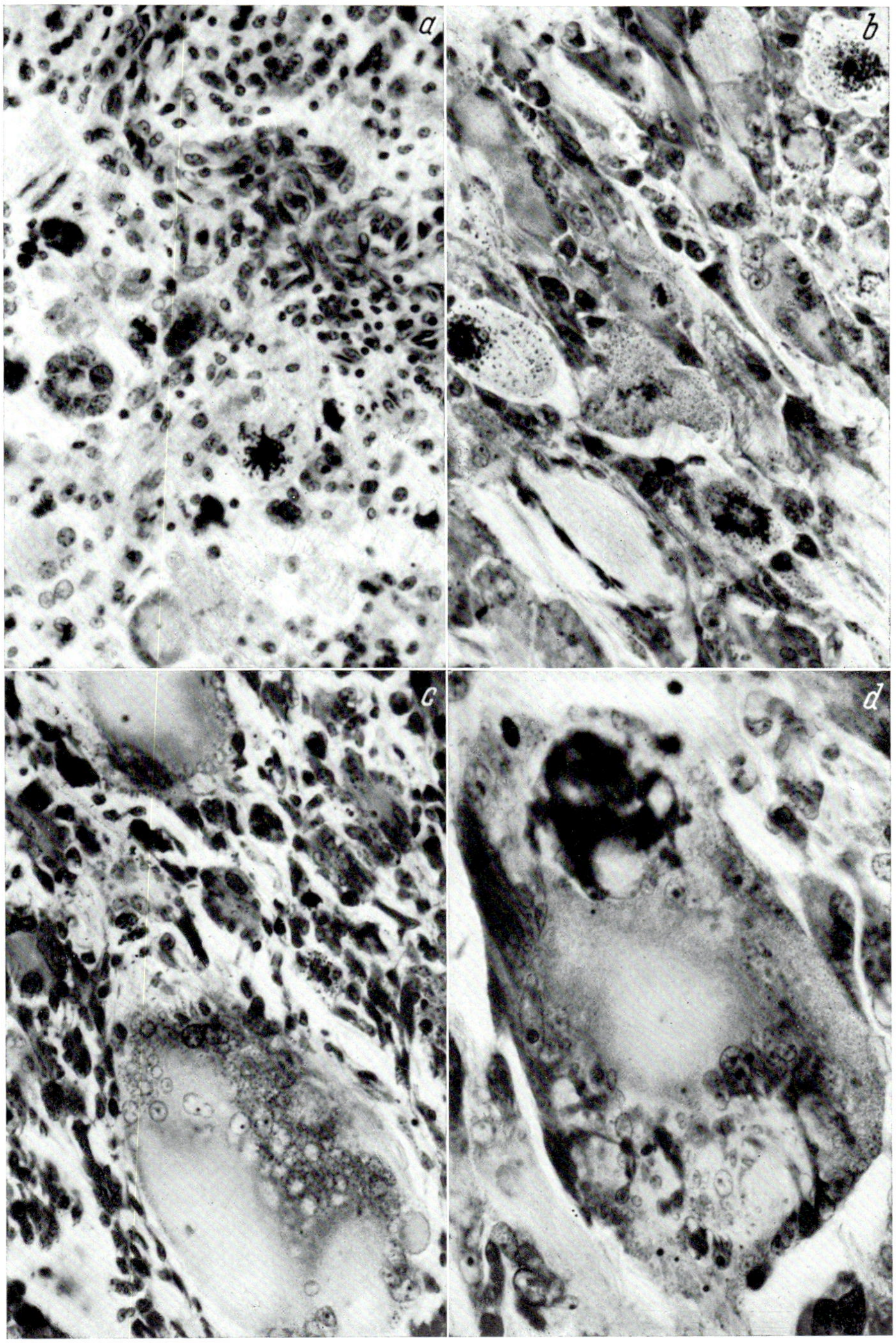

Fig. 85a—d: a ×176, b—d ×224
Cresyl violet stain

Fig. 86 — Sarcoma, Monstrocellular

The tissue pattern of the "monstrocellular sarcoma":

a) Necrotic portion in a predominantly spindle-celled area.

b) Vascular proliferation at the margin of a zone of necrosis with peculiar papillary formations. One recognizes a monstrous giant cell.

c) and d) Location of the tumor cells with reference to the vascular lumen: Sometimes the tumor cells seem to border directly on the blood vessel without any special endothelium.

Das Gewebsbild des ,,monstrocellulären Sarkoms":

a) Nekrotische Partie in einem vorwiegend spindelzelligen Teil.

b) Gefäßproliferation am Rande einer Nekrose mit eigenartig papillären Bildungen. Man erkennt eine monströse Riesenzelle.

c) u. d) Lage der Geschwulstzellen zum Gefäßlumen: Manchmal scheinen die Geschwulstzellen ohne besonderes Endothel direkt an die Blutbahn zu grenzen.

L'aspect histologique du «sarcome monstrocellulaire».

a) Zone nécrotique dans une région constituée principalement de cellules fusiformes.

b) A la périphérie d'une nécrose, prolifération vasculaire et formation de curieuses images papillaires. On reconnaît une cellule géante monstrueuse.

c) et d) Couche de cellules tumorales autour de la lumière vasculaire: on a souvent l'impression que les cellules tumorales arrivent au contact direct du contenu sanguin, sans qu'il y ait de limite endothéliale.

Imagen del sarcoma monstrocelular:

a) Zonas necróticas en una parte predominantemente fusiforme.

b) Proliferación vascular en los bordes de una necrosis con características formaciones papilares. Se reconoce una célula gigante monstruosa.

c) y d) Disposición de las células tumorales en el lumen vascular: a veces las células tumorales parecen limitar directamente la corriente sanguínea, sin que exista ningún endotelio especial.

Строение «уродливоклеточной саркомы»:

a) очаг некроза в преимущественно веретеноклеточной части опухоли (окраска крезилвиолетом).

b) Пролиферация сосудов в окружности некроза со своеобразными папиллярными образованиями. Видна уродливая гигантская клетка.

c) и d) Расположение опухолевых клеток по отношению к просвету сосуда. Иногда опухолевые клетки непосредственно граничат с кровотоком.

「Monstrozelluläres Sarkom」の組織像。

a) 主として紡錘細胞よりなる腫瘍部。その一部に壊死をみとめる。

b) 壊死周辺における特有な乳頭状構造をもった血管の増殖。異様な巨細胞がみられる。

c) および d) 血管腔にたいする腫瘍細胞の位置的関係。腫瘍細胞は、しばしば内皮細胞のごとく直接血流に接している。

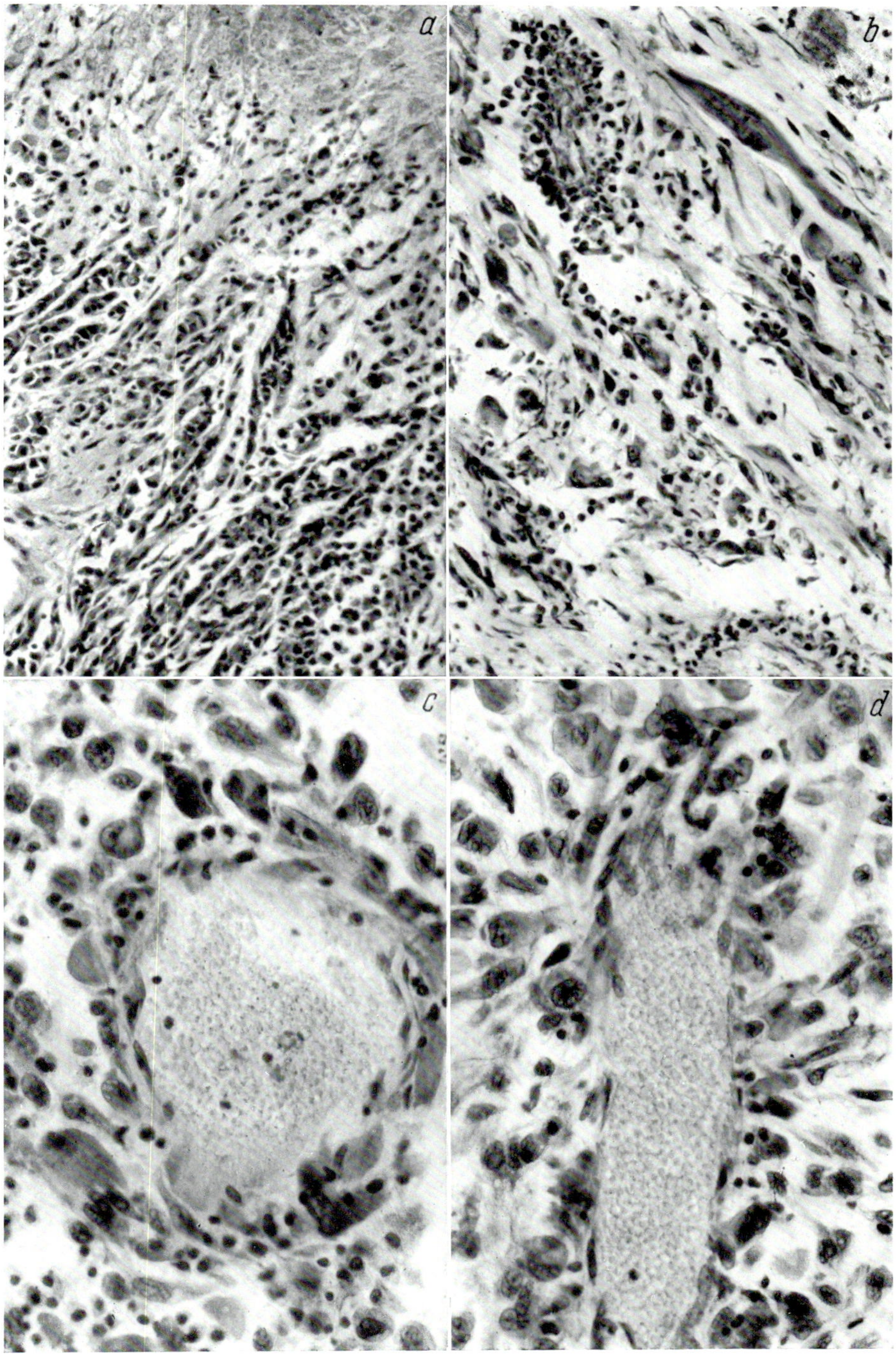

Fig. 86a—d: a ×136, b ×144, c and d ×240
Cresyl violet stain

Fig. 87 — Sarcoma, Monstrocellular

a) and b) Penetration of the tumor into the surrounding tissue by means of papilliform processes from which large, undifferentiated tumor cells detach.
c) and d) Concentric layers of tumor cells around vessels.

a) u. b) Vordringen der Geschwulst in der Randzone mit papillenförmigen Fortsätzen, von denen sich monströse Geschwulstzellen ablösen.
c) u. d) Konzentrische Anordnung der Geschwulstzellen um die Gefäße in mehreren Lagen.

a) et b) Pénétration de la tumeur dans le tissu environnant par des bourgeons de forme papillaire, dont se détachent des cellules géantes monstrueuses.
c) et d) Disposition concentrique des cellules tumorales en plusieurs couches autour des vaisseaux.

a) y b) Crecimiento en la zona periférica con formas papilares, desprendiéndose células tumorales monstruosas.
c) y d) Disposición concéntrica de las células tumorales en los vasos en varios puntos.

a) и b) Проникновение опухоли в краевую зону сосочковидными отростками, от которых отделяются уродливые опухолевые клетки.
c) и d) Многослойное концентрическое расположение опухолевых клеток вокруг сосудов.

a) および b) 腫瘍は乳頭状の突起をもって周囲組織に浸入し、その部位から異様な形の腫瘍細胞が分離する。
c) および d) 腫瘍細胞が血管を層状にとり囲む。

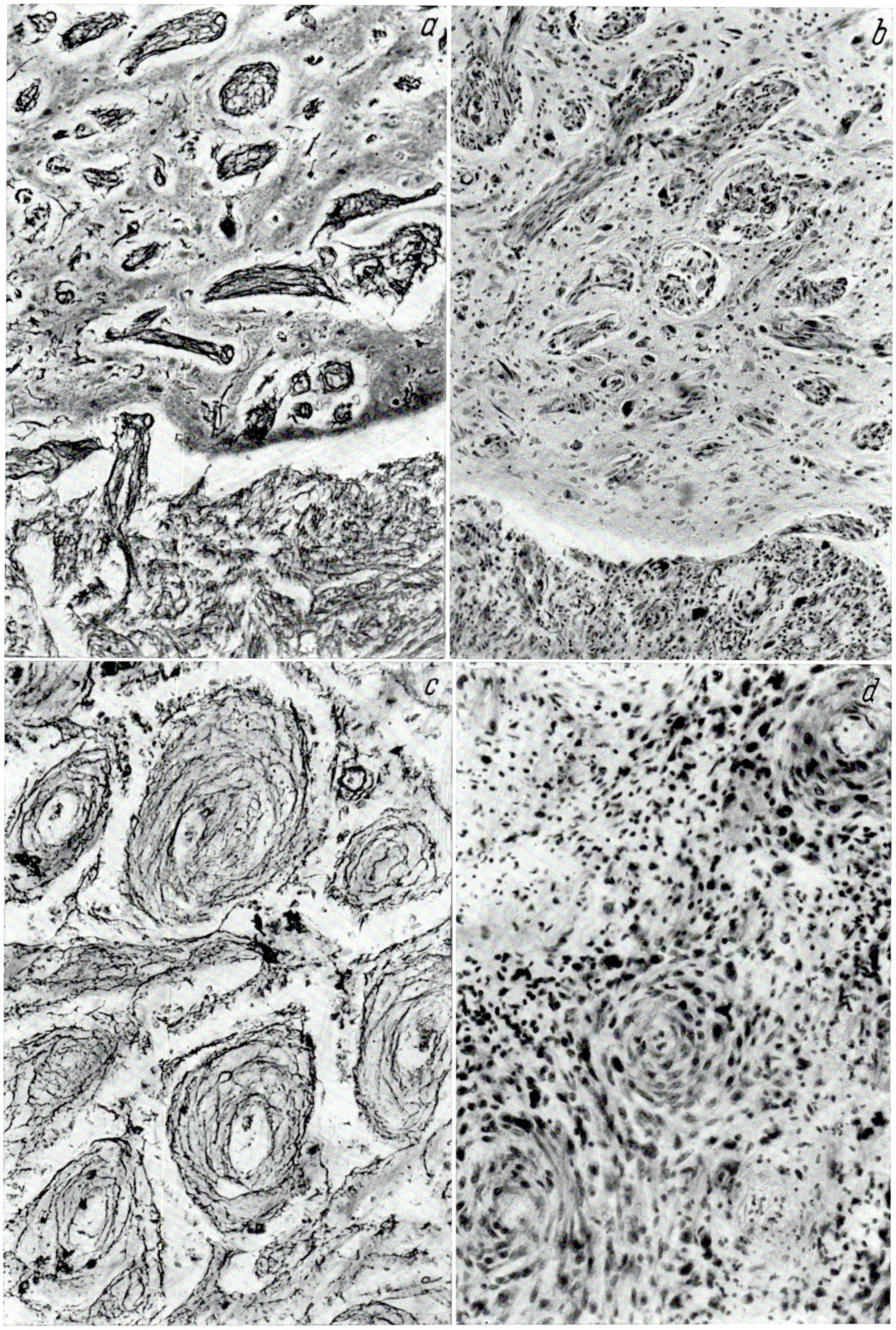

Fig. 87a—d: a ×78, c ×104. Perdrau's method
b ×78, d ×104. Cresyl violet stain

Fig. 88 — Sarcomas, Various Types

So-called "arachnoidal sarcoma".

a) Typical architecture demonstrating islets containing few cells lying within the highly cellular tissue of the tumor.
b) Similar architecture following silver impregnation: there is hardly any fiber production within the cells although such fibers are present abundantly in the tumor.
c) and d) Reticulum cell sarcoma.
c) Tumor cells are situated on the fibers like "buds on a pussy willow twig".
d) More alveolar architecture, likewise, containing numerous silver impregnated fibers.

Sog. „Arachnoidalsarkom".

a) Typische Architektur mit zellärmeren Inseln in dem zellreicheren Normalgewebe der Geschwulst.
b) Gleiche Architektur mit Silberimprägnation: in den Zellen keinerlei Produktion von Silberfasern, die sonst reichlich in der Geschwulst vorhanden sind.
c) u. d) Retothelsarkom.
c) Die Geschwulstzellen sitzen den Fasern auf wie „Weidenkätzchen auf den Ruten".
d) Mehr alveoläre Architektur, ebenfalls mit reichlich Silberfasern.

Tumeur appelée «sarcome de l'arachnoïde».

a) Architecture typique due à la présence d'îlots pauvres en cellules au sein du tissu tumoral, qui est par ailleurs très cellulaire.
b) Même architecture après imprégnation argentique: dans les îlots, les fibres réticuliniques sont absentes alors qu'elles sont très abondantes dans le reste de la tumeur.
c) et d) Réticulosarcome.
c) Les cellules tumorales sont situées le long des fibres «comme des chatons sur des branches».
d) Architecture plus alvéolaire, également riche en fibres argentophiles.

Los llamados «sarcomas de la aracnoides»:

a) Típica arquitectura con conglomerados pobres en células en tejido normal del tumor.
b) La misma arquitectura con impregnación argéntica. En las células ninguna producción de fibras argentófilas tan ricas por otro lado en el tumor.
c) y d) Retotelsarcoma.
c) Las células tumorales están localizadas en las fibras como racimos.
d) Arquitectura más alveolar, pero más rica en fibras argentófilas.

Так называемая «арахноидальная саркома».

a) Типичные строение опухоли. В нормальной богатой клетками ткани опухоли видны островки бедные клетками.
b) Такая же структура при импрегнации серебром. Полное отсутствие продуцирования аргирофильных волокон, обилием которых обычно отличается эта опухоль.
c) и d) Ретотельсаркома.
c) Опухолевые клетки сидят на волокнах как «сережки на ветке».
d) Более альвеолярные строения так же с многочисленными аргирофильными волокнами.

いわゆる〝クモ膜肉腫〞

a) 定型的腫瘍は、細胞成分に富んだ腫瘍組織内に、細胞成分の少い島をみとめる。
b) 鍍銀を行なった同一腫瘍。腫瘍組織は好銀線維に富む。
c) および d) 細網肉腫。
c) 腫瘍細胞は線維に密着している。
d) 好銀線維を豊富にもった胞状構造。

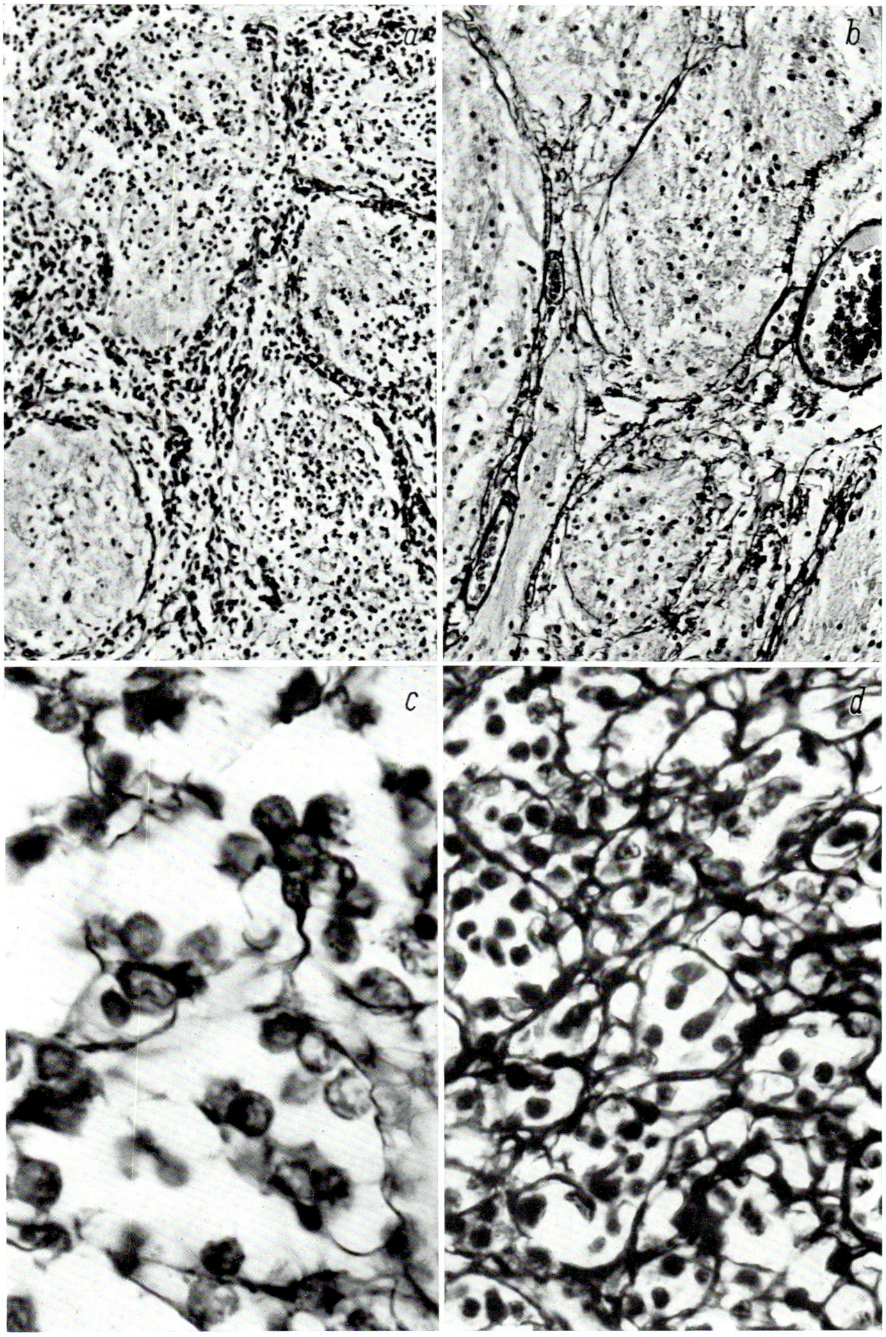

Fig. 88a—d: a and b × 125. H. & E. stain
c × 500, d × 250. Perdrau's method

Pinealomas

Pineocytoma, pineoblastoma, germinoma of the pineal gland, adenoma, adenocarcinoma, psammoma or psammosarcoma of the pineal body

Fig. 89 — Pinealomas

The various forms of pinealomas:

a) Typical juxtaposition of the large clear cells and the small "lymphoid" elements in the anisomorphic pinealoma.
b) Markedly striated architecture in an anisomorphic pinealoma with multinucleated giant cells and only a few lymphoid elements.
c) Same tissue as in a), but impregnated with gold sublimate.
d) Isomorphic type of a pinealoma. The cells are medium-sized and round or oval. Only single, somewhat larger, hyperchromatic nuclei can be seen. The small lymphoid cells are lacking.

Die verschiedenen Formen der Pinealome:

a) Typisches Nebeneinander der großen hellen Zellen und der kleinen „lymphoiden" Elemente im anisomorphen Pinealom.
b) Ausgesprochen streifenförmige Architektur in einem anisomorphen Pinealom mit einzelnen mehrkernigen Riesenzellen und nur wenig lymphoiden Elementen.
c) Gleiches Gewebe wie a), aber bei Imprägnation mit Goldsublimat.
d) Isomorpher Typ eines Pinealoms. Die Zellen sind mittelgroß, rundlich oder oval. Nur einzelne etwas größere hyperchromatische Kerne sind zu sehen. Es fehlen die kleinen lymphoiden Zellen.

Les différentes formes du pinéalome.

a) Mélange caractéristique de grandes cellules claires et de petits éléments «lymphoïdes» dans le pinéalome anisomorphe.
b) Nette disposition architecturale sous forme de cordons dans un cas de pinéalome anisomorphe, qui contient quelques cellules géantes, multinucléées, et un petit nombre seulement d'éléments lymphoïdes.
c) Même tissu que dans a), mais après une imprégnation à l'or sublimé.
d) Type isomorphe du pinéalome. Les cellules ont une taille moyenne et sont arrondies ou ovalaires. Il existe seulement quelques noyaux un peu plus volumineux et hyperchromatiques. On ne voit pas de petits éléments lymphoïdes.

Las distintas formas de los pinealomas:

a) Típica asociación en el pinealoma anisomorfo de las células grandes y claras con los pequeños elementos linfoideos.
b) Acusada arquitectura en bandas en un pinealoma anisomorfo con algunas células gigantes multinucleadas y escasos elementos linfoides.
c) El mismo tejido que a) pero impregnado por el oro sublimado.
d) Pinealoma de tipo isomorfo. Las células son de mediano tamaño, redondas u ovales. Sólo se ven algunos núcleos hipercromáticos algo mayores. Las pequeñas células linfoideas faltan.

Различные формы пинеаломы:

a) Типичное сочетание крупных светлых клеток и мелких «лимфоидных» элементов в анизоморфной пинеаломе.
b) Выраженное тяжистое строение анизоморфной пинеаломы с отдельными многоядерными гигантскими клетками и немногочисленными лимфоидными элементами.
c) Та же ткань, что и на рис. a), окрашенная золото-сулемовым методом.
d) Изоморфный тип пинеаломы. Округлые или овальные клетки средней величины. Единичные крупные гиперхромные ядра. Мелкие лимфоидные клетки отсутствуют.

松果体腫の各型。

a) 不同形性松果体腫にみられる、大形淡明な細胞と小「リンパ球様」細胞の定型的な配列。
b) 不同形性松果体腫にみられた著明な索状配列。数個の多核巨細胞がある。リンパ球様細胞は少ない。
c) a) と同じ組織の鍍金像。
d) 同形性松果体腫。細胞は中等大で、円形あるいは楕円形。ところどころに、やゝ大きい濃染性の核がみられる。リンパ球様細胞はない。

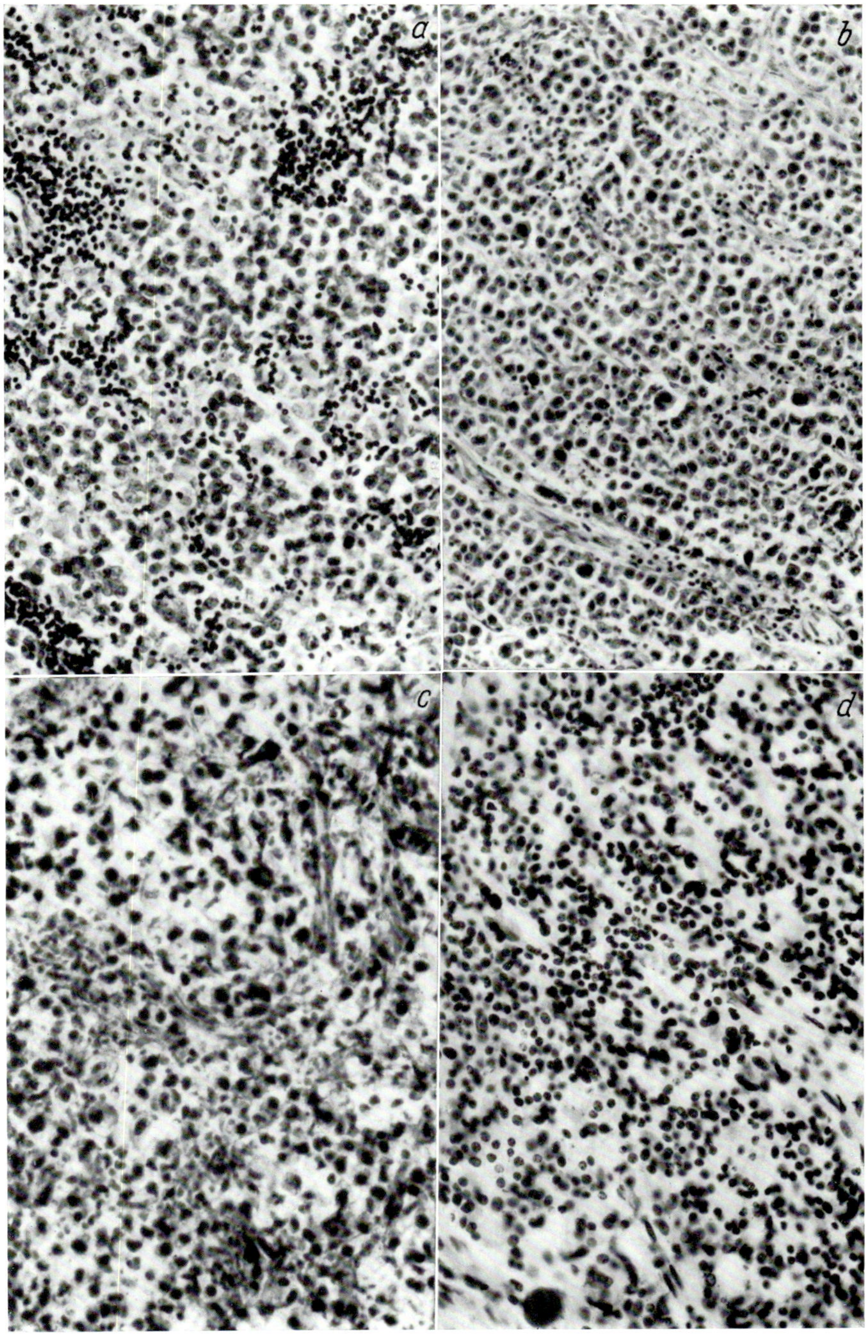

Fig. 89a—d: a ×144, b ×168. Cresyl violet stain
c ×224. Gold sublimate impregnation
d ×144. Nissl stain

Fig. 90 — Pinealomas

a) Large clear cells in the typical anisomorphic pinealoma.
b) Microscopic picture of a cyst in a pinealoma. One recognizes the non-keratinizing pavement epithelium, from which epithelial cells are peeling off toward the interior of the cyst.
c) In differential diagnosis the seminoma is occasionally important: One can discern also here the juxtaposition of large, usually clear epithelial cells in a nest-shaped arrangement and, running in between them, pathways with dark, small lymphoid cells.
d) From a pinealoma metastasis to the cauda equina.

a) Große helle Zellen im typischen anisomorphen Pinealom.
b) Mikroskopisches Bild einer Cyste in einem Pinealom. Man erkennt das nicht verhornende Plattenepithel, von dem aus nach dem Cysteninneren Epithelien abschilfern.
c) Für die Differentialdiagnose ist gelegentlich das Seminom wichtig: Man erkennt auch hier das Nebeneinander großer, meist heller Epithelien in nestförmiger Anordnung und dazwischen Straßen mit dunklen, kleinen lymphoiden Zellen.
d) Aus einer Pinealommetastase ins Caudagebiet.

a) Grandes cellules claires dans un pinéalome anisomorphe typique.
b) Aspect microscopique d'un kyste dans un pinéalome: on reconnaît l'épithélium pavimenteux non cornifiant dont les cellules desquament dans la cavité.
c) Il est parfois important de faire le diagnostic différentiel avec le séminome: on reconnaît ici des cellules épithéliales volumineuses, généralement claires et groupées en amas, entre lesquels on note des accumulations de cellules lymphoïdes, petites et denses.
d) Métastase d'un pinéalome dans la queue de cheval.

a) Células grandes, claras en un típico pinealoma anisomorfo.
b) Cuadro microscópico de un quiste en un pinealoma. Se observa el epitelio plano estratificado no queratinizante. A partir del canal, se desprenden células en el interior del quiste.
c) Para el diagnóstico diferencial en ocasiones es importante tener en cuenta el seminoma: aquí se reconoce la asociación de células epiteliales grandes, la mayoría de las veces claras, dispuestas en nidos y entre medio regueros de pequeñas células oscuras linfoideas.
d) Metástasis de un pinealoma en el territorio de la cauda.

a) Крупные светлые клетки в типичной анизоморфной пинеаломе.
b) Микроскопическая картина кисты в пинеаломе. Виден неороговевший плоский эпителий, слущивающийся в полость кисты.
c) В дифференциально-диагностическом отношении придается значение семиноме: здесь наряду с крупными гнездно-расположенными эпителиальными клетками видны тяжи темных мелких лимфоидных клеток.
d) Участок метастаза пинеаломы в область конского хвоста.

a) 定型的不同形性松果体腫にみられた大型淡明細胞。
b) 松果体腫にみられた嚢胞。内壁は非角化性扁平上皮でおおわれていて、内腔に向い上皮細胞が鱗落している。
c) 鑑別診断上、時に精細胞腫が問題になる。精細胞腫でも、巣状に配列した大形、多くは明るい上皮様細胞と、その間に介在する濃染、リンパ球様細胞からなる。
d) 馬尾神経部への松果体腫転移。

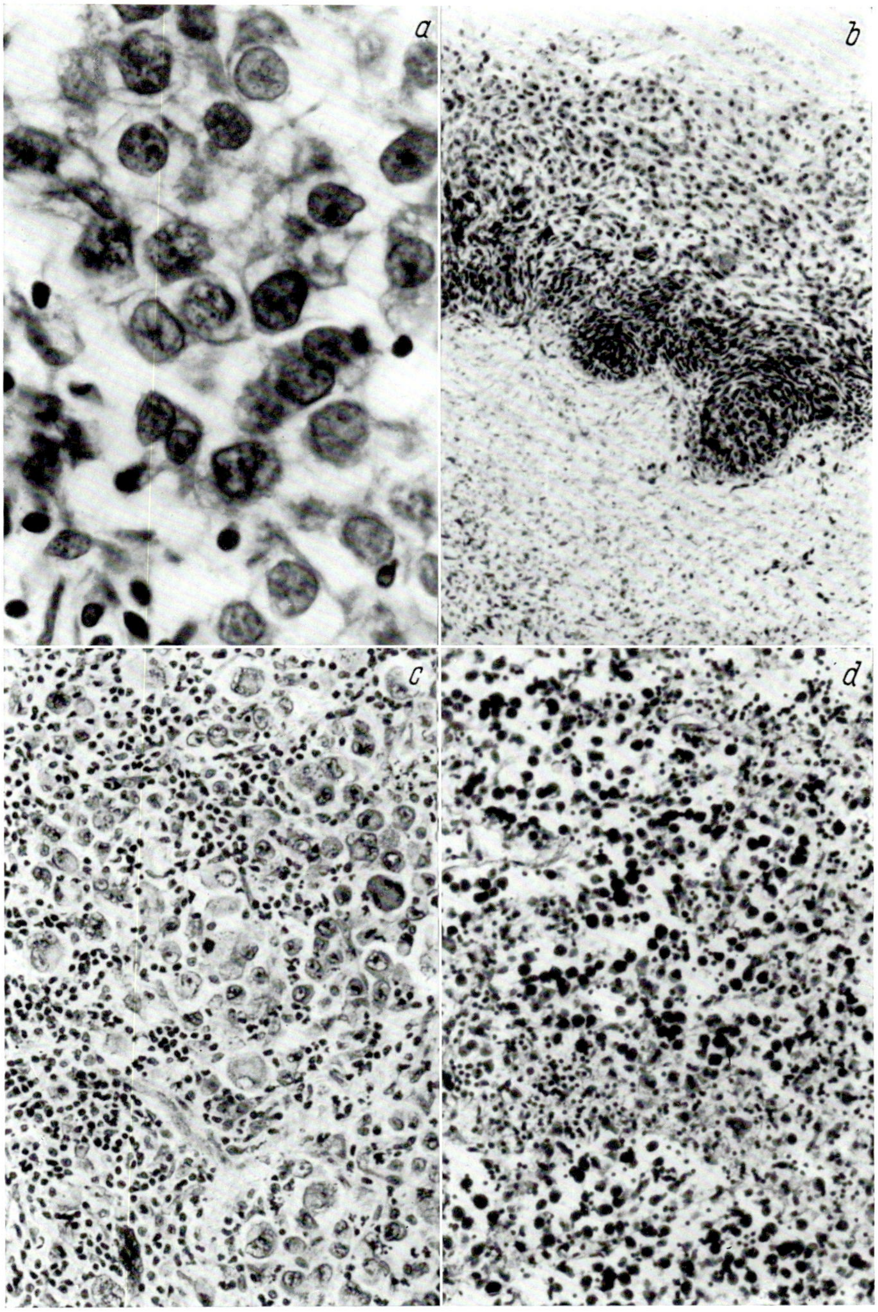

Fig. 90a—d: a ×528. Cresyl violet stain
b ×224. Gold sublimate impregnation
c ×324, d ×136. H. & E. stain

Fig. 91 — Pinealomas

a) Infiltrative growth of a pinealoma in the marginal zone:
Usually there are large cells with numerous mitoses, between which only single lymphoid elements are found.
b) From an atypical malignant pinealoma: The cells are multinucleated, the nuclei are vesicular with one or more nucleoli, and the cell body is very large. *Bottom right:* A psammoma kernel, probably stemming from the infiltrated pineal gland.
c) In a pinealoma lie epithelial tubules (*top*), from which the tumor cells (*bottom*), apparently have developed by metaplasia.
d) Several cavities with ependyma-like epithelial cysts in the case of a pineal cyst.

a) Infiltratives Wachstum eines Pinealoms in der Randzone:
Meist handelt es sich um große Zellen mit zahlreichen Mitosen, zwischen denen nur einzelne lymphoide Elemente liegen.
b) Aus einem atypischen malignen Pinealom: Die Zellen sind vielkernig, die Kerne bläschenförmig mit einem oder vielen Nucleolen, der Zelleib ist sehr groß. Rechts unten ein Psammomkorn, wahrscheinlich aus der infiltrierten Pinealis stammend.
c) In einem Pinealom liegen Epithelschläuche (oben), von denen sich anscheinend durch Metaplasie die Tumorzellen entwickelt haben (unten).
d) Mehrere Hohlräume mit ependymartigen Epithelcysten im Falle einer Zirbelcyste.

a) Caractère infiltrant de la prolifération tumorale à la périphérie d'un pinéalome.
Le plus souvent, il s'agit de cellules volumineuses, fréquemment en mitose, entre lesquelles on voit peu d'éléments lymphoïdes.
b) Dans un pinéalome malin atypique, les cellules sont multinucléées, les noyaux gonflés contiennent un ou plusieurs nucléoles et le cytoplasme est très abondant. Dans le coin inférieur droit, il existe un grain psammomateux, qui provient vraisemblablement de la glande pinéale infiltrée.
c) Dans un pinéalome, on peut voir des tubes épithéliaux (au-dessus), à partir desquels les cellules tumorales se sont développées apparemment par un processus métaplasique (au-dessous).
d) Présence de plusieurs cavités kystiques bordées par un épithélium de type épendymaire, dans un cas de kyste épiphysaire.

a) Crecimiento infiltrante de un pinealoma por sus bordes:
La mayoría de las veces se trata de células grandes con numerosas mitosis, entre las cuales sólo hay algunos elementos linfoideos.
b) Pinealoma atípico maligno: Las células son multinucleadas, los núcleos vesiculosos con uno o varios nucleolos. El cuerpo célular es muy grande. Abajo y a la derecha se ve un cuerpo psamomatoso lo más seguro proveniente de la pineal infiltrada.
c) En un pinealoma se ven túbulos epiteliales (arriba), de los que aparentemente se han desarrollado las células tumorales por metaplasia (abajo).
d) Varios espacios claros con quistes epiteliales de tipo ependimario en el caso de un quiste pineal.

a) Инфильтративный рост пинеаломы в краевой зоне:
В основном крупные клетки с многочисленными митозами. Между ними расположены лишь отдельные лимфоидные элементы.
b) Атипическая злокачественная пинеалома: очень крупные многоядерные клетки, пузырьковидные ядра с одним и многими ядрышками. Справа внизу псаммоматозное зерно, исходящее, по-видимому из инфильтрированной шишковидной железы.
c) Пинеалома с эпителиальными канальцами (вверху), из которых, по-видимому, в процессе метаплазии развились опухолевые клетки (внизу).
d) Киста шишковидной железы. Многочисленные полости с эпендимоподобными эпителиальными кистами.

Continued on page 238

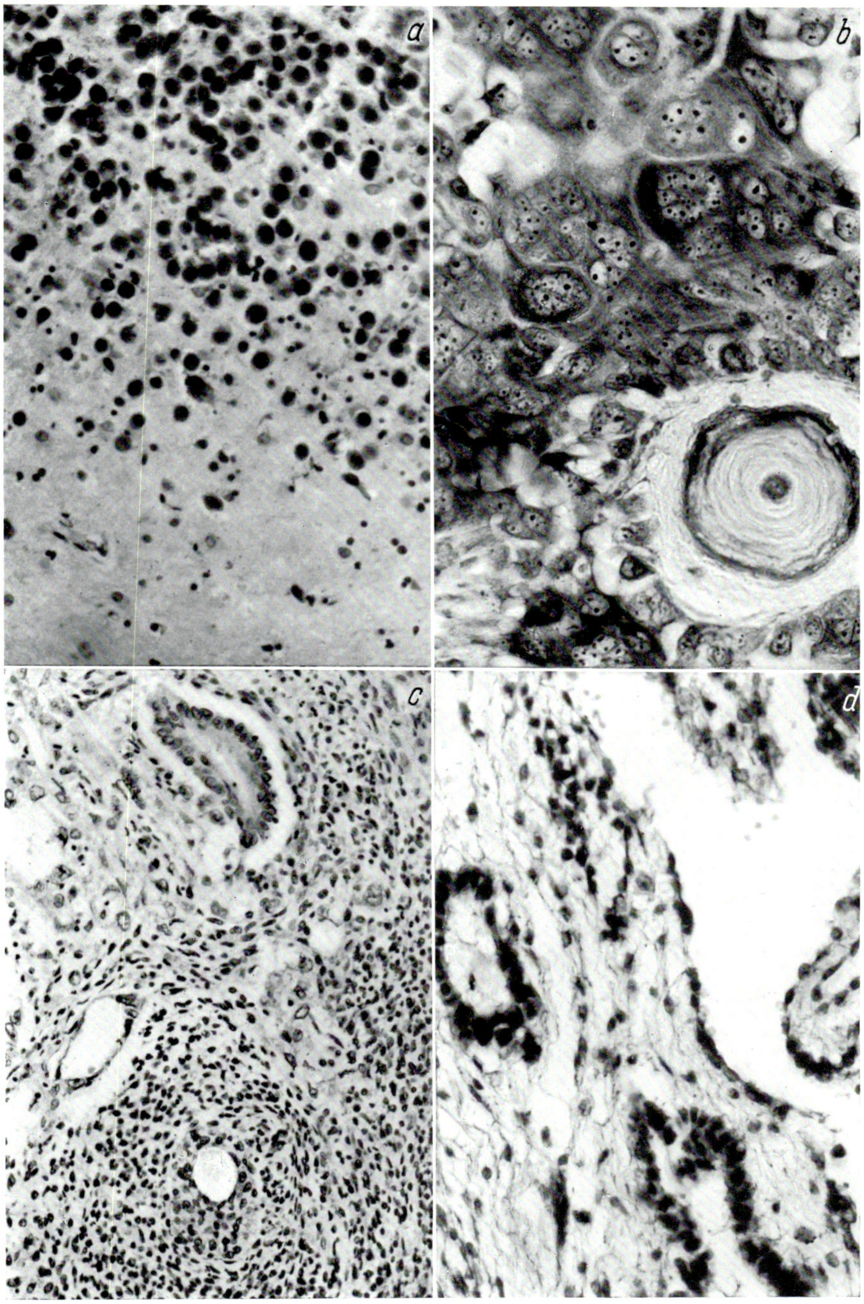

Fig. 91a—d: a ×128, d ×296. H. & E. stain
b ×192, c ×112. Cresyl violet stain

Fig. 91 — Pinealomas (continued)

a) 松果体腫辺縁部の浸潤性増殖。
浸潤部を占める細胞の多くは大形で、多数の核分裂が見られる。リンパ球様細胞は少数散在しているにすぎない。

b) 異型的悪性松果体腫の一部。細胞は多核性、核は胞状で、1ないし数個の核小体をもつ。細胞体は非常に大きい。右下に砂粒腫顆粒が1個ある。これは腫瘍に浸潤された松果体組織のものと思われる。

c) 松果体腫にみられた、上皮性腺管（図上)。腫瘍細胞は、前者から化生によって発生してきたとも考えられる（図下)。

d) 松果体囊胞例では、脳室上衣様細胞でおおわれた多数の管腔がある。

Pituitary Adenomas

Fig. 92 and 93

Acidophile, (oxyphile), basophile, mixed, chromophobe adenomas, pituitary cancer, hypophyseal struma

Craniopharyngiomas

Fig. 94 and 95

Tumors or cysts of the hypophyseal duct, cysts or tumors of Rathke's pouch, tumors of Rathke's cleft, craniopharyngeal pouch tumors, suprasellar epidermoid cysts, pituitary stalk tumors, Erdheim's tumors, adamantinomas or ameloblastomas of the pituitary region. Malpighion epithelioma

Glomus Tumors

Fig. 96

Carotid body tumors, glomus caroticum tumors, glomus jugulare tumors, chemodectomas, glomangiomas

Epidermoids — Dermoids — Teratomas

Fig. 97

Epidermoid cysts, pearly tumors, tumeurs perlées, cholesteatomas without hair, sebaceous cysts — Dermoid cysts, cholesteatomas with hair

Chordomas

Fig. 98

Chondromas — Lipomas — Xanthomas

Fig. 99

Cylindromatous Epitheliomas — Cylindromas

Fig. 100a, b

Cavernoma — Cavernous Angioma

Fig. 100c

Arteriovenous Angioma or Malformation

Fig. 100d

Fig. 92 — Pituitary Adenomas

a) The epithelium of a chromophobe adenoma of the hypophysis appears aligned along blood vessels.
b) Polymorphous eosinophilic adenoma of the hypophysis. Note the giant cells with hyperchromatic nuclei and the mitotic figures.
c) Moderately polymorphous epithelium in an eosinophilic adenoma of the hypophysis.
d) Marked basophilia and true polymorphic epithelium of an adenoma of the hypophysis.

a) Entlang den Gefäßen reihen sich die Epithelien des chromophoben Hypophysenadenoms auf.
b) In dem polymorphen eosinophilen Hypophysenadenom kommen einzelne Riesenzellen mit hyperchromatischem Kern vor. Zahlreiche Mitosen.
c) Große, mäßig polymorphe Epithelien aus einem eosinophilen Hypophysenadenom.
d) Große basophile, recht polymorphe Epithelien eines basophilen Hypophysenadenoms.

a) Les cellules épithéliales de l'adénome chromophobe de l'hypophyse se rangent le long des vaisseaux.
b) Dans l'adénome éosinophile polymorphe de l'hypophyse, on rencontre quelques cellules géantes à noyau hyperchromatique et de nombreuses mitoses.
c) Grand épithélium moyennement polymorphe dans un adénome éosinophile de l'hypophyse.
d) Grand épithélium basophile et très polymorphe d'un adénome basophile de l'hypophyse.

a) Las células epiteliales cromófobas del adenoma hipofisario se ordenan a lo largo de los vasos.
b) En el adenoma hipofisario aparte de células acidófilas aparecen células grandes con núcleos hipercromáticos. Varias mitosis.
c) Epitelio grande ligeramente polimorfo de un adenoma hipofisario eosinófilo.
d) Intensa basofilia y polimorfismo del epitelio en un adenoma hipofisario basófilo.

a) Наличие единичных гигантских клеток с гиперхромным ядром в полиморфной эозинофильной аденоме гипофиза. Многочисленные митозы.
b) Полиморфная аденома гипофиза с многочисленными гигантскими клетками и митозами.
c) Крупные, умеренно полиморфные эпителиальные клетки эозинофильной аденомы гипофиза.
d) Ряды эпителиальных клеток вдоль сосудов хромофобной аденомы гипофиза.

a) 血管に沿って色素嫌性下垂体腺腫の上皮細胞がならぶ。
b) 多形性酸好性下垂体腺腫内で、濃染核をもった二三の巨細胞がみられる。分裂像も多い。
c) 酸好性下垂体腺腫内の大形、軽度に多形性を示す上皮細胞。
d) 塩基好性下垂体腺腫にみられた大形、多形性塩基好性細胞。

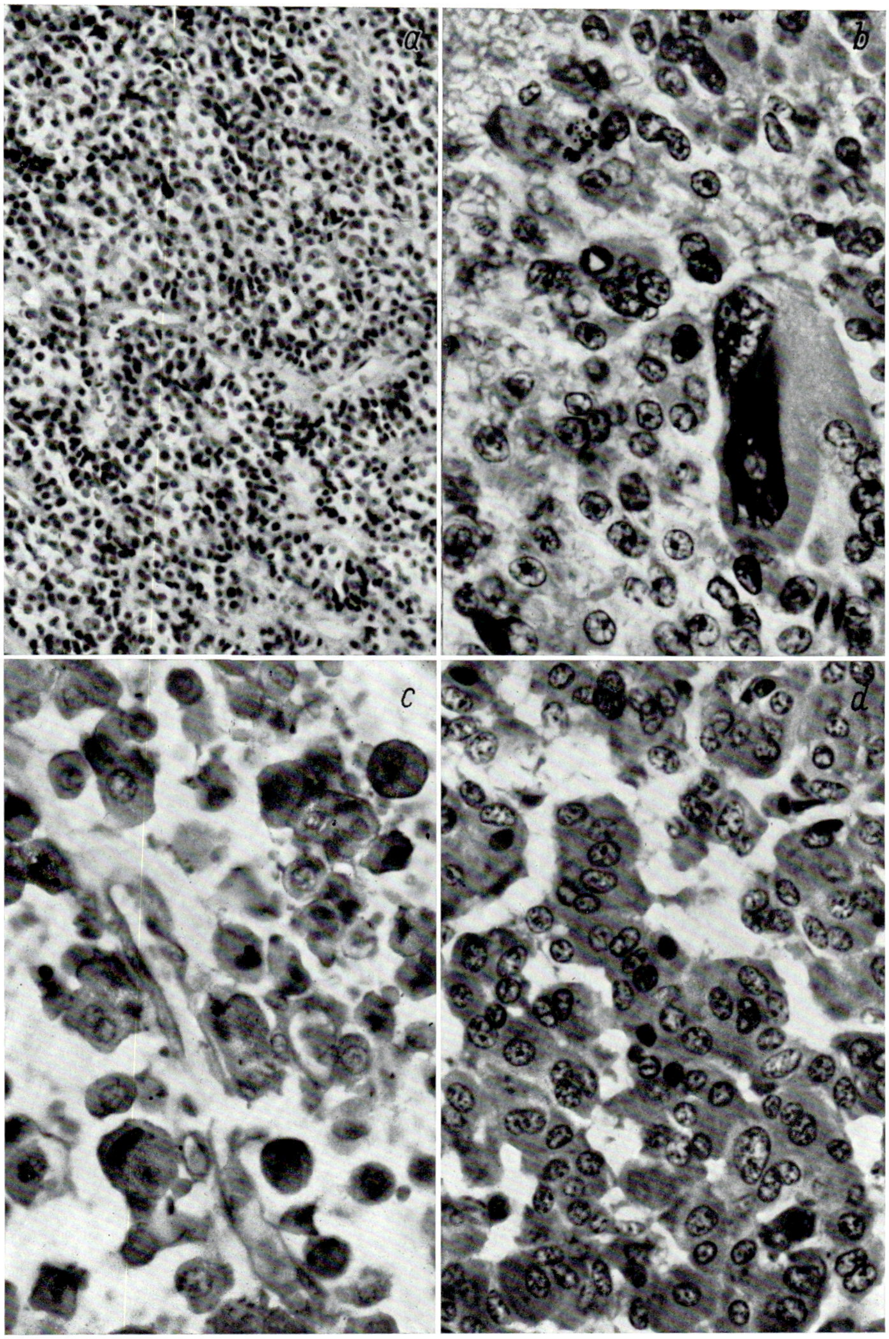

Fig. 92a—d: a ×125, c ×350, b and d ×500
H. & E. stain

Fig. 93 — Pituitary Adenomas

a) and b) Typical chromophobe adenoma: The large cells with moderately chromatin-rich nuclei lie along the capillaries.
c) Through liquefaction, small cavities arise in the tissue. *Top right:* A colloid concrement.
d) Liquefaction and the inception of a cyst formation. Although some of the cells are "clear", others show nuclear pyknosis as a preliminary stage of liquefaction. Narrow streaks of albumin-rich fluid traverse the tissue from bottom right to top left. In the vicinity the cells have undergone marked regressive changes.

a) u. b) Typisches chromophobes Adenom: die großen Zellen mit mäßig chromatinreichen Kernen liegen entlang den Capillaren.
c) Durch Verflüssigung entstehen im Gewebe kleine Hohlräume. Oben rechts ein kolloides Konkrement.
d) Starke Verflüssigung und Beginn einer Cystenbildung. Während ein Teil der Zellen „hell" ist, sieht man bei anderen als Vorstufe der Verflüssigung die Kernpyknose. Schmale Streifen von eiweißreicher Flüssigkeit ziehen von rechts unten nach links oben durch das Gewebe. In ihrem Bereich sind die Zellen deutlich regressiv verändert.

a) et b) Adénome chromophobe typique: les grandes cellules, à noyaux moyennement riches en chromatine, se disposent le long des capillaires.
c) De petites cavités de liquéfaction se forment dans le tissu. L'une d'elles (au-dessus et à droite) contient une substance colloïde.
d) Liquéfaction importante et début de transformation kystique. Alors qu'une partie des cellules ont un aspect «clair», le premier stade de la liquéfaction des autres cellules se manifeste par la pycnose des noyaux. Des coulées de liquide riche en albumine s'infiltrent dans le tissu, depuis l'angle inférieur droit vers la région supérieure gauche. Le long de ces coulées, les cellules présentent d'importantes altérations régressives.

a) y b) Adenoma cromófobo típico: las grandes células con núcleos medianamente ricos en cromatina se disponen a lo largo de los capilares.
c) En el tejido se forman pequeños quistes, por liquefacción. Arriba y a la derecha una formación coloide.
d) Intensa liquefacción e inicio de formación de quistes. Mientras una parte las células son «claras», en otras zonas se ven, como estadio preliminar de la liquefacción, núcleos picnóticos. Delgadas fran jas de líquido rico en albúmina cruzan el tejido desde la derecha y abajo hacia la izquierda y arriba. En estos territorios las células estan manifiestamente degeneradas.

a) и b) Типичная хромофобная аденома: крупные клетки и ядра с умеренным содержанием хроматина расположены вдоль капилляров.
c) Появление мелких полостей вследствие разжижения. Справа вверху коллоидный конкремент.
d) Выраженное разжижение и начало кистообразования. Часть клеток «светлые», в то время в других отмечается пикноз ядер — предварительная ступень разжижения. Узкие полоски богатой белком жидкости тянутся справа снизу налево кверху. В этих учатсках клетки подверглись четким регрессивным изменениям.

a) および b) 定型的な色素嫌性腺腫。やゝクロマチンに富む核をもつ大形の細胞が、毛細血管にそってならんでいる。
c) 腫瘍組織の液化によって小嚢胞ができる。右上にコロイド凝塊がある。
d) 高度の液化と嚢胞形成のはじまり。一部の細胞は淡明であるが、他の細胞に液化の前段階として核濃縮がおこっている。蛋白に富む液体が、右下から左上に、線状に組織をつらぬいて滲出している。この部分で、細胞の退行変性が著明である。

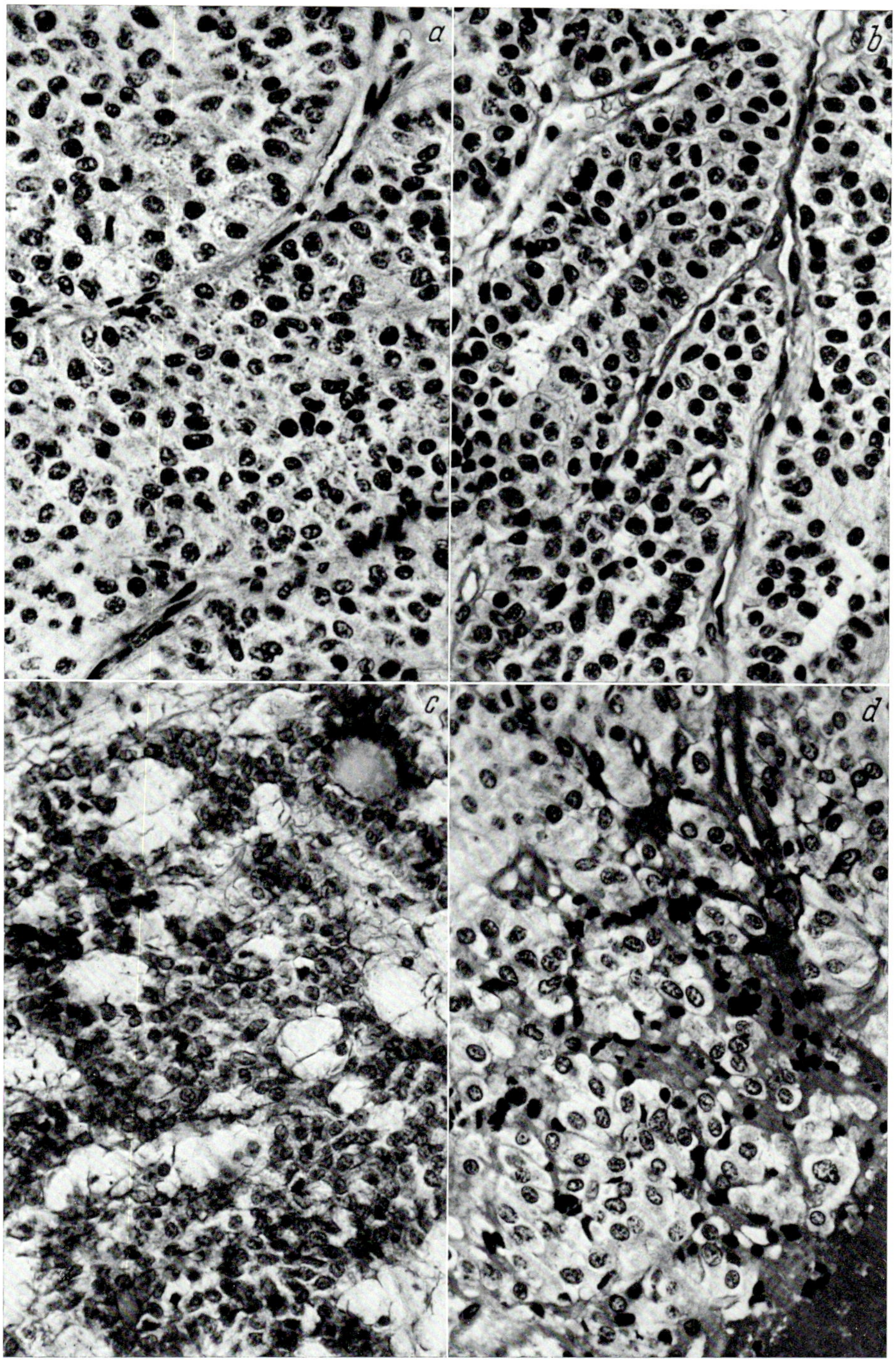

Fig. 93a—d: a and d ×272. H. & E. stain
b and c ×272. Cresyl violet stain

Fig. 94 — Craniopharyngiomas

Various patterns of a craniopharyngioma:

a) The tumor consists of epithelial bands and stroma. In the interior, one sees liquefaction, and nearly "prickle cells" arise. The marginal epithelial cells are rather columnar.

b) Here, in epithelial bands, the central transformation into "prickle cells" can be clearly discerned. The stroma is considerably increased and is undergoing mucoid degeneration. Individual capillaries are still clearly apparent. In the stroma lie round cells and macrophages.

c) and d) Considerable liquefaction in the interior of the epithelial bands. Entire cystic systems have arisen.

Verschiedene Bilder eines Kraniopharyngeoms:

a) Der Tumor besteht aus Epithelbändern und Stroma. Im Inneren sieht man eine Verflüssigung, wobei ,,Stachelzellen" entstehen. Die Randepithelien sind mehr säulenförmig.

b) Hier ist in Epithelbändern die zentrale Umwandlung zu ,,Stachelzellen" besonders deutlich zu erkennen. Das Stroma ist erheblich vermehrt und verschleimt. Einzelne Capillaren sind noch deutlich zu erkennen. Im Stroma liegen Rundzellen und Makrophagen.

c) u. d) Erhebliche Verflüssigung im Inneren der Epithelbänder. Es entstehen ganze Cystensysteme.

Différents aspects du crânio-pharyngiome.

a) La tumeur se compose de cordons épithéliaux et de stroma. L'intérieur des cordons tend à se liquéfier et contient des «cellules en aiguille». En bordure des cordons, les cellules épithéliales ont davantage le type cylindrique.

b) On voit très bien la transformation du centre des cordons épithéliaux en «cellules en aiguille». Dans le stroma, qui est fort gonflé et œdématié, il existe quelques capillaires bien visibles ainsi que des cellules rondes et des macrophages.

c) et d) Réseau kystique, causé par la liquéfaction importante à l'intérieur des cordons épithéliaux.

Diferentes imágenes de un craneofaringioma:

a) El tumor consta de bandas epiteliales y estroma. En el interior se observa una fluidificación, por la que se constituyen células espinosas. Los epitelios marginales son más columnares.

b) Aquí es especialmente evidente la transformación central en células espinosas. El estroma está considerablemente aumentado y liquefacto. En el estroma hay células redondas y macrófagos.

c) y d) Notable fluidificación en el interior de las bandas epiteliales. Se constituyen sistemas quísticos completos.

Различные картины краниофарингеомы:

a) Опухоль состоит из эпителиальных тяжей и стромы. Внутри опухоли разжижение. Появление «шиповидных клеток». Краевой эпителий столбовиден.

b) Четко видно превращение эпителиальных тяжей в «шиповидные клетки». Строма обильна и подверглась мукоидному перерождению. Еще видны отдельные капилляры. В строме видны круглые клетки и макрофаги.

c) и d) Значительное разжижение внутри эпителиальных тяжей. Появление целых кистозных систем.

頭蓋咽頭腫のいろいろな組織像。

a) 腫瘍は、上皮細胞索と間質から構成されている。上皮細胞索の内部に液化がおこり、その結果「棘状細胞」ができる。上皮索最外層の細胞は円柱状である。

b) 上皮索中心部は棘状細胞化が明瞭である。間質結合組織は多くなり粘液様に変化している。若干の毛細血管がまだはっきりみとめられる。間質内には、円形細胞、貪喰細胞がある。

c) および d) 上皮細胞索の内部に液化がおこり、多数の嚢胞がつくられる。

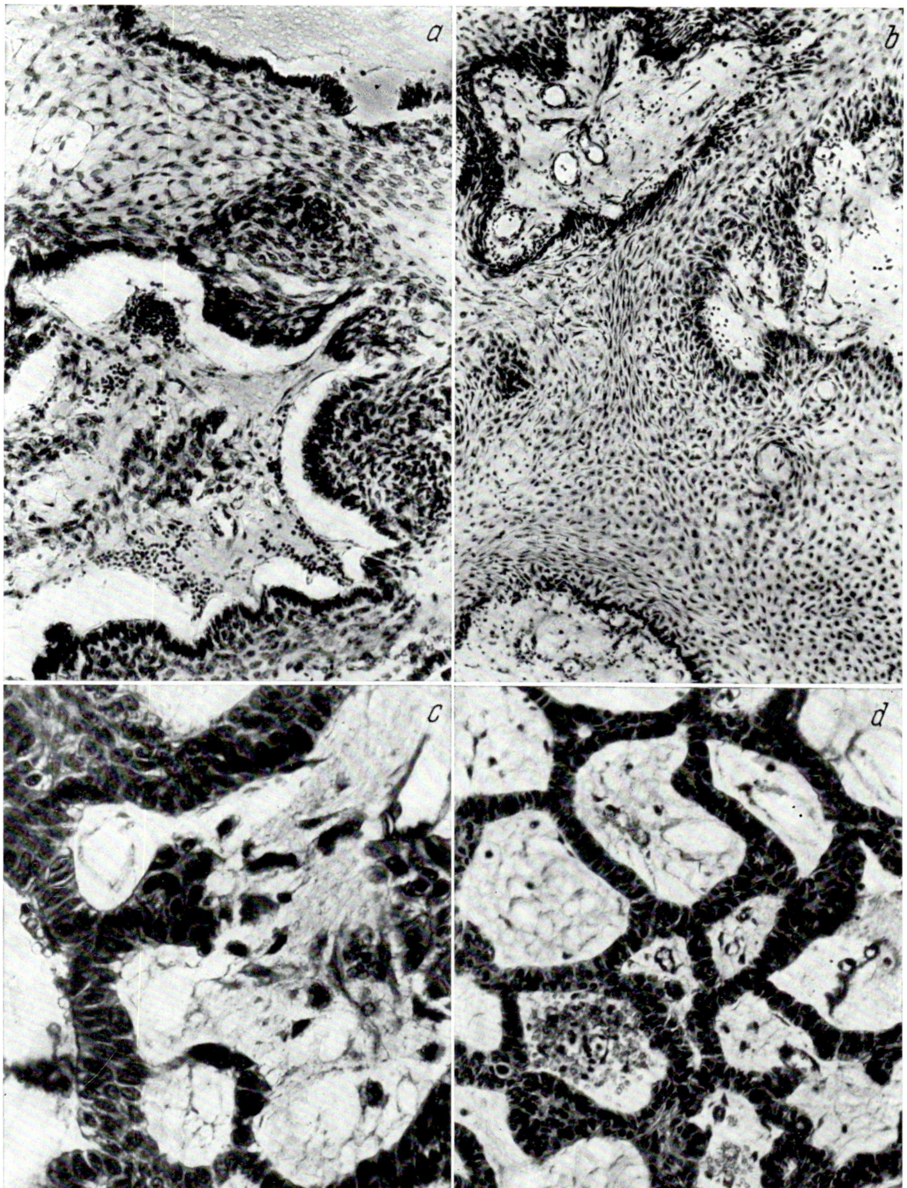

Fig. 94a—d: a ×112, c ×272, d ×136. H. & E. stain
b ×84. Cresyl violet stain

Fig. 95 — Craniopharyngiomas

a) In the stroma are numerous leucocytes.
b) Within the epithelial bands occur large cysts. The marginal epithelium has transformed itself into a columnar shape.
c) and d) Growth of a craniopharyngioma in the marginal zone with single cones toward the brain. These cones are found lying partly longitudinally and partly obliquely. One cone, d) *top right,* has already become keratoid.

a) Im Stroma liegen hier zahlreiche Leukocyten.
b) Hier entstehen auch innerhalb der Epithelbänder große Cysten. Das Randepithel hat sich säulenförmig umgebildet.
c) u. d) Wachstum eines Kraniopharyngeoms in der Randzone mit einzelnen Zapfen gegen das Hirn, die teils längs, teils quer getroffen sind. Ein Zapfen (d rechts oben) ist bereits keratoid umgewandelt.

a) Le stroma contient ici de nombreux leucocytes.
b) De grands kystes se forment également à l'intérieur des cordons épithéliaux. En bordure, les cellules épithéliales se sont transformées en cellules cylindriques.
c) et d) Invasion du tissu cérébral par le crânio-pharyngiome sous forme de languettes, qui apparaissent coupées longitudinalement ou transversalement. Dans la portion supérieure droite de d) une languette a déjà subi une transformation kératoïde.

a) En el estroma hay numerosos leucocitos.
b) Aquí tambien entre las bandas de epitelio se constituyen grandes quistes. El epitelio marginal es de tipo columnar.
c) y d) Crecimiento periférico de un craneofaringioma. Se ven algunas prolongaciones hacia el cerebro cortadas unas a lo largo, otras transversalmente. Una prolongación (a la derecha y arriba) ha sufrido ya una transformación queratoidea.

a) Многочисленные лейкоциты в строме.
b) Возникновение больших кист в эпителиальных тяжах. Краевой эпителий стал столбовидным.
c) и d) Рост краниофарингеомы в краевой зоне с отдельными выростами в сторону мозга. Один вырост, d) справа вверху, подвергся кератоидной дегенерации.

a) 間質の白血球浸潤。
b) 上皮細胞索内に生じた大きな嚢胞。辺縁の上皮細胞は、柱状に変化している。
c) および d) 頭蓋咽頭腫の辺縁の一部は栓状に脳実質へ侵入している。これは縦断あるいは横断された上皮索として示されている。図 d) の右上にある腫瘍侵入部は角化傾向を示している。

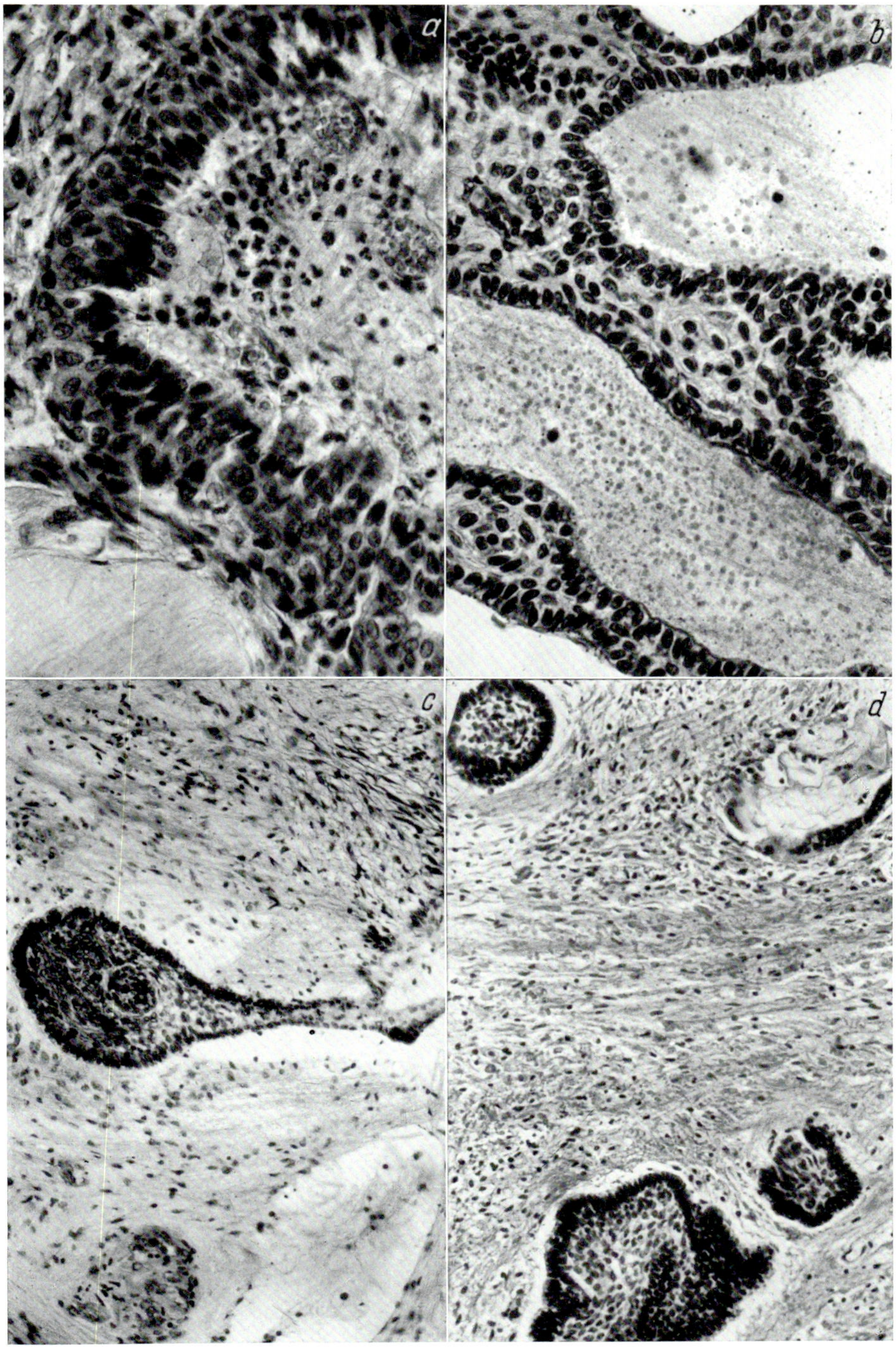

Fig. 95a—d: a and b ×272, c and d ×136
H. & E. stain

Fig. 96 — Glomus Tumors

Glomus tumors consist of large epithelial cells which lie in islets and are separated by a coarse collagen or hyaline framework.

a) General view demonstrating the various sizes and staining affinities of the nuclei.
b) Enlargement of a).
c) In another case, the cells are isomorphic and the islets ("cell packets") are small.
d) Fine reticular fibers as demonstrated by silver impregnation.

Die Glomustumoren bestehen aus großen epithelialen Zellen, die in Inseln gelagert und durch grobes kollagenes oder hyalines Balkenwerk unterteilt sind.

a) Übersichtsbild, wo man die verschiedene Größe und Färbbarkeit der Kerne gut erkennt.
b) Vergrößerung von a).
c) In einem anderen Falle sind die Zellen isomorpher und die Inseln kleiner („Zellballen").
d) Mit Silber stellen sich feine Retikulinfasern dar.

Les tumeurs du glomus sont constituées de grandes cellules épithéliales qui s'assemblent en îlots séparés les uns des autres par d'épais faisceaux collagènes.

a) Vue d'ensemble: on reconnaît bien les variations de taille et de colorabilité des noyaux.
b) Agrandissement de a).
c) Dans un autre cas, les cellules sont plus isomorphes et les îlots plus petits («boules cellulaires»).
d) L'imprégnation argentique met en évidence de fines fibres de réticuline.

Los tumores glómicos aparecen con grandes células epiteliales formando grupos separados por una estructura colágena o hialina.

a) Panorámica que muestra la variedad de tamaño y coloración de los núcleos.
b) Mayor aumento del campo anterior.
c) En otros casos las células son isomorfas y las islas pequeñas «aglomerados de células».
d) Con la plata aparecen finas fibras de reticulina.

Опухоли гломуса состоят из крупных эпителиальных клеток, расположенных в виде островков и разделенных грубыми коллагеновыми и гиалиновыми тяжами.

a) Обзорный снимок, на котором хорошо прослеживаются ядра различной величины и окрашиваемости.
b) Рисунок a) под 500-кратным увеличением.
c) В другом случае клетки более изоморфны и островки меньше («клеточные комья»).
d) Серебрением выявлены тонкие ретикулиновые волокна.

頸動脈洞腫瘍は大形の上皮様細胞よりなる。この細胞は粗大な膠原性または硝子様の網状索でわけられ、島様に配列している。

a) この概観像では、種々の大きさと染色性をもった核がみられる。
b) a)図の強拡大、
c) 他の例では細胞は同形性で、島は小さい(細胞塊)。
d) 鍍銀で微細な細網線維が染まる。

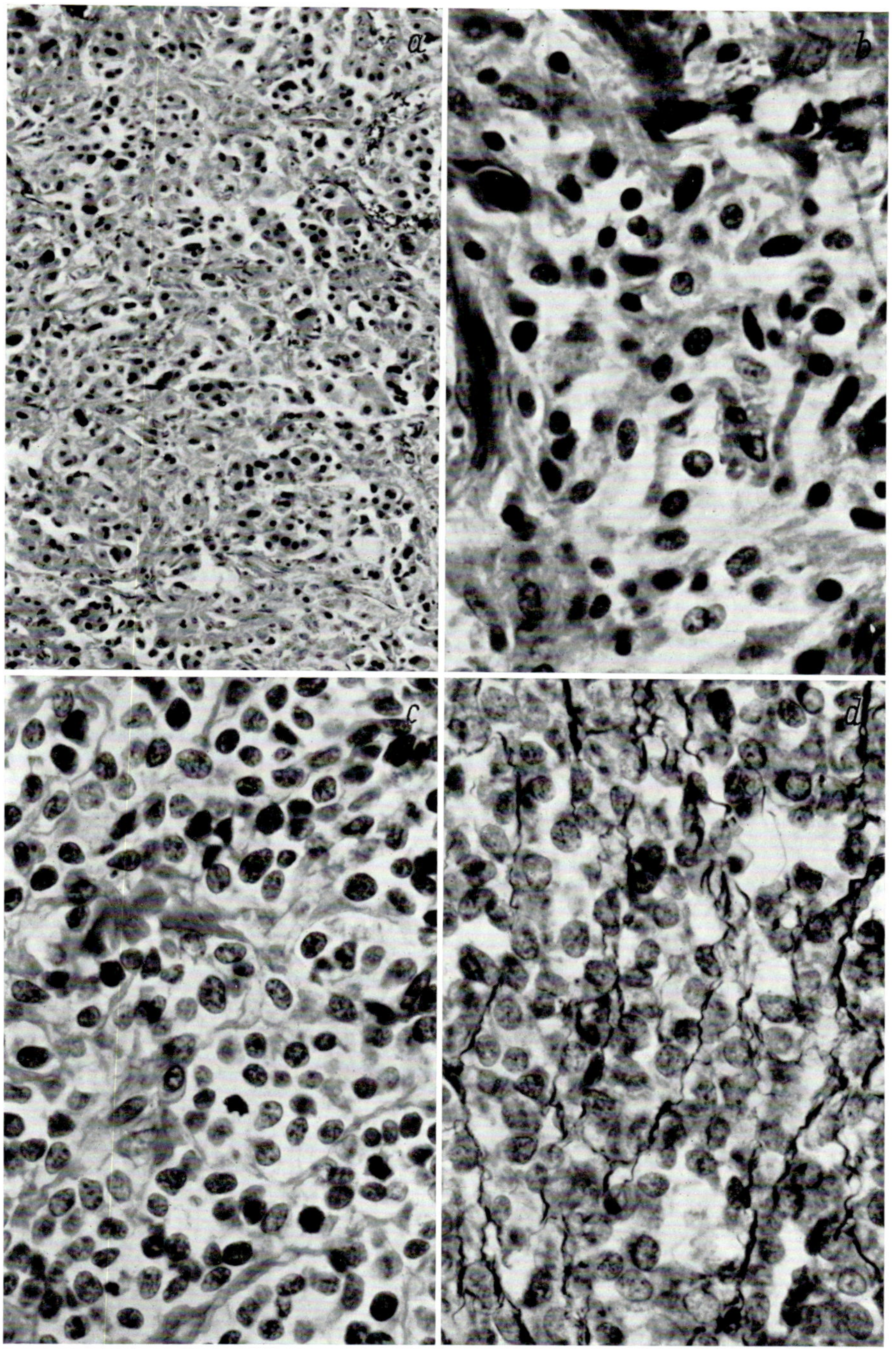

Fig. 96a—d: a ×125, b and c ×500. H. & E. stain
d ×500. Gomori method

Fig. 97 — Epidermoids — Dermoids — Teratomas

a) Typical layers in the capsule of an epidermoid: *Bottom right:* Stroma with some chronic inflammatory cells. Then follow the three layers: the stratum germinativum, granulosum, and corneum. Finally, one recognizes (*top left*) the exfoliated and keratinized epithelial cells, which first lie next to each other in layers, then (further out) in a somewhat mosaic-like pattern.
b) Fine kerato-hyaline granules of the stratum germinativum at higher magnification.
c) The dermoid shows, apart from the somewhat thicker layers described in a), also ceruminal and occasionally sebaceous glands and hair follicles.
d) Metaplastic change from cylindric to squamous epithelium in a teratoma.

a) Typische Lagen der Kapsel eines Epidermoids: rechts unten Stroma mit einigen chronischen Entzündungszellen. Dann folgen die drei Lagen des Str. germinativum, granulosum, corneum. Man erkennt schließlich links oben die abgeschilferten und verhornten Epithelien, die zuerst geschichtet, dann (ganz außen) mehr mosaikartig nebeneinander liegen.
b) Eine höhere Vergrößerung zeigt die feinen Keratohyalinkörnchen des Stratum granulosum noch besser.
c) Beim Dermoid sieht man neben den eben geschilderten Epidermislagen — die gewöhnlich etwas dicker sind — auch noch Talgdrüsen und gelegentlich Haarfollikel.
d) Metaplastische Umwandlung eines Zylinderepithels in Plattenepithel in einem Teratom.

a) Couches typiques constituant la capsule d'un kyste épidermoïde. Dans le coin inférieur droit, le stroma contient quelques cellules inflammatoires chroniques. Ensuite, on reconnaît successivement les couches germinative, granuleuse et cornée. Dans la partie supérieure gauche, les cellules épithéliales, desquamées et cornifiées, se disposent d'abord en couches stratifiées, puis (tout en haut) elles se tassent l'une contre l'autre à la façon d'une mosaïque.
b) A un plus fort grossissement, on reconnaît mieux les granules de kératohyaline dans la couche granuleuse.
c) Dans le kyste dermoïde, on observe des glandes sébacées et parfois des follicules pileux, sous les couches épidermiques décrites plus haut et habituellement plus épaisses.
d) Transformation métaplasique d'un épithélium cylindrique en épithélium pavimenteux, dans un cas de tératome.

a) Disposición típica de la cápsula de un epidermoide: abajo y a la derecha estroma con algunas células propias de la inflamación crónica. Siguen entonces las tres capas de los estratos germinativo, granuloso y córneo. Finalmente arriba y a la izquierda se ven los epitelios queratinizados y exfoliados, dispuestos en capas (arriba esquierda) o también en forma de mosaico.
b) A mayor aumento, se observan finos granulos de keratohialina en el estrato germinativo.
c) El dermoide presenta, a parte de las delgadas capas descritas en la figura a), algunas glandulas ceruminosas, y escasos foliculos pilosos y glandulas sebaceas.
d) Se destingue, dentro de un teratoma, una metaplasia de epitelio clilindrico en epitelio pavimentoso.

a) Типичное расположение капсулы эпидермоида: справа внизу строма с клетками хронического воспаления. Затем следуют три слоя: зародышевый, зернистый, роговой. Слева вверху виден слущившийся и ороговевший эпителий, имеющий то слоистое, то мозаичное строение.
b) При большом увеличении керато-гиалиновые зерна лучше отличаются в зернистом слое.
c) Кроме высше указанных, обычно более толстых, эпидермических слоях, в дермоиде так же видны сальные железы и волосные фолликулы.
d) Метаплазная трансформация в тератоме циллиндрического эпителия в плоский.

Continued on page 252

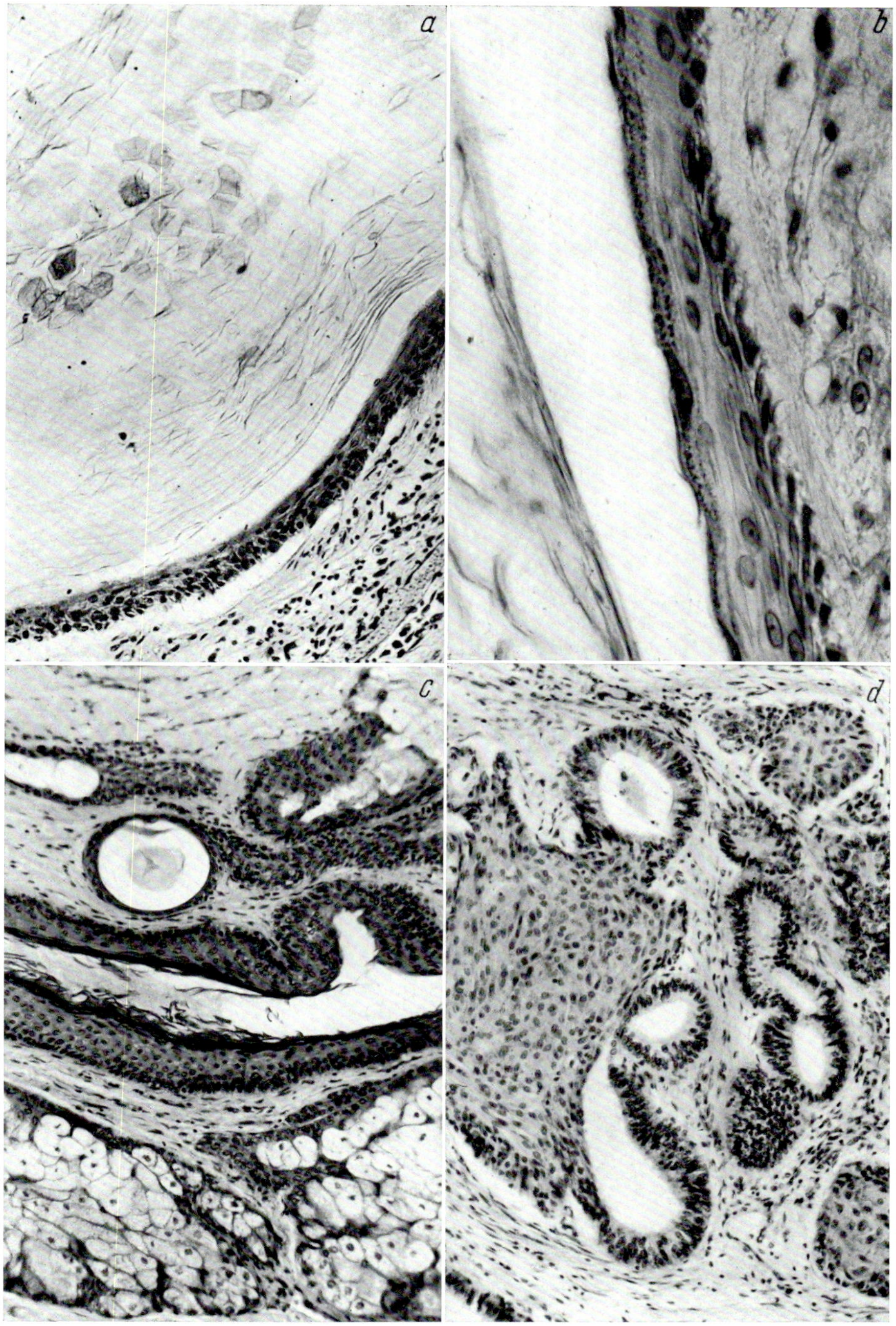

Fig. 97a—d: a ×112, b ×324, c ×136, d ×104. H. & E. stain

Fig. 98 — Chordomas

Various types of a chordoma:

a) and b) Show predominantly vesicular cells in between trabeculae consisting of a mucous material.

c) Very polymorphic cells, whose boundary lines are permeated by very fine, mucous-filled vacuoles. Single trabeculae of chondroid tissue.

d) Here the cell bodies are densely stained and not clear. Individual cells are regressively altered.

Verschiedene Typen eines Chordoms:

a) und b) zeigen vorwiegend bläschenförmige Zellen zwischen Balken aus einem mukösen Material.

c) Sehr polymorphe Zellen, deren Grenzlinien von mit feinstem Mucus gefüllten Vacuolen durchsetzt sind. Einzelne Balken chondroiden Gewebes.

d) Hier sind die Zelleiber deutlich angefärbt und nicht hell. Einzelne Zellen sind regressiv verändert.

Différents types de chordome.

a) et b) La plupart des cellules sont ballonnées et disposées entre des amas de matériel muqueux.

c) Cellules très polymorphes, dont s'échappent de petites vacuoles remplies de mucus. Présence de quelques amas de tissu chondroïde.

d) A cet endroit, le cytoplasme des cellules n'est pas clair, mais bien coloré. Quelques cellules ont subi des modifications régressives.

Distintos tipos de cordomas:

a) y b) muestran células predominantemente vesiculosas entre franjas de un material mucoso.

c) Células muy polimorfas, cuyos márgenes están separados por vacuolas rellenas de un muco muy fino. Algunas bandas de tejido condroideo están presentes.

d) Aquí se han teñido de manera clara los cuerpos celulares. Algunas células han sufrido procesos regresivos.

Различные типы хордомы:

a) и b) Преимущественно пузырьковидные клетки между перекладинами из мукоидного вещества.

c) Очень полиморфные клетки, по краям которых видны заполненные муцином вакуоли, единичные перекладины хондроидной ткани.

d) Тела клеток четко, но не светло окрашены. В отдельных клетках регрессивные изменения.

脊索腫の諸型。

a) および b) こゝでは空胞状細胞が主で、その間に梁状に粘液様物質が介在している。

c) 腫瘍細胞は非常に多形で、その境界部に粘液をいれた多数の空胞がみられる。梁状の軟骨様組織が、細胞間に散在している。

d) こゝでは細胞体は淡明でなく、明瞭に染まっている。若干の細胞は退行変性におちいっている。

Fig. 97 — Epidermoids — Dermoids — Teratomas (continued)

a) 表皮嚢腫の被膜部の定型的な組織構造。右下に、慢性炎症性細胞浸潤をともった間質、つづいて表皮基底層、顆粒層、角化層がある。内部には、剝離した角化上皮がみられ、これは最初重層状、左上にいくにつれモザイク状にならんでいる。

b) 強拡大で、顆粒層の微細なケラトヒアリン顆粒が明瞭に観察される。

c) 皮様嚢腫の表皮層は、一般に表皮嚢腫のそれよりいくぶん厚く、さらに皮脂腺とときに毛嚢が存在する。

d) 奇型腫にみられた円柱上皮の扁平上皮化生。

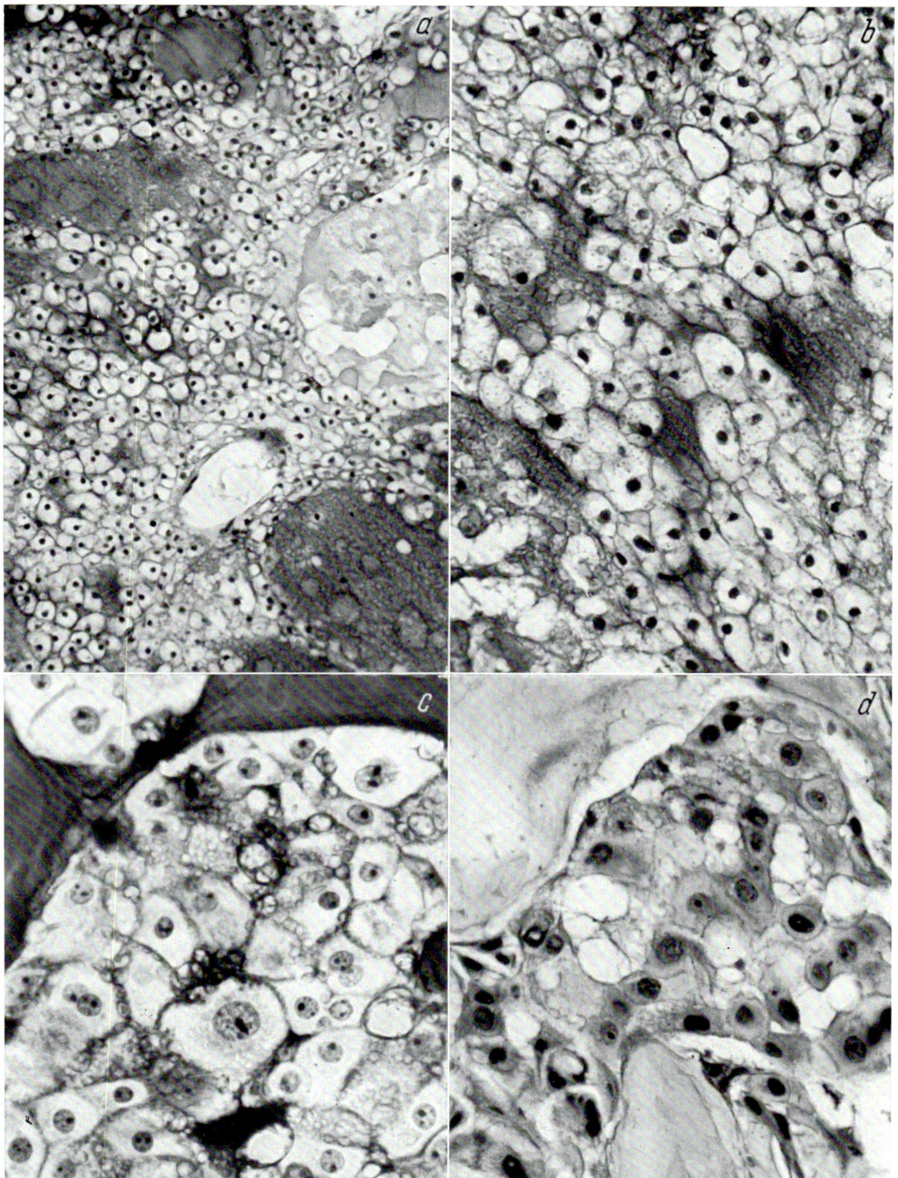

Fig. 98a—d: a ×136, b and d ×272. H. & E. stain
c ×272. Cresyl violet stain

Fig. 99 — Chondromas — Lipomas — Xanthomas

a) Typical chondroma of the middle cranial fossa.
b) Lipoma of the chiasm with considerable angiomatous components.
c) Lipoma, which has grown around the caudal roots.
d) Xanthoma of the choroid plexus: One recognizes everywhere the large "foam cells" filled with fine drops. This is probably not a genuine infiltration, but rather an autochthonous occurrence of fat cells from the vascular connective tissue.

a) Typisches Chondrom der mittleren Schädelgrube.
b) Lipom (Chiasma) mit erheblicher angiomatöser Komponente.
c) Lipom, das die Caudawurzeln umwachsen hat.
d) Xanthom des Plexus chorioideus: Man erkennt überall die großen, feintropfig gefüllten ,,Schaumzellen". Es handelt sich hier wohl nicht um eine echte Infiltration, sondern um eine autochthone Entstehung von Fettzellen aus dem Gefäßbindegewebe.

a) Chondrome typique de la fosse cérébrale moyenne.
b) Lipome du chiasma avec composante angiomateuse prononcée.
c) Lipome entourant les racines de la queue de cheval.
d) Xanthome du plexus choroïde: on voit beaucoup de grosses cellules «spumeuses», qui sont bourrées de petites gouttelettes. Il ne s'agit pas d'une infiltration véritable, mais bien d'une prolifération locale de cellules graisseuses à partir du tissu conjonctif vasculaire.

a) Típico condroma de la fosa media.
b) Lipoma (quiasma) con un notable componente angiomatoso.
c) Lipoma que ha rodeado las raices caudales.
d) Xantoma del plexo coroideo: por todas partes se ven las grandes células «espumosas» llenas de finas gotas. Aquí no se trata sin embargo de una verdadera infiltración, sino de una formación autóctona de células grasas a partir del conectivo vascular.

a) Типическая хондрома средней черепной ямы.
b) Липома хиазмы с выраженными ангиоматозными компонентами.
c) Липома корешков конского хвоста.
d) Ксантома хориоидного сплетения: везде видны крупные мелкокапельные «пенистые клетки». Здесь нет истинной инфильтрации, а аутохтонное происхождение жировых клеток из сосудистой соединительной ткани.

a) 中頭蓋窩の定型的軟骨腫。
b) 血管腫様要素の多い、視束交叉の脂肪腫。
c) 馬尾神経周囲に発生した脂肪腫。
d) 脈絡叢の黄色腫。小滴を含んだ大型の「泡沫細胞」が多数みられる。この細胞は浸潤してきたものでなく、血管結合組織の脂肪細胞から変化したものである。

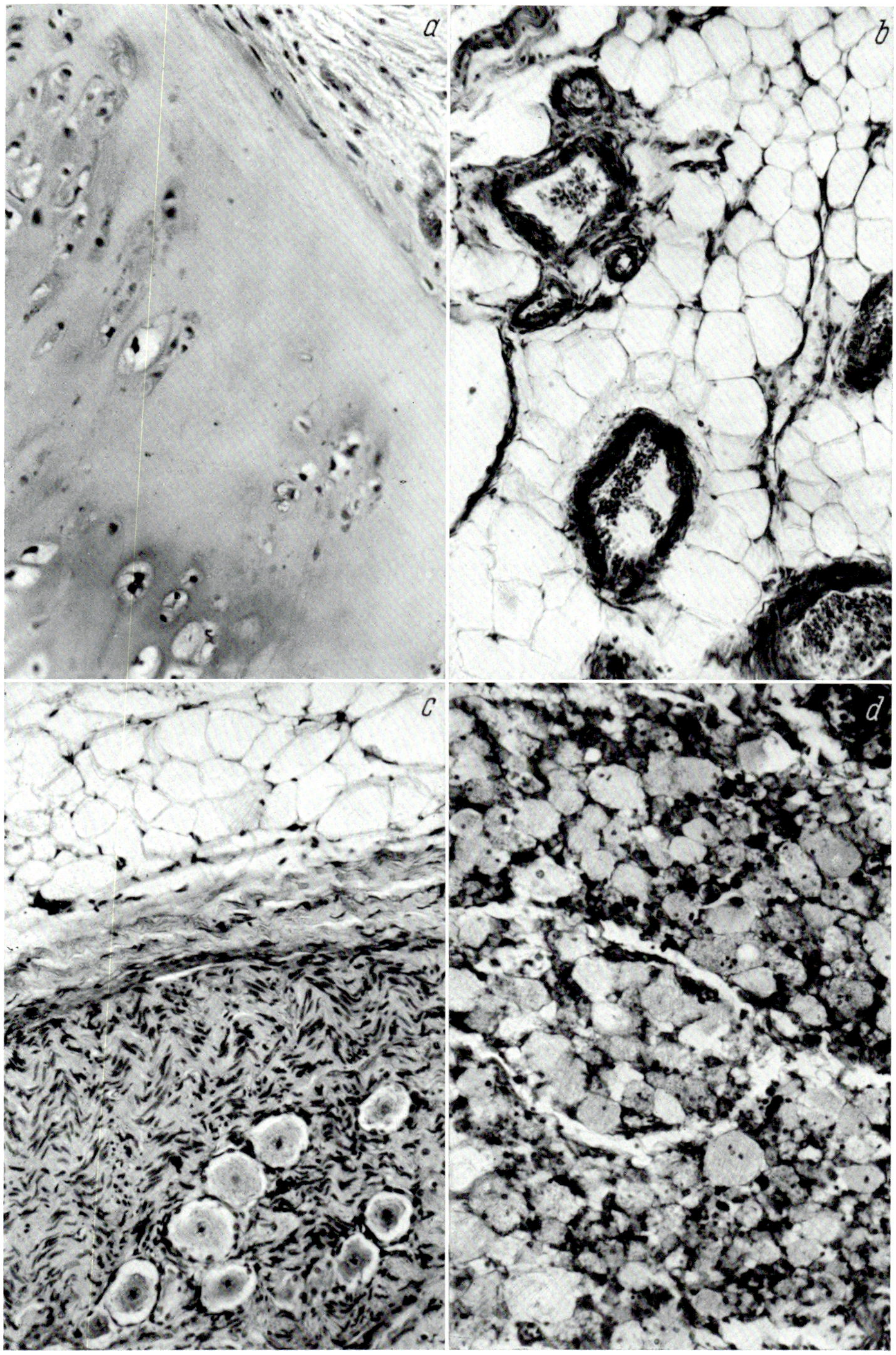

Fig. 99a—d: a ×236, b—d ×136
H. & E. stain

Fig. 100 — Cylindromatous Epitheliomas — Vascular Malformations

a) Typical cylindrical epithelioma of the Gasserian ganglion. The commencement of regressive changes can be recognised in the centre of the field and later leads to the cylindrical formations. Below there appears the same in a very small region like a miniature process occurring.
b) The cylinder formation has reached a maximum degree. It has developed colloid filled cysts which are covered with only a single layer of epithelium as in a colloid tumour of the thyroid glands.
c) Typical cavernous haemangioma of the brain with moderately swollen walls.
d) Thin walled vessels in an arteriovenous angioma. The vessel walls consist in parts of a single layer and in parts of two layers of cells.

a) Typisches cylindromatöses Epitheliom am Ganglion Gasseri. Man erkennt zentral den Beginn der regressiven Veränderungen im Zentrum der Balken, die später zur Zylinderbildung führen. Unten scheint sich das gleiche in einem sehr kleinen Balken als Miniaturvorgang abzuspielen.
b) Die Zylinderbildung ist zum Höchstmaß fortgeschritten: es haben sich mit Kolloid gefüllte Cysten gebildet, die nur von einem einschichtigen Epithel ausgekleidet sind. Ähnlichkeit mit einer Kolloidstruma der Schilddrüse.
c) Typisches Kavernom des Großhirns mit mäßig verquollenen Wänden.
d) Dünnwandige Gefäße in einem arteriovenösen Angiom. Die Gefäßwand besteht teils aus einer, teils aus zwei Lagen von Zellen.

a) «Epithélioma cylindromateux» typique du ganglion de Gasser. Des altérations régressives commencent à apparaître au centre des cordons, ce qui aboutira à la formation de «cylindres». En bas, le même processus semble se produire en miniature dans un très petit faisceau.
b) Les cylindres sont devenus manifestes: des kystes remplis de matière colloïde se sont formés et sont entourés par une simple assise de cellules épithéliales. Il existe une ressemblance avec le stroma colloïde de la thyroïde.
c) Cavernome typique, à parois modérément gonflées, dans l'hémisphère cérébral.
d) Vaisseaux à parois minces dans un angiome artério-veineux. La paroi vasculaire ne comporte qu'une ou deux couches cellulaires, selon les endroits.

a) Típico «epitelioma cilindromatoso» de un ganglio de Gasser. Se ve en el centro el inicio de la transformación regresiva que más tarde tomará la forma cilindromatosa. Abajo se ve lo mismo en proporción menor.
b) La formación cilindromatosa evoluciona formando masas con quistes coloides revestidos por una sola capa epitelial, de modo semejante al coloide del tiroides.
c) Típico cavernoma del cerebro con paredes ligeramente hinchadas.
d) Paredes delgadas en un angioma arteriovenosa. Las paredes vasculares están formadas por un estrato celular que puede ser simple o doble.

a) Типичная «цилиндроматозная эпителиома» гассерова узла. В центральной части видны начинающиеся регрессивные изменения в центре балок, приводящие позднее к образованию цилиндров. Внизу та же ситуация повторяется в миниатюре в небольшой балке.
b) Интенсивное образование цилиндров: сформировались заполненные коллоидом кисты, выстланные лишь однослойным эпителием. Сходство с коллоидной струмой щитовидной железы.
c) Типичная кавернома больших полушарий головного мозга с умеренно разбухшими стенками.
d) Тонкостенные сосуды в артериовенозной ангиоме. Сосудистая стенка состоит то из одного, то из двух слоев клеток.

a) Gasser 神経節にみられた定型的な〝円柱腫〟。上皮索の中央部に退行変化の初期像をみとめる。この上皮索は後に円柱上皮化する。下方には類似の経過をたどる小上皮索がある。
b) 円柱上皮形成が急速に進み、コロイドを含む嚢胞が形成されている。この嚢胞は一層の上皮によって囲まれ、甲状腺腫に似ている。
c) 大脳の定型的海綿腫。軽度に膨化した壁をみとめる。
d) 動静脈性血管腫内の薄い壁をもった血管。血管壁は一層ないし二層の細胞層よりなる。

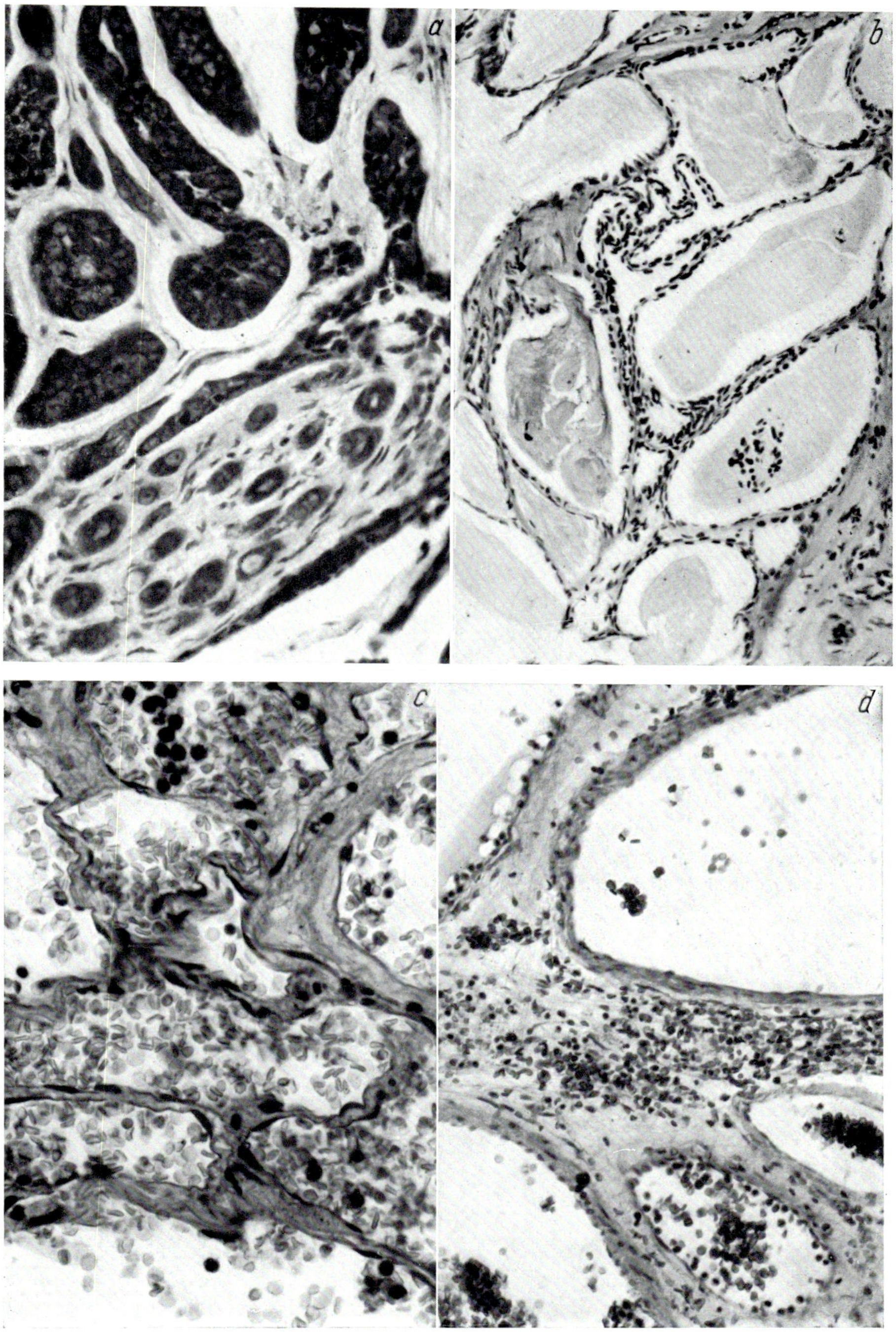

Fig. 100 above: a and b $\times$ 136, Cresyl violet stain,
below: c and d $\times$ 272, Cresyl violet stain

Bibliography

Bailey, P.: Histological atlas of gliomas. Arch. Path. **4**, 871—921 (1927).

— Intracranial tumors. Springfield: Thomas 1933.

— Die Hirngeschwülste. Stuttgart: Ferd. Enke 1936.

— Cushing, H.: A classification of the tumors of the glioma group on a histogenetic basis with a correlated study of prognosis. J. E. Lippincott Comp., Philadelphia, London & Montreal, 1926

— — Die Gewebsverschiedenheit der Gliome und ihre Bedeutung für die Prognose. G. Fischer, Jena, 1930.

Bergstrand, H.: Über das Gliom in den Großhirnhemisphären. Virchows Arch. path. Anat. **287**, 797—822 (1933).

— Weiteres über sogenannte Kleinhirnastrozytome. Virchows Arch. path. Anat. **299**, 725—739 (1937).

Costero, I.: Pathology of glial neoplasms. In: The biology and treatment of intracranial tumors, p. 178—211. Springfield, Illinois: Ch. C. Thomas 1962.

Cushing, H.: Intracranial tumors. Springfield: Thomas 1932.

— Intrakranielle Tumoren. Berlin: Springer 1935.

Globus, J. H., Strauss, I.: Spongioblastoma multiforme. Arch. Neurol. Psychiat. (Chic.) **14**, 139—151 (1925).

Hortega, del Rio P.: Estructura y systematisacion de los gliomas y paragliomas. Arch. esp. Oncol. **2**, 411—677 (1932).

— Nomenclatura y clasificacion de los tumores del sistema nervioso. Buenos Aires: Lopez & Etchegoyen S.R.L. 1945.

Kernohan, J. W., Mabon, R. F., Svien, H. J., Adson, A. W.: A simplified classification of the gliomas. Symp. on a new simplified concept of gliomas. Proc. Mayo Clin. **24**, 71—75 (1949).

— Sayre, G. P.: Tumours of the central nervous system. Armed Forces Inst. of Pathology, Washington, 1952.

Olivecrona, H.: The surgical treatment of intracranial tumors. In: Handbuch der Neurochirurgie, vol. IV, S. 1—301. Berlin-Göttingen-Heidelberg: Springer 1967.

Penfield, W.: Principles of the pathology of neurosurgery, chapt. VI, p. 303—347. New York: Nelson & Sons 1927 (Suppl. 1932).

Penfield, W.: Tumors of the sheaths of the nervous system. Chapt. 1 in: Penfields cytology and cellular pathology of the nervous system, p. 955—990. New York: Hoeber 1932.

Pick, L., Bielschowsky, M.: Über das System der Neurome und Beobachtungen an einem Ganglioneurom des Gehirns nebst Untersuchung über die Genese der Nervenfasern in „Neurinomen". Z. ges. Neurol. Psychiat. **6**, 391—437 (1911).

Polak, M.: Blastomas del Sistema Nervioso Central y periferico, Patologia y Ordenacion Histogenética. Buenos Aires: Lopez Libreros Edit. 1966.

Roussy, G., Oberling, Ch.: Atlas du cancer. Paris: Felix Alcan. 1931.

Russell, D. S., Rubinstein, L. J.: Pathology of tumours of the nervous system. London: Edward Arnold (Publishers) Ltd. 1959.

Tönnis, W.: Diagnostik der intrakraniellen Geschwülste. In: Handbuch der Neurochirurgie, vol. IV/3, p. 1—579. Berlin-Göttingen-Heidelberg: Springer 1962.

UICC (Unio Internationalis Contra Cancrum): Histological nomenclature of human tumors. Abstract of „Acta" vol. XIV, No 3 (1958).

— Histologische Nomenklatur menschlicher Tumoren. Z. Krebsforsch. **63**, 75—98 (1959).

— Illustrierte Tumor-Nomenklatur. Springer-Verlag, Berlin-Heidelberg-New York, 1965/1969.

Zülch, K. J.: Biologie und Pathologie der Hirngeschwülste. Handbuch der Neurochirurgie, vol. III. Berlin-Göttingen-Heidelberg: Springer 1956.

— Mikroskopischer Farbatlas der Hirngeschwülste. Max-Planck-Institut für Hirnforschung, Köln, 1956.

— Brain tumors, their biology and pathology. Berlin-Heidelberg-New York: Springer 1957; 2nd edit. 1965.

— Die Hirngeschwülste in biologischer und morphologischer Darstellung. Leipzig: Joh. Ambr. Barth, 1. Aufl. 1951; 3. Aufl. 1958.

— Geschwülste und Parasiten des Nervensystems. In: Kaufmann u. Staemmler, Lehrbuch der speziellen pathologischen Anatomie, S. 427—574. Berlin: Walter de Gruyter 1958. Italian Edition with Editor Dr. Francesco Vallardi, Milano.

Zülch, K. J.: The present state of the classification of intracranial tumors and its value for the neurosurgeon. In: The biology and treatment of intracranial tumors, p. 157—177. Springfield, Ill.: Ch. C. Thomas 1962.

— Soll man den Begriff des (unipolaren) Spongioblastoms beibehalten? Beitr. Neurochir. **15**, p. 373—382. Joh. Ambr. Barth, Leipzig, 1968.

Zülch, K. J., Wechsler, W.: Pathology and classification of gliomas. Progr. in Neurol. Surg., vol. II, p. 1—84. Basel-New York: S. Karger 1968.

— Woolf, A. L.: Classification of brain tumors. Report of the Internat. Symposion at Cologne 1961. In: Acta neurochir. (Wien), Suppl. 10 (1964).

Subject Index